Bone Marrow Failure Syndromes

Bone Marrow Failure Syndromes

Neal S. Young, MD
National Institutes of Health
Bethesda, Maryland

W.B. SAUNDERS COMPANY
A Harcourt Health Sciences Company
Philadelphia London New York St. Louis Sydney Toronto

W.B. SAUNDERS COMPANY
A Harcourt Health Sciences Company

The Curtis Center
Independence Square West
Philadelphia, Pennsylvania 19106

Library of Congress Cataloging-in-Publication Data

Bone marrow failure syndromes / [edited by] Neal S. Young.—1st ed.

p.   cm.

Includes index.

ISBN 0–7216–7174–8

1. Bone marrow—Diseases.   2. Myelodysplastic syndromes.
   3. Myeloproliferative disorders.   I. Young, Neal S.

[DNLM: 1. Bone Marrow Diseases. WH 380 B7114 2000]
RC645.7.B66   2000

616.4′1—dc21   00-023872

Acquisitions Editor: Marc Strauss
Designer: Paul Fry
Production Manager: Peter Faber
Illustration Specialist: Walt Verbitski

BONE MARROW FAILURE SYNDROMES   ISBN 0–7216–7174–8

Copyright © 2000 by W.B. Saunders Company.

All rights reserved. No part of this publication may be reproduced or transmitted in any form or by any means, electronic or mechanical, including photocopy, recording, or any information storage and retrieval system, without permission in writing from the publisher.

Printed in the United States of America.

Last digit is the print number: 9   8   7   6   5   4   3   2   1

To my father, who was denied a career in
medicine but inspired me to a life of clinical research.

Our blood to us, this to our blood is born;
It is the show and seal of nature's truth.

What is infirm from your sound parts shall fly,
Health shall live free and sickness freely die.

All's Well That Ends Well

Contributors

John Barrett, M.D.
Chief, Bone Marrow Transplant Unit, Hematology Branch, National Heart, Lung, and Blood Institute, National Institutes of Health, Bethesda, Maryland
Myelofibrosis (Agnogenic Myeloid Metaplasia)

Cynthia E. Dunbar, M.D.
Senior Investigator, Hematology Branch, National Heart, Lung, and Blood Institute, National Institutes of Health, Bethesda, Maryland
Myelodysplastic Syndromes

Daniel E. Dunn, M.D., Ph.D.
Assistant Professor, Blood and Marrow Transplant Program, University of Utah, Salt Lake City, Utah
Paroxysmal Nocturnal Hemoglobinuria

Elizabeth M. Kang, M.D.
Senior Staff Fellow, Molecular and Clinical Hematology Branch, NIDDK (National Institute of Diabetes and Digestive and Kidney Diseases), National Institutes of Health, Bethesda, Maryland
Pure Red Cell Aplasia

Johnson M. Liu, M.D.
Senior Investigator, Hematology Branch, National Heart, Lung, and Blood Institute, National Institutes of Health, Bethesda, Maryland
Fanconi's Anemia; Paroxysmal Nocturnal Hemoglobinuria

Jaroslow P. Maciejewski, M.D.
Clinical Associate, Hematology Branch, National Heart, Lung, and Blood Institute, National Institute of Health, Bethesda, Maryland
Human Immunodeficiency Virus–Related Bone Marrow Failure

Dimitrios Mavroudis, M.D.
Visiting Fellow, Hematology Branch, National Heart, Lung, and Blood Institute, National Institutes of Health, Bethesda, Maryland
Myelofibrosis (Agnogenic Myeloid Metaplasia)

Jeffrey J. Molldrem, M.D.
Chief, Section of Transplantation Immunology Department of Blood and Marrow Transplantation, University of Texas M.D. Anderson Cancer Center, Houston, Texas
T Cell Large Granular Lymphocyte Lymphoproliferative Disorder

Stephen Rosenfeld, M.D.
Deputy Chief Investigative Officer for Clinical Informatics, Warren Grant Magnuson Clinical Center, National Institutes of Health, Bethesda, Maryland
Acquired Amegakaryocytic Thrombocytopenic Purpura

Yogen Saunthararajah, M.B.B.Ch.
Fellow in Hematology and Oncology, National Institutes of Health, Bethesda, Maryland
Myelodysplastic Syndromes

Elaine M. Sloand, M.D.
Assistant to Director, National Heart, Lung, and Blood Institute, National Institutes of Health, Bethesda, Maryland; Assistant Professor, Georgetown University Hospital, Washington, D.C.
Human Immunodeficiency Virus–Related Bone Marrow Failure

John F. Tisdale, M.D.
Senior Investigator, Molecular and Clinical Hematology Branch, National Institute of Diabetes and Digestive and Kidney Disorders, National Institutes of Health, Bethesda, Maryland
Pure Red Cell Aplasia

Neal S. Young, M.D.
Chief, Hematology Branch, National Heart, Lung, and Blood Institute, National Institutes of Health, Bethesda, Maryland
Acquired Aplastic Anemia; Paroxysmal Nocturnal Hemoglobinuria; Agranulocytosis

Preface

Related but incompletely understood diseases invite war between "lumpers," who stress common clinical and pathologic processes, and "splitters," who emphasize the differences. In a monograph published a few years ago, I reviewed clonal hematologic diseases and isolated forms of bone marrow failure in the context of aplastic anemia, but this oblique unifying effort would be unfairly contrasted to the separation of these syndromes in the current volume. Grouping of these diseases in a single text should instead be compared to their confusing ordering in standard textbooks of medicine and hematology, where some appear in sections devoted to anemia, others among the lymphoid or myeloid malignancies, or as aspects of infectious disease or pharmacology.

While the true relationship of each of these syndromes to the other is not yet clear, they all frequently and very dramatically result in low blood counts, with the bone marrow at fault. Classic clinical and pathologic presentations, of course, assist the student in the first approach to a complex subject, guide the differential diagnosis of the experienced practitioner, and are required for the comparison and interpretation of published reports of therapeutic outcomes and underlying pathophysiologies. Simple approaches, especially those based on bone marrow morphology alone, have become less reliable, however. In hypocellular myelodysplasia, which dominates: the destructive process producing an empty bone marrow or the "preleukemic" chromosomal abnormality? With greatly improved survival of affected patients, we are increasingly confounded by the apparent evolution of one process to another, as for example marrow aplasia to dysplasia. A further complication is that more sensitive and specific clinical tests leave the hematologist grasping to explain frequent and sometimes concurrent findings of paroxysmal nocturnal hemoglobinuria cells, missing or extra chromosomes, or clonal lymphoid populations in diverse marrow failure syndromes or even in a single patient—dilemmas that are not only nosologically unsatisfying and clinically confusing but, due to the precisely defined biochemical and genetic lesions, of potentially much biologic significance. Progress in the study of these diseases ultimately rests on explication of the regulation of the stem cell compartment; on human autoimmunity and the role of environmental factors in its initiation; on the nature of genomic instability, particularly the relationship of inflammation and malignancy. In turn, observations of human disease will inform our understanding of these processes. The proper classification—and better treatments—of bone marrow failure will be based on a close tie between basic biology and clinical behavior.

The Hematology Branch of the National Heart, Lung, and Blood Institute is a major referral center for patients with bone marrow failure, where also laboratory studies, applied and basic, are devoted to these diseases. I am very grateful to my NIH colleagues, with whom I have happily worked closely and at close quarters for years, for stimulating discussions of individual cases, productive collaborative clinical protocols, and shared laboratory investigations, as well as for their contributions to this volume. Many thanks also to Marc Strauss of the W.B. Saunders Company, an exemplary editor; without his persistent efforts, this book could not have been produced. Finally, I express the gratitude of all the authors to patients who participate in research protocols at the Clinical Center and at other institutions. Their courageous generosity in the face of frightening and occasionally overwhelming symptoms, in the setting of an unfamiliar diagnosis, is heroic, and we as scientists and physicians are in their debt.

Neal S. Young, M.D.

NOTICE

Hematology and Oncology are ever-changing fields. Standard safety precautions must be followed, but as new research and clinical experience broaden our knowledge, changes in treatment and drug therapy become necessary or appropriate. The editors of this work have carefully checked the generic and trade drug names and verified drug dosages to ensure that the dosage information in this work is accurate and in accord with the standards accepted at the time of publication. Readers are advised, however, to check the product information currently provided by the manufacturer of each drug to be administered to make certain that changes have not been made in the recommended dose or in the contraindications to administration. This is of particular importance in regard to new or infrequently used drugs. It is the responsibility of treating physicians, relying on experience and knowledge of the patient, to determine dosages and the best treatment for their patients. The editors cannot be responsible for misuse or misapplication of the information in this work.

THE PUBLISHER

Contents

Color Plates

1
Acquired Aplastic Anemia   **1**
Neal S. Young, M.D.

2
Fanconi's Anemia   **47**
Johnson M. Liu, M.D.

3
Myelodysplastic Syndromes   **69**
Cynthia E. Dunbar, M.D.,
and Yogen Saunthararajah, M.B.B.Ch.

4
Paroxysmal Nocturnal
Hemoglobinuria   **99**
Daniel E. Dunn, M.D., Ph.D.,
Johnson M. Liu, M.D.,
and Neal S. Young, M.D.

5
Myelofibrosis   **122**
Dimitrios Mavroudis, M.D.,
and John Barrett, M.D.

6
Pure Red Cell Aplasia   **135**
Elizabeth M. Kang, M.D.,
and John F. Tisdale, M.D.

7
Agranulocytosis   **156**
Neal S. Young, M.D.

8
Acquired Amegakaryocytic
Thrombocytopenic Purpura   **183**
Stephen Rosenfeld, M.D.

9
Human Immunodeficiency
Virus–Related Bone Marrow
Failure   **187**
Elaine M. Sloand,
and Jaroslow P. Maciejewski

10
T Cell Large Granular
Lymphocyte Lymphoproliferative
Disorder   **207**
Jeffrey J. Molldrem

Index   **217**

Color Plates

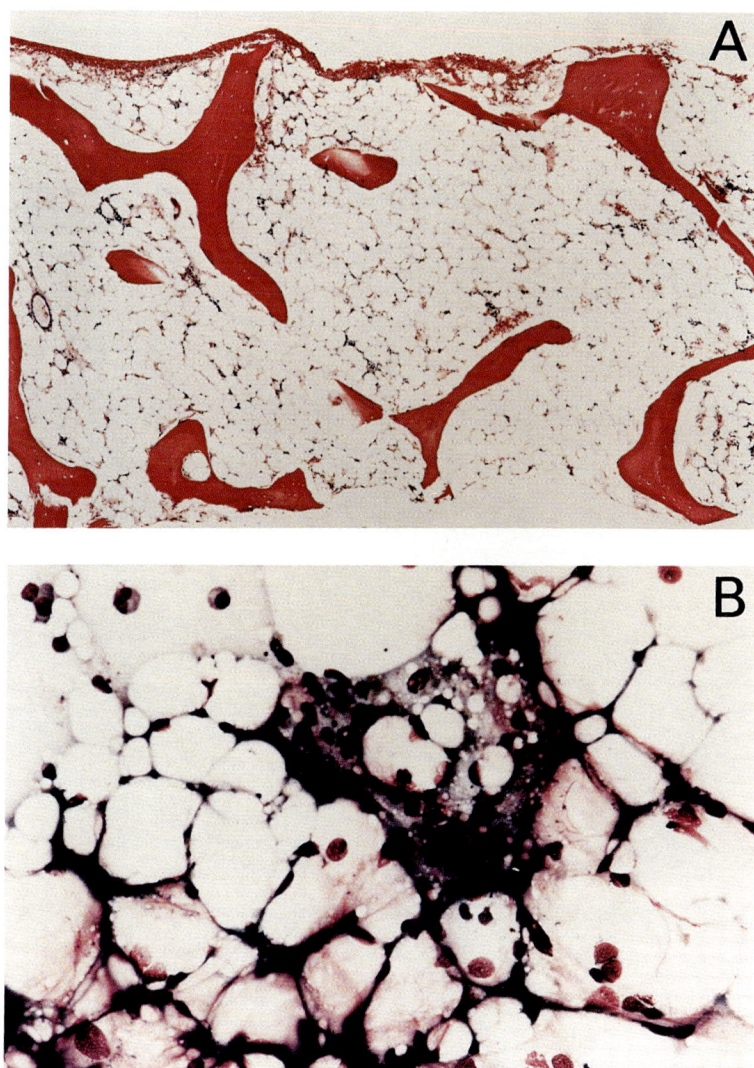

Plate 1 Bone marrow biopsy (low magnification) **(A)** and aspirate (high magnification) **(B)** in severe aplastic anemia.

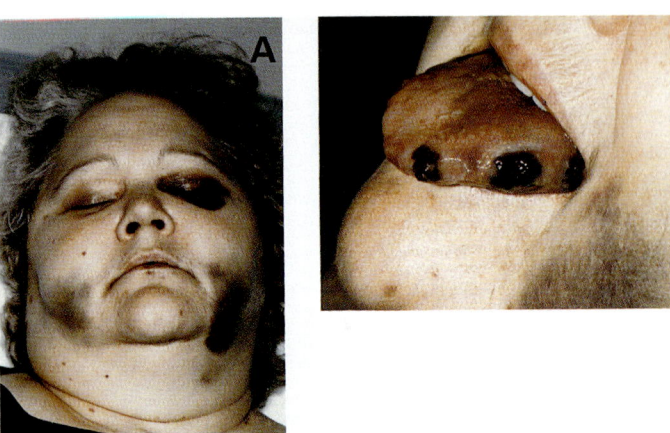
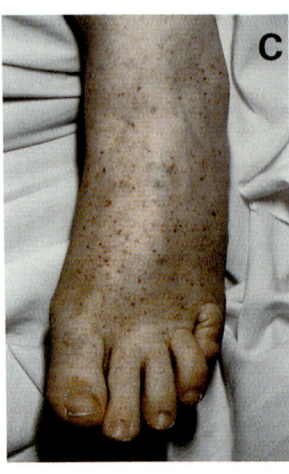

Plate 2 Bleeding manifestations in a patient with severe thrombocytopenia due to aplastic anemia: facial ecchymoses **(A)**, lingual hemorrhage **(B)**, and petechiae **(C)**.

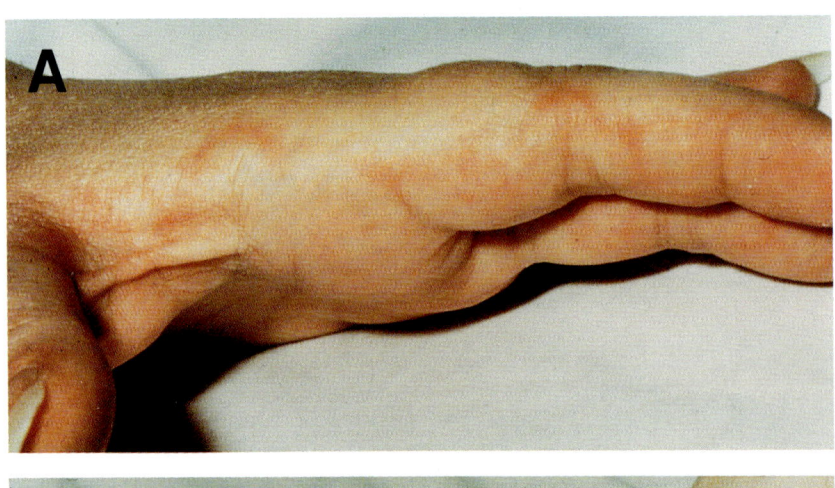
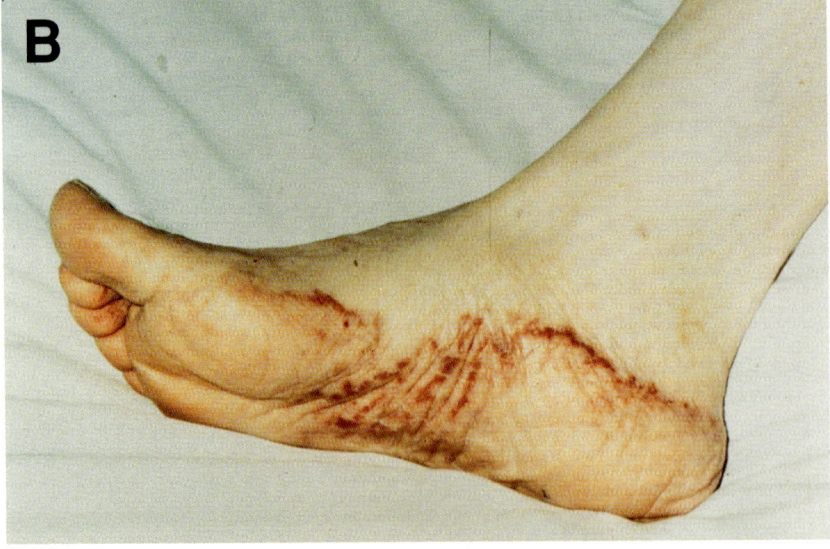

Plate 3 Characteristic cutaneous eruptions of serum sickness; see Bielory et al.[448]

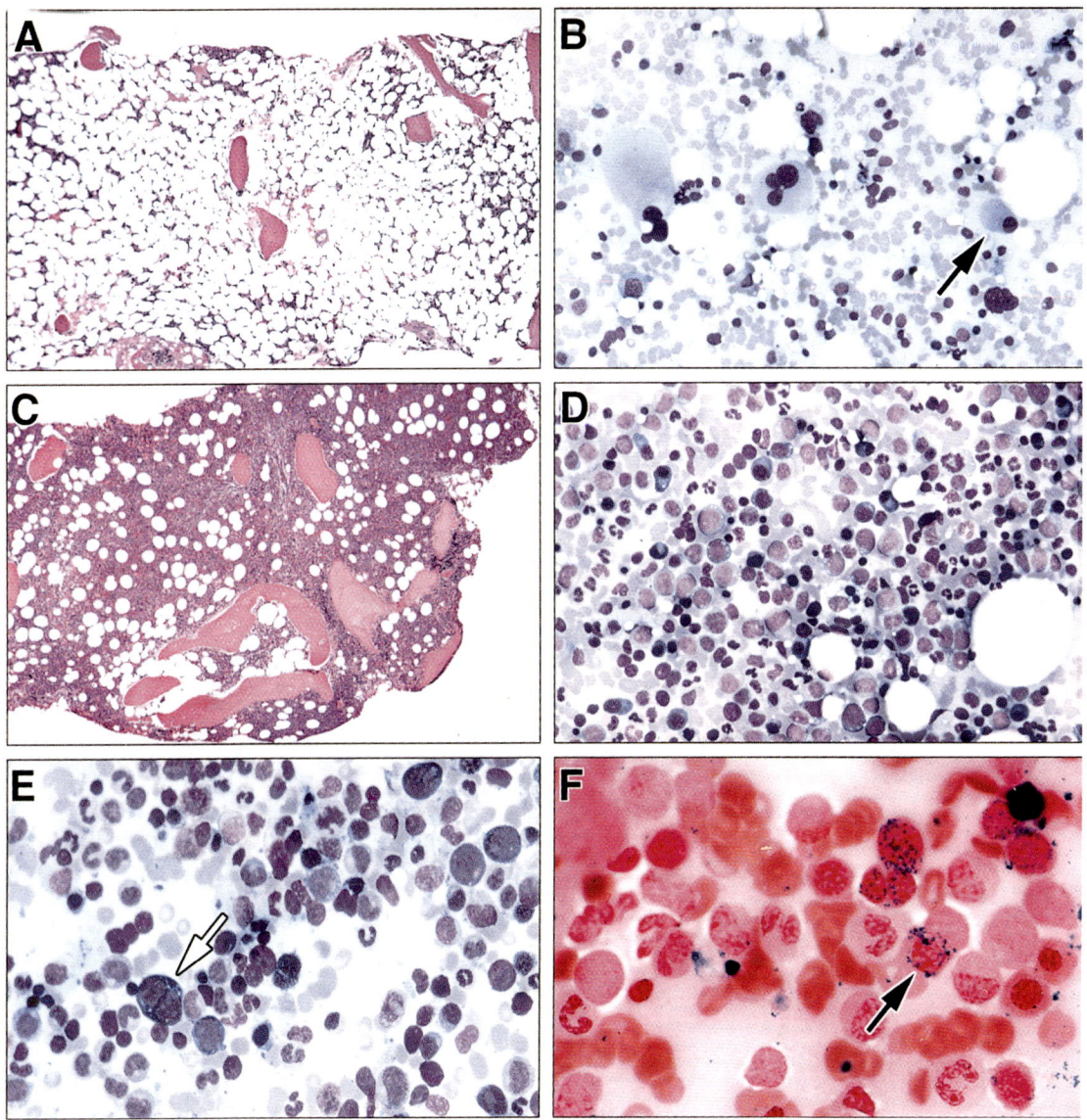

Plate 4 **Photomicrographs of marrow aspirates and biopsy specimens from patients with myelodysplastic syndromes.**
(A) Biopsy section from the marrow of a young female patient with isolated anemia, shown at low magnification. Note the marked hypocellularity initially believed to be consistent with aplastic anemia. **(B)** Aspirate marrow smear from the same patient, shown at high magnification. Note the uninuclearity and other dysplastic features of the abundant megakaryocytes *(arrow)*. The relative number of lymphocytes is increased, and the myeloid cells are left-shifted. There is a paucity of erythroid precursors. Cytogenetics on this marrow sample revealed the 5q– abnormality in 100% of metaphases. This patient falls into the refractory anemia category in the French-American-British (FAB) classification. **(C)** Biopsy section from an elderly man with profound thrombocytopenia and moderate anemia and neutropenia, shown at low magnification. Note the marked hypercellularity for his age, with replacement of fat. **(D)** Aspirate marrow smear from the same patient, shown at high magnification. Note the marked left shift in the myeloid series, with easily identified blasts. The myeloid cells are also hypogranulated and have various nuclear abnormalities. The erythroid precursors are megaloblastic. This patient falls into the refractory anemia with excess blasts (RAEB) category in the FAB classification. Cytogenetics revealed complex cytogenetic abnormalities, including deletion of chromosome 7. **(E)** Aspirate marrow smear from a middle-aged man with transfusion-dependent anemia with normal platelet and neutrophil counts, shown at high magnification. Note the marked erythroid hyperplasia, with multiple dysplastic features of the erythroid precursors, including binuclearity *(arrow)*. **(F)** Iron stain of the marrow aspirate from the same patient, shown at high magnification. Note the blue granules surrounding the nucleus of the erythroid precursor cell *(arrow)*; this cell is a ringed sideroblast, and the blue particles are iron-laden mitochondria.

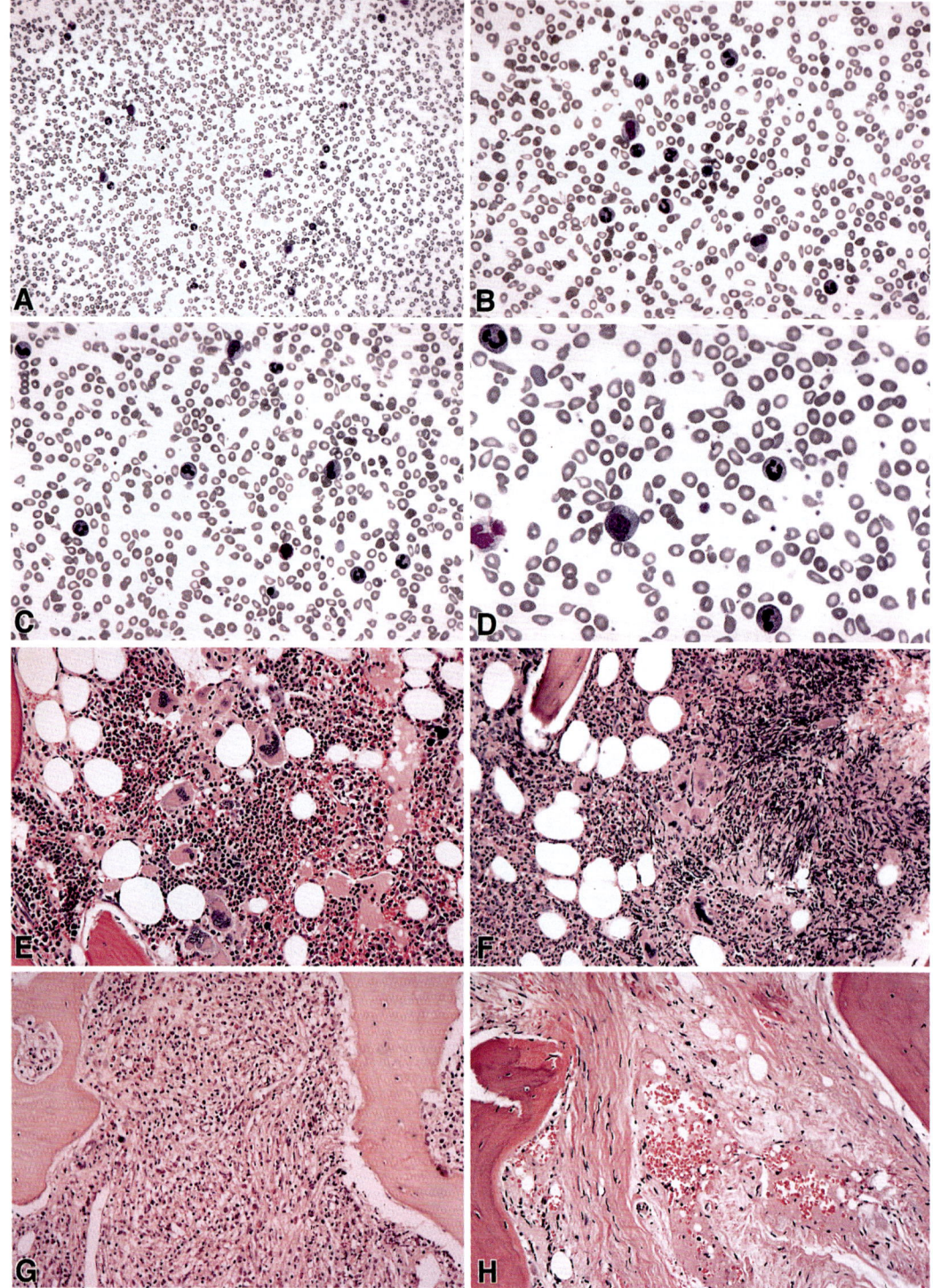

Plate 5   Blood and bone marrow morphology in agnogenic myeloid metaplasia (AMM).   **(A–D)** Peripheral blood morphology in smears from patients with AMM showing teardrop poikilocytosis, nucleated red blood cells, immature myeloid cells, and giant platelets. **(E–H)** Bone marrow morphology in biopsy specimens from different stages of AMM: **E** shows a hypercellular marrow with clusters of dysplastic megakaryocytes; **F** and **G** show more advanced stages of AMM with decreased cellularity and increased fibrosis; **H** shows replacement of bone marrow by fibrous tissue in advanced AMM.

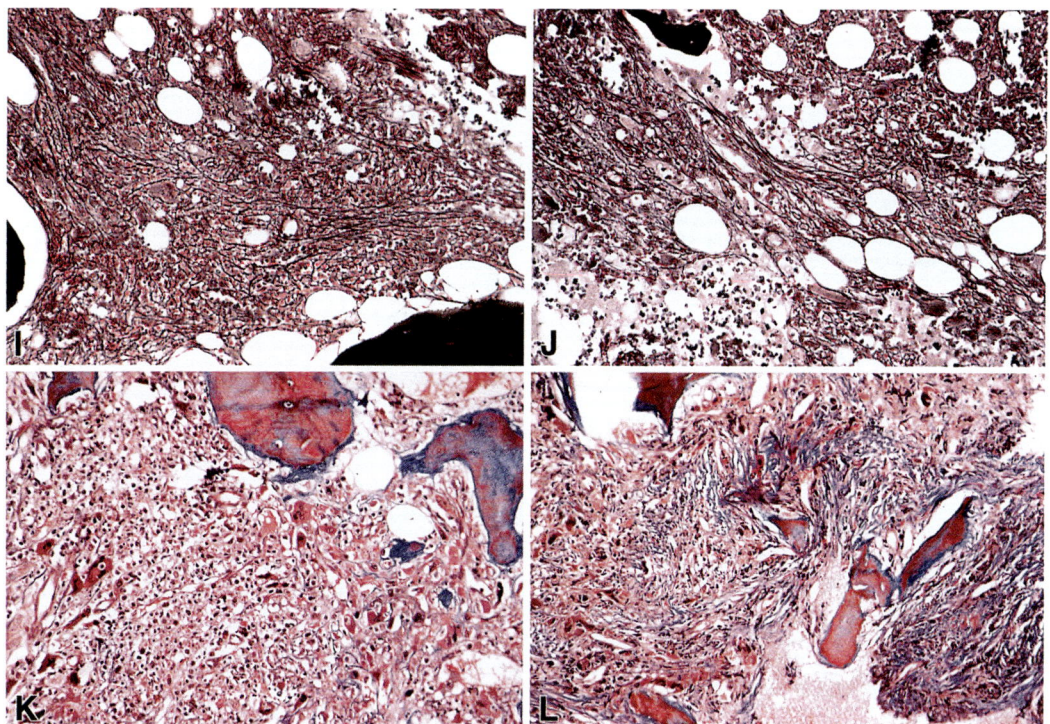

Plate 5—*Continued* **(I–L)** Fibrosis of the bone marrow on biopsy specimens in AMM: increased reticulin in early **(I)** and advanced disease **(J)**; lack of collagen in early disease **(K)**; accumulation of collagen in later stage disease **(L)**.

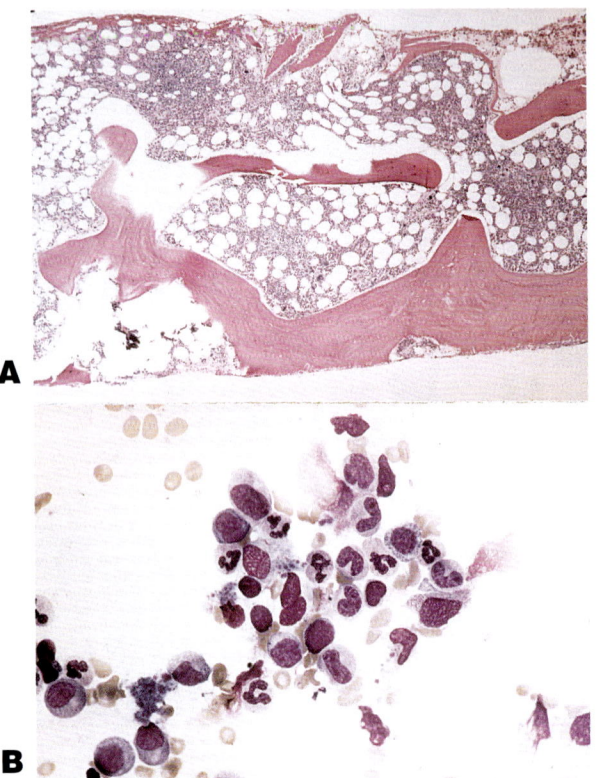

Plate 6 Bone marrow morphology in pure red blood cell aplasia. **(A)** Normal bone marrow cellularity on biopsy (low magnification). **(B)** Erythroid precursor cells are absent on aspirate smear from the same patient (high magnification).

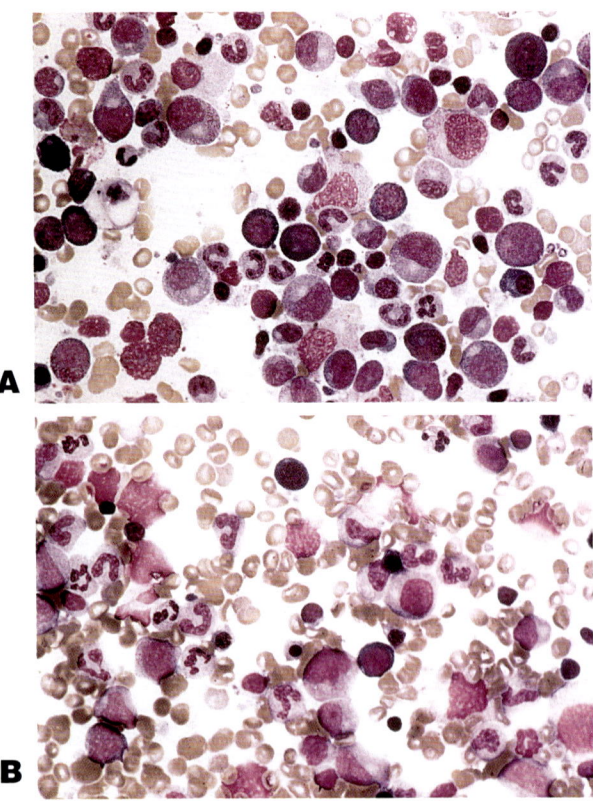

Plate 7 Bone marrow morphology in pure red blood cell aplasia secondary to large granular lymphocytosis and after treatment with cyclosporine: **(A)** at diagnosis (high magnification); **(B)** after treatment.

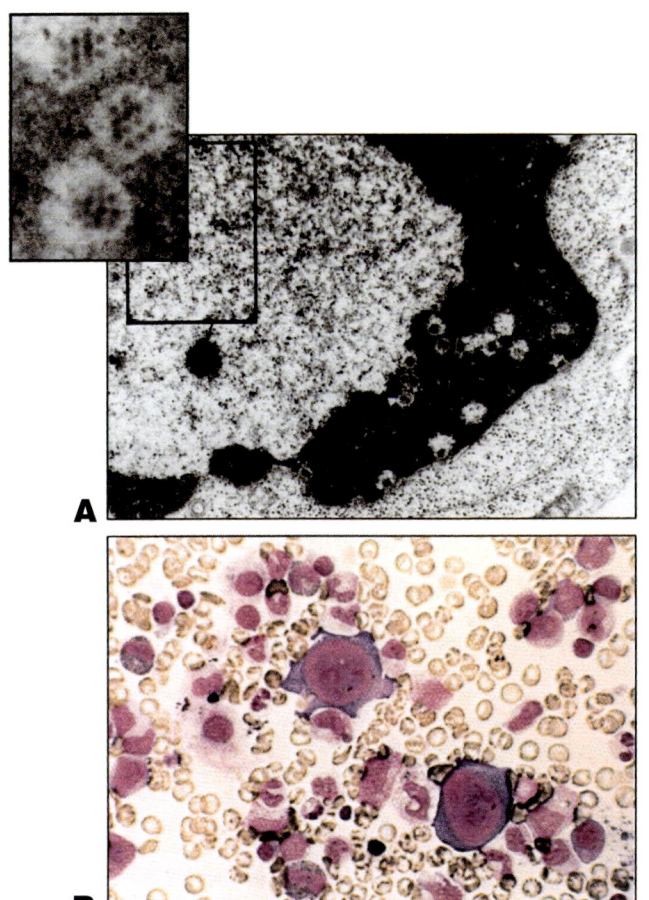

Plate 8 B19 parvovirus infection of human bone marrow cells in tissue culture. **(A)** Erythroid precursor cell nucleus showing marginated chromatin and lacunae that contain assembling viral particles *(inset)*, as detected by electron microscopy. **(B)** Giant pronormoblasts stained by Wright's-Giemsa, as seen by light microscopy under high magnification. (Courtesy of N. S. Young.)

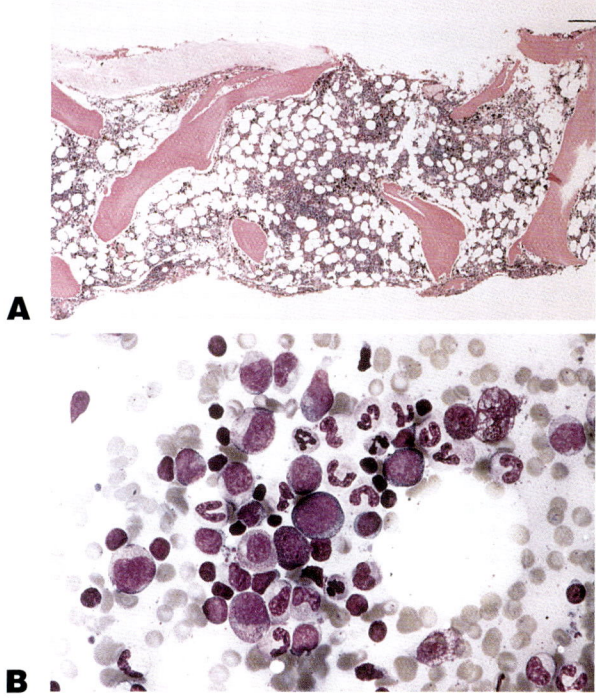

Plate 9 Bone marrow aspirate and biopsy specimen from a patient with Diamond-Blackfan anemia. **(A)** Normocellular biopsy (low magnification). **(B)** Aspirate showing absence of mature erythroid elements (high magnification).

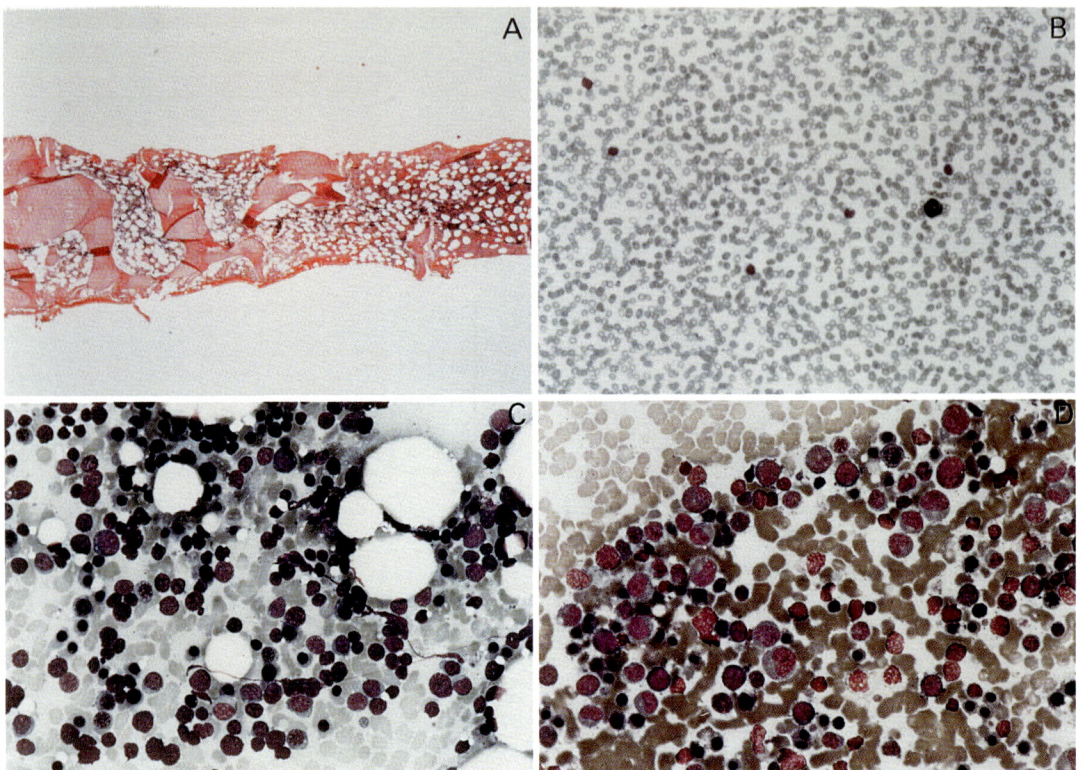

Plate 10 Blood and bone marrow appearance in agranulocytosis. **(A)** Bone marrow biopsy showing well-preserved total cellularity (low magnification). **(B)** Peripheral blood smear in which granulocytes are absent (low magnification). **(C)** Typical appearance of marrow aspirate smear with absent recognizable myeloid precursor cells (high magnification). **(D)** In another patient, preservation of early myeloid cells, so-called "maturation arrest", consistent with either early recovery or a pathophysiologic mechanism in which more mature cells are targets.

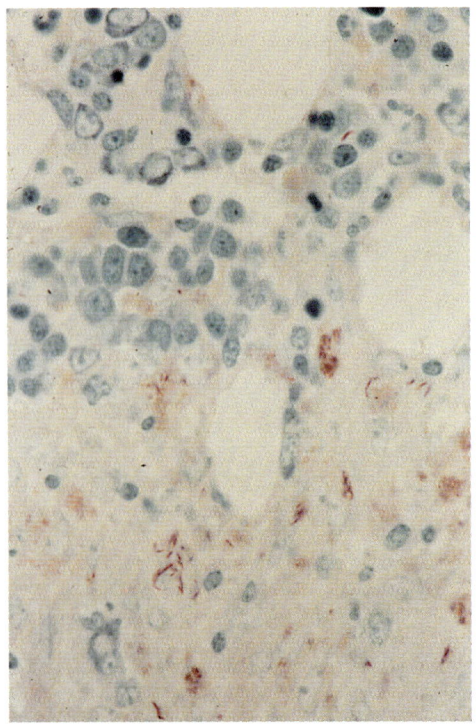

Plate 11 Mycobacterial infection of the bone marrow in a patient with acquired immunodeficiency syndrome (AIDS). Acid-fast bacilli are seen in bone marrow of an AIDS patient with fever and weight loss.

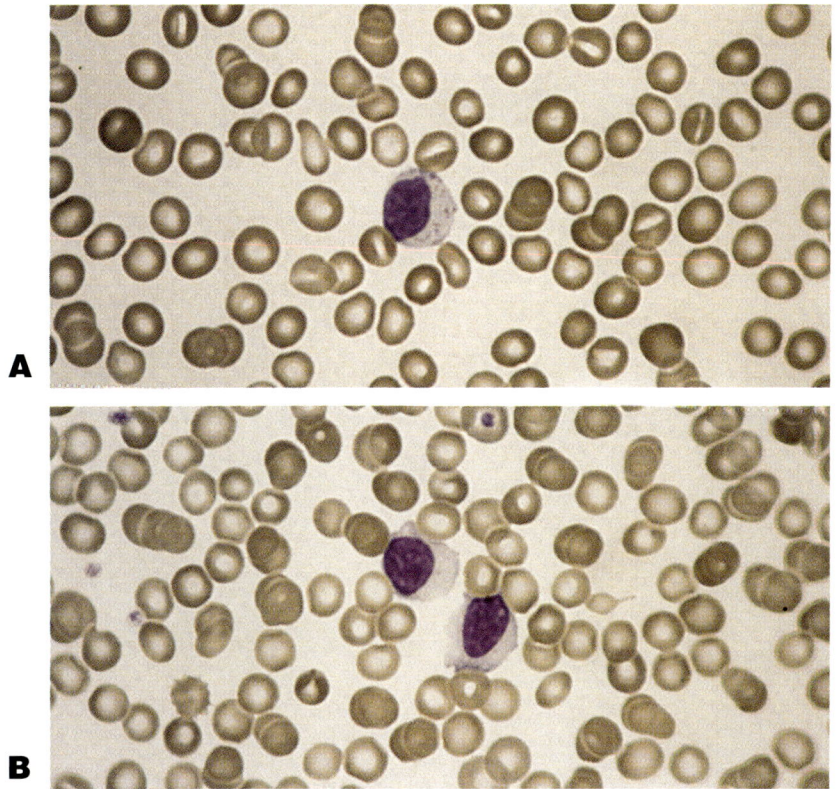

Plate 12A and B Large granular lymphocytes in the peripheral blood of a patient with T-LGL leukemia. Note the heterogeneity of the lymphocyte granules, which is typical in this disorder.

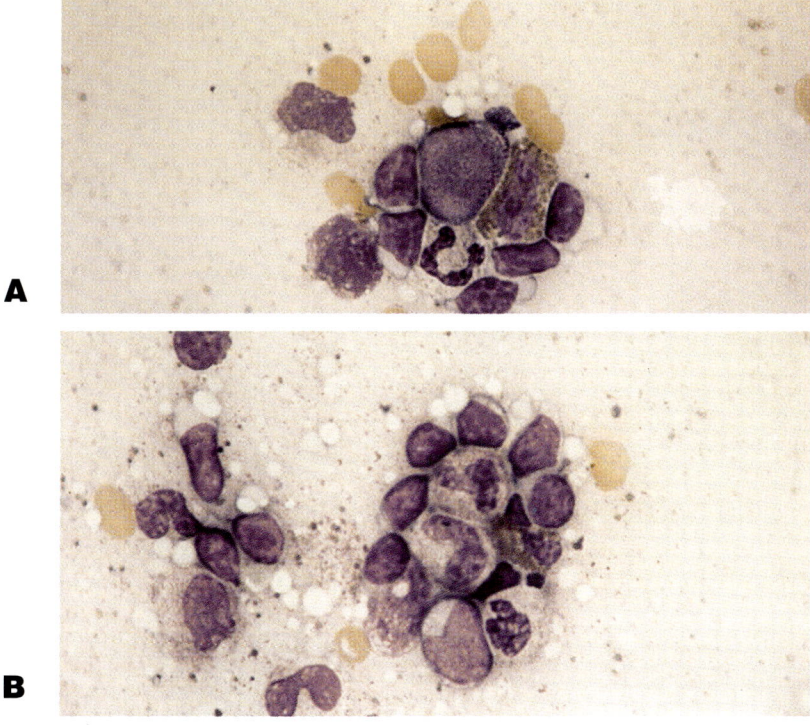

Plate 13A and B Bone marrow aspirate showing large granular lymphocytes in a patient with T-LGL leukemia. Clustering of the lymphocytes around hematopoietic progenitors can be seen.

1

Acquired Aplastic Anemia

Neal S. Young, M.D.

HISTORY

In 1888 Paul Ehrlich[1] first described aplastic anemia (AA) in his report of an autopsy of a young woman who died after a brief, catastrophic illness marked by severe anemia, bleeding, and high fever (Fig. 1–1A). As a pathologist, Ehrlich was struck by the absence of nucleated red blood cells and the fatty quality of the femoral marrow, quite the reverse of the appearance of the marrow compensating for severe anemia, and he inferred from morphology a mechanism of failed blood cell regeneration. Vaquez and Aubertin[2] in their 1904 case report of "pernicious anemia with yellow marrow" first used the term aplastic anemia (Chauffard has been inaccurately credited with naming the disease because his own case report, published 2 weeks later and referring to Vaquez and Aubertin's discussion, included *aplastique* in its title!) (Fig. 1–1B). The literature of the early twentieth century emphasized the clinical course of the disease, the laboratory findings of reticulocytopenia, despite severe anemia, and thrombocytopenia, as well as the consistent pathologic findings. Cabot[3] stressed the marrow's distinctive pathologic changes and the requirement of its examination for diagnosis, but before the development of techniques for marrow extraction by aspiration and biopsy in living patients, the diagnosis was made at autopsy. The hematologist's, or more commonly the pathologist's, task was the differentiation of AA by clinical evidence and ultimately tissue appearance from the pernicious anemias, thrombocytopenic purpuras, and secondary forms of marrow failure. Pathologically, the watery yellow marrow seen at autopsy defined aplasia, but in practice pancytopenia was often equated with AA.

Vaquez and Aubertin presciently emphasized a pathophysiology of failed blood cell production ("anhematopoiesis"); indeed, the etymology of "aplastic" is the Greek verb πλάϑω *(plassein)* to create and give shape to ἀπλαστκή *(aplastileos,* unformed). Although AA was viewed as an intrinsic marrow disease, a relationship to the environment was inferred from important clinical associations.[4] Chemical exposure, particularly to benzene, was linked to marrow failure by Santesson's studies of bicycle tire workers in Sweden at the end of the nineteenth century.[5] The role of dipyrone in the closely related syndrome of agranulocytosis, publicized in the 1930s by Kracke and Parker,[6] and an apparent epidemic of AA that followed the introduction of chloramphenicol as an antibiotic in the 1960s[7] dramatized the relationship of medical drugs to marrow failure. Marrow aplasia also was appreciated as the idiosyncratic outcome not only of chemical and drug exposure but as a rare complication of other environmental agents: infection, as in the stereotypic posthepatitis syndrome; during pregnancy; and in association with other diseases such as systemic lupus.

The almost invariably fatal course of AA was a theme of the literature of the early twentieth century (Fig. 1–2A). Corticosteroids, in retrospect of uncertain benefit, were employed in the 1950s; androgens, with apparent efficacy, were used in the 1960s. Bone marrow transplantation was obviously ideal for a disease of failed hematopoiesis, and after unsuccessful attempts at intraosseous infusion and across major histocompatibility barriers, in the 1970s this procedure was increasingly curative in patients who survived without graft rejection, graft-versus-host disease (GvHD), and other complications.[8] Antilymphocyte sera was first pioneered by Mathé at about the same time; hundreds of patients were treated in Basel, Paris, and London before American hematologists recognized the value of the commercially available antithymocyte globulin (ATG).[9] The 1990s saw further refinements in stem cell transplantation, so

VII.

Ueber einen Fall von Anämie mit Bemerkungen über regenerative Veränderungen des Knochenmarks.

Von

Professor Dr. **P. Ehrlich,**
Assistent der II. medicinischen Klinik.

Die Literatur der perniciösen Anämie ist eine ausserordentlich grosse, sodass die Veröffentlichung einzelner Fälle, soweit sie nicht erheblich von der Norm abweichen, nur noch ein mehr lexicographisches Interesse darbietet.

Ich habe aus diesem Grunde aus der überreichen Casuistik, die ich im Laufe der Jahre sammeln konnte, nur 2 Fälle veröffentlicht, weil diese durch besondere Eigenheiten ausgezeichnet waren. Der eine von ihnen betraf die sehr seltene Combination von perniciöser Anämie mit periostalem Sarcom, während der zweite durch ein eigenartiges und ganz isolirt dastehendes Verhalten der Leucocyten, in specie der polynucleären Form, mir von principieller Bedeutung zu sein schien.[1]

Auch in den letzten Jahre habe ich an der Klinik des Herrn Geheimrath Gerhardt unter anderen einen Fall beobachten können, der einen bemerkenswerthen Blutbefund darbot und den ich deswegen mittheilen zu müssen glaube, weil er beweist, bis zu welcher Feinheit mittelst der mikroskopischen Untersuchung die Diagnostik der Bluterkrankungen gebracht werden kann.

Ausserdem dürfte sich hierbei auch Gelegenheit bieten, den Stand-

[1]) Siehe Charité-Annalen Jahrgang V. p. 198. und Charité-Annalen Jahrgang XII.

A

L'ANÉMIE PERNICIEUSE D'APRÈS LES CONCEPTIONS ACTUELLES,

par M. H. Vaquez
Agrégé, médecin de l'hôpital Saint-Antoine,

et Ch. Aubertin,
Interne des hôpitaux.

L'attention de la Société médicale des hôpitaux a été récemment appelée sur les modalités diverses et la signification de l'anémie pernicieuse. Nous avons observé l'année dernière un cas très particulier, dans ses manifestations cliniques et anatomiques, de cette affection. Nous le rapporterons seul, à cause du caractère exceptionnel qu'il a présenté, bien, que nous ayons eu l'occasion d'en examiner d'autres de forme plus commune, cette maladie étant, à notre avis, moins rare qu'on ne l'a admis jusqu'ici, mais plutôt facilement méconnue. Ce cas suffira d'ailleurs à nous permettre d'exposer nos considérations personnelles, relatives aux données nouvelles que nous ont fournies les connaissances actuelles sur l'état anatomique du sang, et relatives aussi à la conception que nous nous faisons de l'anémie pernicieuse. Voici cette observation :

Observation (résumée) (3). — S..., Léon, comptable, âgé de dix-neuf ans, vient le 29 mai 1903 à notre consultation, se plaignant de faiblesse et de palpitations. Frappés tout d'abord par la pâleur de ses téguments et de ses muqueuses, et ayant constaté l'absence de tuméfaction splénique et ganglionnaire, nous pratiquons immédiatement un examen de sang qui donne le résultat suivant : 850.000 globules rouges et 6.000 leucocytes : on pose donc immédiatement le diagnostic d'anémie grave, pernicieuse ou symptomatique.

Les cas de cet ordre sont encore assez exceptionnels. Ehrlich a bien rapporté une seconde observation, dont nous n'avons pu avoir la relation *in extenso*. Engel a exposé une observation analogue présentant les mêmes lésions. Billings n'a pas apporté d'examens nécropsiques à l'appui des cas dont il fait mention. Plus récemment, une observation de M. A. Cade (*Bulletin médical*, 1903) est à coup sûr plus complète, malgré quelques particularités qui la différencient de l'exemple rapporté par Ehrlich.

Si l'on examine la valeur de notre observation, en s'aidant de ces données, on sera frappé du rapport qu'il y a entre l'aspect du sang et celui de la moelle. Ici, la forme aplastique apparaît dans toute sa pureté. La moelle épiphysaire des os longs est comme frappée de stérilité, à peine la moelle des côtes a-t-elle conservé une coloration légèrement rosée. Et ce ne sont pas seulement les globules rouges qui ne se régénèrent plus, mais les éléments blancs eux-mêmes. Du moins les éléments granuleux ont considérablement diminué de nombre. La moelle n'en fabrique pas plus que d'hématies, et le chiffre des polynucléaires du sang est réduit au minimum.

On serait, dès lors, tenté de diviser, au point de vue fonctionnel, les anémies pernicieuses en deux groupes : dans le premier, le travail médullaire, bien qu'anormal, serait encore visible ; dans le second, il serait complètement aboli. Dans le premier groupe, on rencontrerait surtout les anémies pernicieuses symptomatiques (anémies bothriocéphaliques, de la grossesse, des cancers, etc.) ; dans le deuxième, prendrait place l'anémie pernicieuse essentielle, celle à laquelle le professeur Hayem a donné le nom d'anémie par anhématopoièse, et à laquelle il serait tenté de réserver presque exclusivement le nom d'anémie pernicieuse.

B

Figure 1-1 Initial pages of two early papers on aplastic anemia. **(A)** Ehrlich's description of the first patient.[1] **(B)** Case report by Vaquez and Aubertin in which the disease was named.[2]

---

that 70% to 90% of sibling recipients now survive long-term; intensification of immunosuppressive regimens to improve hematologic response rates to approximately 70% and provide outcomes comparable to replacement treatments; and the introduction of hematopoietic growth factors as adjunctive therapies.[10] AA remains a serious disease but, if managed appropriately, in most patients marrow failure can be effectively ameliorated or cured (Fig. 1–2B and C).

External factors were linked pathophysiologically to hematopoietic failure by recognition of the immune system in mediating marrow suppression, first clearly formulated in the 1970s when in vitro culture systems for hematopoietic progenitor cells entered clinical use. At the same time, patients were observed to respond to therapies aimed at the immune system. Laboratory studies have established that destruction of the hematopoietic compartment probably occurs in most cases as a result of T cell attack on stem and progenitor cells, mediated at least in part by cytokines such as interferon-γ (IFN-γ) and through cell surface and intracellular pathways of programmed cell

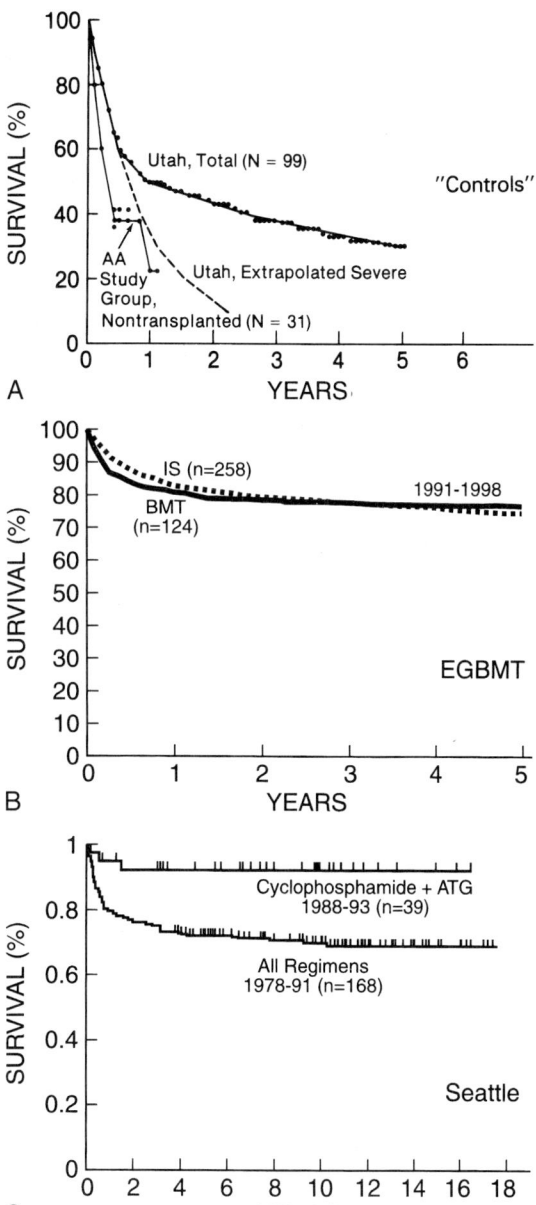

Figure 1–2 Actuarial survival in aplastic anemia. **(A)** "Natural history"— in reality, survival with supportive care and other treatments. Extrapolated survival curves for patients with severe disease are derived from retrospective reviews at the University of Utah of 101 records collected from the late 1940s to early 1970.[446] Patients received blood transfusions and later in this period also platelets; almost all were treated with corticosteroids and half with androgens as well. Data for the nontransplanted patients come from a multicenter study of the efficacy of marrow transplantation, performed in the early 1970s[335]; this control group was variably treated with androgens. **(B)** Similar long-term survival following either bone marrow transplantation (BMT) (various conditioning regimens) or immunosuppression (IS), mainly with ALG in the most recent analysis from the European Group for Bone Marrow Transplantation (EGBMT).[204] However, certain subgroups do better with transplant (children, severely neutropenic cases) or immunosuppression (older or less neutropenic patients). **(C)** Bone marrow transplantation outcomes at a single center (University of Washington[199, 325]). The larger experience includes some of the more recently treated patients (ATG a component of the regimen, 13% of the total cases) as well as patients who received supplemental peripheral blood white cells (46% of the total), which increased graft-versus-host disease.

death, or apoptosis. Although these insights derived from clinical observations, such as the observation of cyclosporine responsiveness and dependence, they in turn provide a basis for the development of novel treatments directed at both more selective or comprehensive immunosuppression and to stem cell preservation. The exact nature of the inciting antigens, the determinants of an aberrant, presumably autoimmune response, and the forces that drive development of the somatic genetic alterations leading to late clonal hematologic diseases remain outstanding questions of clinical and biologic importance.

DEFINITION

Aplastic anemia, the paradigm of bone marrow failure syndromes, is simply defined as peripheral blood pancytopenia and a hypocellular bone marrow (Plate 1). From its clinical features and epidemiology, responsiveness to therapy, and pathophysiology, AA is a distinctive disease. The typical patient, young and previously well, presents with symptoms of mild bleeding or easy fatigue; the peripheral blood shows severe reductions in platelets, and red and white blood cells, and the marrow is partly or entirely replaced by fat. Although usually characterized by diminished marrow function that affects all the hematopoietic lineages, granulocyte, platelet, and red blood cell levels may not be uniformly lowered, and less drastic degrees of marrow hypoplasia and odd combinations of bicytopenias and even monocytopenias occur. With early diagnosis, pancytopenia may not be complete, with relative preservation of red blood cell numbers or adequate neutrophils, which will decline over a week or two of observation. The degree of marrow hypocellularity is variable and need not correlate with the blood counts: hematopoietic cells may be seen in the marrow, especially on aspirations from a central site like the sternum, even with the severest pancytopenia, and conversely marrow aplasia may be profound in AA that is only moderate by blood count criteria. Even typical AA may vary in its clinical presentation and course, from a fulminant illness marked by continuous or recurrent hemorrhage and major infections to an indolent process manageable by transfusions alone.

Accurate diagnosis requires exclusion of other causes of pancytopenia (Table 1–1). Although of less importance in practice, AA is conventionally classified by presumed etiology as a primary hematologic disease, almost invariably idiopathic, or apparently secondary to various proximate causes, including obvious physical and chemical toxins but also medical drugs and viruses that may act indirectly through the immune system.

EPIDEMIOLOGY

Incidence

The largest and most comprehensive approach to the epidemiology of bone marrow failure is the International Aplastic Anemia and Agranulocytosis Study (IAAAS), which was conducted in Europe and Israel from 1980 to 1984[11] to examine the rate and general drug use associations with both agranulocytosis and AA. This study was performed prospectively, used strict case definition, and required pathologic confirmation of all cases. By such stringent criteria, the overall incidence rate was determined to be two new cases of acquired AA per million population each year. The

TABLE 1–1 A Classification of Aplastic Anemia

Acquired Aplastic Anemia	Inherited Aplastic Anemia
Secondary Aplastic Anemia	Fanconi's anemia
Radiation	Dyskeratosis congenita
Drugs and chemicals	Shwachman syndrome
Regular effects:	Reticular dysgenesis
Cytotoxic agents	Amegakaryocytic thrombocytopenia
Benzene	Familial aplastic anemias
Idiosyncratic reactions:	Preleukemia (monosomy 7, etc.)
Chloramphenicol	Nonhematologic syndromes (Down, Dubowitz,
Nonsteroidal anti-inflammatory drugs	Seckel's)
Antiepileptics	
Gold	
Others (see Table 1–5)	
Viruses	
Epstein-Barr virus (infectious mononucleosis)	
Hepatitis (non-A, non-B, non-C hepatitis)	
Parvovirus (rare; usually transient aplastic crisis, pure red cell aplasia)	
Human immunodeficiency virus (rare; more commonly dysplasia, multifactorial marrow failure)	
Immune diseases	
Eosinophilic fasciitis	
Hypoimmunoglobulinemia	
Thymoma and thymic carcinoma	
Graft-versus-host disease in immunodeficiency	
Paroxysmal nocturnal hemoglobinuria	
Pregnancy	
Idiopathic Aplastic Anemia	

TABLE 1-2 Epidemiology of Aplastic Anemia

Study	Dates	Method, Database	Population Size (10⁶)	N	Incidence (10⁶)
United Kingdom[435]	1985	Prospective survey of hematologists	21.0	49	2.3
Denmark[436]	1967–1982	Retrospective registry (children only)	1.13	39	2.2
Europe[437]	1980–1984	Population-based case control survey	22.3	168	2.2
Buenos Aires[438]	1966–1977	Retrospective; medical records	0.45	35	6
France[439]	1984–1987	Prospective; medical records	81.5	250	1.4
China[20]	1986–1988	Case collection	17.3	387	7.4
Bangkok[19]	1989	Population-based case control survey	8.8	32	3.7
Nordic countries[440]	1982–1993	Retrospective-prospective registry (children <15 yr)	4.31	101	1.95
Northern England[441]	1983–1995	Physician reports; reference bone marrow examinations (children <15 yr)	0.58	14	2.0
Saskatchewan[442]	1982–1991	Retrospective; administrative healthcare database	—	257	2.7

incidence figure from the IAAAS is considerably lower (three- to fourfold) than rates obtained in many earlier, mainly retrospective, and less well-designed surveys (Table 1–2). Although an apparent increase in incidence during the 1950s and 1960s was reported by some authors, such a trend is not supported by data collected during the last 20 years, in which rates have been stable.

Age Distribution

AA often affects young persons (Fig. 1–3). Most patients present at 15 to 25 years or over 60 years

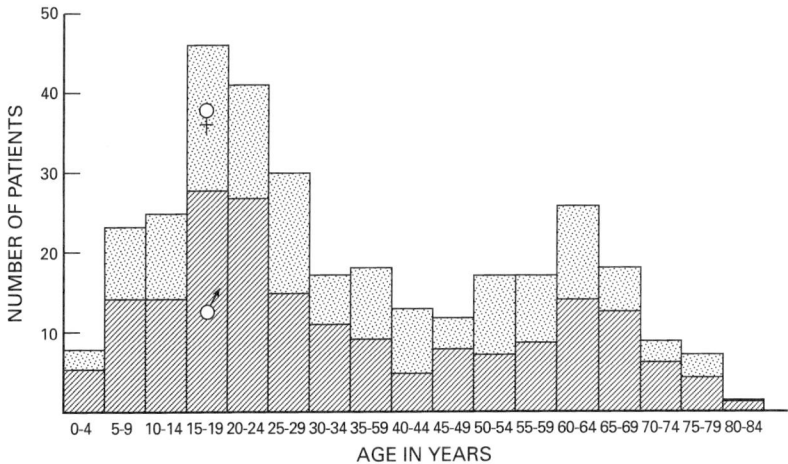

Figure 1-3 Distribution of age at diagnosis of over 300 patients with an admitting diagnosis of severe aplastic anemia, seen at the Clinical Center of the National Institutes of Health between 1978 and 1998.

of age, with a trough in middle life. (The early age of occurrence from hospital series conflicts with mortality data showing a single major peak in deaths from AA in late middle age[12]; the explanation for this discrepancy is probably misdiagnosis of aplasia for the far commoner syndrome of myelodysplasia in older persons.[13])

Geographic Distribution

The most remarkable feature of the epidemiology of AA is the marked geographic variation in its incidence.[14] A long-standing impression of physicians in the Orient and their European and American visitors has been that AA is more common in Asia compared with the West. In hematology clinics in China or Thailand, the frequency of AA as an admitting diagnosis may rival that of acute myelogenous leukemia (AML), whereas in most American hospitals acute leukemia is 5 to 10 times more common as an admitting diagnosis. National surveys in Japan[15] and China[16] reported extraordinarily high prevalence rates. Autopsy series[17] and mortality statistics[18] suggested that the annual death rate from AA might be more than three times higher in the Far East than in the West. More recently, the incidence of AA in Bangkok and two rural regions of Thailand has been rigorously determined, using the same methods as employed by the IAAAS in Europe and Israel: the annual incidence was $4.0/10^6$ in the capital and $5.6/10^6$ in the northeastern province of Khonkaen.[19] A large study[20] of 21 Chinese provinces yielded an estimated annual incidence rate of $7.4/10^6$; in Sabah province of Malaysia a retrospective analysis[21] found a rate of $5/10^6$. From published, hospital-based series of patients and from personal communications and first-hand observations, AA is almost certainly at similarly high prevalence in Vietnam and Indonesia; in Russia and the former Soviet republics; in Iran, Iraq, Pakistan, and India; in Mexico and other regions of Latin America[22]; and in Africa, where it is likely much underdiagnosed.[23, 24]

In the United States, there are no major sex or racial differences in the occurrence of AA.[25]

Environmental Risk Factors

Population-based studies have investigated possible causal associations. Drugs were implicated in only about 25% of European cases identified in the IAAAS,[11] where the major drug associations were with gold salts (relative risk [RR] of 29), antithyroid drugs (RR = 11), and nonsteroidal anti-inflammatory agents (NSAIDs; e.g., RR = 8.2 for indomethacin); benzene, insecticides, and petrochemicals were only modestly related[11] (Table 1–3). Other, smaller studies have shown associations with chemical exposures and to viruses through

TABLE 1–3 Drugs Associated With Aplastic Anemia in the International Aplastic Anemia and Agranulocytosis Study[11]

Drug	Stratified Risk Estimate (95% Confidence Interval)	Multivariate Relative Risk Estimate* (95% Confidence Interval)
Nonsteroidal analgesics		
Butazones	3.7 (1.9–7.2)	5.1 (2.1–12)
Indomethacin	7.1 (3.4–15)	8.2 (3.3–20)
Piroxicam	9.8 (3.3–29)	7.4 (2.1–26)
Diclofenac	4.6 (2.0–11)	4.2 (1.6–11)
Antibiotics		
Sulfonamides†	2.8 (1.1–7.3)	2.2 (0.6–7.4)
Antithyroid drugs	16 (4.8–54)	11 (2.0–56)
Cardiovascular drugs		
Furosemide	3.3 (1.6–7.0)	3.1 (1.2–8.0)
Psychotropic drugs		
Phenothiazines	3.0 (1.1–8.2)	1.6 (0.4–7.4)
Corticosteroids	5.0 (2.8–8.9)	3.5 (1.6–7.7)
Penicillamine	∞	
Allopurinol	7.3 (3.0–17)	5.9 (1.8–19)
Gold	29 (9.7–89)	

*The multivariate model included the following factors: age, sex, geographic area, date of interview, reliability of the patient, person interviewed, transfer from another hospital, history of blood disorder or tuberculosis, exposure to benzene and related chemicals, and use of other suspected drugs.
†Other than trimethoprim-sulfonamide combination.

transfusions, hepatitis, and occupation.[26] In Thailand, significant and high relative risk ratios have been established for a number of independent variables, including low income,[27] rural residence, and prior exposure to hepatitis A virus; perhaps most provocative is a link to farming.[28] In Thailand, contrary to expectations, medical drug use accounted for only about 15% of cases, and neither chloramphenicol nor household pesticide exposure was significantly related.[29] "Clusters" of AA have been reported only rarely.[30] The explanation for the geographic variation in AA is probably mainly environmental rather than genetic, as Japanese in Hawaii seem to have AA at the American rate.[18] Conversely, American soldiers in the Pacific theater during World War II had a high incidence of AA (blamed on exposure to the antimalarial quinacrine).[31]

Genetic Factors

The occurrence of more than one case of acquired AA in families is very rare. In children and young adults, acquired disease must be distinguished from the inherited bone marrow failure syndrome of Fanconi's anemia: patients with Fanconi's anemia may not manifest typical physical anomalies, and pancytopenia can develop in adulthood (see Chapter 2). In occasional instances, AA that is not Fanconi's anemia by chromosome analysis has been observed in multiple families members.[32]

The host immune response is genetically regulated, and for many autoimmune diseases susceptibility has been linked to specific HLA antigens. A few histocompatibility types have also been associated with AA, most consistently HLA-DR2: in one study, among 75 patients, HLA-DR2 was twice as frequent as in the general population.[33] Other associated antigens include A2,[34,35] B14,[35] and Cw7[36] of class I loci and DR4[37] and Dpw3[38] class II antigens; HLA-B8 and other antigens have been specifically linked to posthepatitis aplasia.[36] In Japanese patients, a class II haplotype (DRB*1501) that determines HLA-DR2 presentation was strongly associated with a hematologic response to cyclosporine,[39] as well as to the probability of relapse[40] and to the dependence of remission on continued administration of cyclosporine.[41] However, HLA-DR2 has been inconsistently correlated with response to immunosuppression in other studies. The haplotypes associated with clozapine agranulocytosis have been linked to heat shock protein variants encoded within the large major histocompatibility gene region.[42] Similar types of genetic predisposition may be responsible for some idiosyncratic reactions to drugs and chemicals (see later).

CLINICAL FEATURES

Symptoms and Signs

History

Patients' complaints derive from their low blood counts. Bleeding is an alarming symptom, even if usually minor in character; gum oozing, nosebleeds, easy bruising, heavy or irregular menses often precipitate the first visit to a physician. Dark urine due to the presence of hemoglobin may accompany paroxysmal nocturnal hemoglobinuria (PNH), but frank blood in the urine or stool is not otherwise observed early in the course of AA. More frequent are the nonspecific symptoms of chronic anemia, especially fatigue or lassitude, shortness of breath, and ringing in the ears; older patients may present with chest pains or congestive heart failure. Surprisingly, serious infection is unusual early in the course of AA. Notably absent also are symptoms of systemic disease like weight loss, appetite loss, or fever, and most patients feel well despite abnormal laboratory values.

In a few instances in which blood counts have been serially monitored, the time interval between exposure to a medical drug or a viral infection and the onset of pancytopenia is about 6 to 8 weeks.[43] The interval may be more prolonged if the resulting symptoms are well tolerated. The IAAAS panel of hematologists and epidemiologists established a window between 1 year and 1 month prior to presentation to establish risk factors, and certainly very distant or almost immediate exposures are difficult to credibly incriminate. A careful and directed history should be obtained to elicit possible inciting events, although their identification rarely has an impact on choice of therapy. Exceptions are the rare cases of acute exposure to high doses of radiation, cytotoxic drugs, and chronic benzene exposure. A past history of chemotherapy points toward secondary myelodysplasia, and familial blood diseases to Fanconi's anemia.

Physical Examination

Findings range from a well-appearing patient with minimal abnormalities to an acutely ill individual with signs of systemic toxicity. Cachexia, lymphadenopathy, and splenomegaly are not seen and should suggest another diagnosis. Petechiae are usually located over dependent regions like the pretibial surface and dorsal aspects of the ankles and wrists, as well as within the oropharynx and on the palate (Plate 2). Ecchymoses of differing sizes and hues may be found on areas that ordinarily suffer minor trauma (see Plate 2). With severe degrees of thrombocytopenia, active hemorrhage may be observed in the retina, from the nares, and as gingival oozing; the stool guaiac test will be positive and blood may be present at the cervical os. Pallor of the mucous membranes and nail beds is common. Less frequently there is fever, but usually without localizing signs of infection. Areas of hyper- or hypopigmentation, as well as typical anomalies, indicate Fanconi's anemia, and peculiarly misshapen nails are pathognomonic of dyskeratosis congenita.

Laboratory Studies

Blood

At presentation, all the blood counts are generally depressed; neutrophil numbers may fall further over a few days of observation. The blood smear lacks platelets and granulocytes but has normal red blood cell morphology. Automated cell counting shows little variation in erythrocyte size, but macrocytosis is the rule; platelets are not enlarged, as they are in peripheral destruction with idiopathic thrombocytopenic purpura. Automated counting has sharpened the accuracy of the reticulocyte count, which is markedly decreased. Monocyte and lymphocyte numbers also are reduced. Prior transfusions temporarily alter platelet and reticulocyte values as well as the hemoglobin. Of the ancillary laboratory studies, Ham's test has historically established PNH but is less useful in the setting of red blood cell transfusions and far less sensitive than flow cytometric methods of assessing glycosylphosphatidylinositol-linked surface proteins.[44] Serum transaminases point to prior or concurrent hepatitis, but specific viral serologies are negative. A fetal pattern of erythrocyte i antigen expression and low sialic acid content, like macrocytosis, reflect stressed erythropoiesis. Lymphocytes cultured in vitro can be analyzed for the characteristic susceptibility of Fanconi's anemia cells to cytogenetic damage in the presence of DNA damaging agents.

Bone Marrow

Cellularity is estimated from a biopsy: core samples obtained using a Jamshidi needle are easily of sufficient length (at least 1 cm) and undistorted by crush artifact (see Plate 1A). Point counting and comparison with age-matched control data are ideal, but visual estimation is the practice; generally the biopsy is so preponderantly fat that precise quantitation is unnecessary. Undecalcified biopsies that are imbedded in plastic may allow a nicer view of morphology than conventionally prepared specimens, especially the appreciation of "abnormally localized immature precursors" (ALIPs), bordering fatty areas rather than ranked at the trabecular bone surface, characteristic of myelodysplasia. Otherwise, the aspirate smear is preferred to assess individual cells (see Plate 1B). Hematopoietic cells are drastically reduced in number and may be totally lacking. Residual erythroid precursors may be megaloblastic or even dysplastic, but there are no myeloblasts and megakaryocytes almost always are absent. Hemophagocytosis may be observed. The few spicules show fibroblastic cells of stromal origin, plasma cells, and lymphocytes.

Cytogenetic analysis of marrow cells is important in bone marrow failure syndromes. In AA at presentation, chromosomes are almost always normal while frequently abnormal in myelodysplasia. Unfortunately, low numbers of mitotic cells limit the applicability of this test in a hypocellular marrow specimen.

DIFFERENTIAL DIAGNOSIS

The differential diagnosis is best considered in two stages, which follow from the blood count results initially and the bone marrow examination later. Pancytopenia has many causes, of which AA is not the most common (Table 1–4). The history and physical examination can quickly lead to an obvious diagnosis: a course of recent chemotherapy for cancer or a long history of systemic lupus; the stigmas of alcoholic liver disease, especially splenomegaly; or overwhelming sepsis. While the typical presentation of AA offers little diagnostic confusion, AA may closely resemble other important hematologic diseases. Leukemia, especially in early childhood and in the elderly, and lymphoma may occasionally present with pancytopenia and a fatty marrow, and without circulating blast cells; abnormal cells must be sought close to the marrow spicule. By sensitive molecular methods, the leukemic clone may be appreciated retrospectively after gene amplification of the original hypocellular marrow specimen.[45] Pancytopenia occurs in myelofibrosis or myeloid metaplasia, and the "dry tap" on marrow aspiration is sometimes mistaken for aplasia; the leukoerythroblastic appearance of the blood smear and fibrosis of the marrow biopsy specimen allow an accurate diagnosis.

Most confusing is the distinction between AA and hypocellular myelodysplasia, for which absolute distinguishing criteria have not yet been developed (see Chapter 3). About 20% of myelodysplasia cases present with a predominantly fatty marrow.[46–48] Morphology, chromosome testing, and radiographic studies are most helpful (see Chapter 3). Marrow morphology in AA is usually normal or shows only erythroid changes. In myelodysplasia, megakaryocytes are preserved and

TABLE 1-4 Differential Diagnosis of Pancytopenia

Pancytopenia With Hypocellular Bone Marrow
    Acquired aplastic anemia
    Inherited aplastic anemia (Fanconi's anemia and others)
    Some myelodysplasia syndromes
    Rare aleukemic leukemia (acute myelogenous leukemia)
    Some acute lymphoblastic leukemia
    Some lymphomas of bone marrow

Pancytopenia With Cellular Bone Marrow
Primary Bone Marrow Diseases
    Myelodysplasia syndromes
    Paroxysmal nocturnal hemoglobinuria
    Myelofibrosis
    Hairy cell leukemia
    Some aleukemic leukemia
    Myelophthisis*
    Bone marrow lymphoma
Secondary to Systemic Diseases
    Systemic lupus erythematosus, Sjögren's syndrome
    Hypersplenism
    Vitamin B_{12}, folate deficiency (familial defect)
    Overwhelming infection
    Alcoholism
    Brucellosis
    Ehrlichiosis
    Sarcoidosis
    Tuberculosis and atypical mycobacteria

Hypocellular Bone Marrow With or Without Cytopenia
    Q fever
    Legionnaires' disease
    Toxoplasmosis
    Mycobacteria
    Tuberculosis
    Anorexia nervosa, starvation
    Hypothyroidism

*Pancytopenia in tuberculosis is only rarely associated with a hypocellular bone marrow at biopsy or autopsy. Marrow failure in the setting of tuberculosis is almost always fatal; exceptional patients probably suffered underlying myelodysplasia or acute leukemia. Metastatic cancer is usually apparent from the appearance of syncytia of malignant, nonhematopoietic cells, but aplasia has been reported as a rare paraneoplastic syndrome.

can be aberrantly micro- and mononuclear. Myeloid precursors are often undergranulated, there may be an increased representation of blasts and other young forms, and nuclear morphology may be abnormal. ALIPs (see earlier) are typical. Extreme megaloblastic changes, bizarre erythroid morphology, and ringed sideroblasts are not consistent with a diagnosis of AA. Chromosomes 5, 7, 9, and others show characteristic abnormalities in myelodysplasia. As noted earlier, cytogenetic abnormalities, at least by conventional testing, are unusual at presentation of AA; more sophisticated assays also suggest that this difference persists at the molecular level, where, for example, p53 expression is normal in aplasia but frequently increased in myelodysplasia.[49] Magnetic resonance imaging (MRI) of a few vertebral bodies can distinguish a uniformly fatty marrow from a spotty mixture of hypo- and hypercellularity.[50] Nevertheless, some degree of shared pathophysiology between aplasia and myelodysplasia has been suggested by similar responses to immunosuppressive drugs[51, 52] and evidence of T cell suppression of hematopoiesis in vitro.[53]

A final difficult differential diagnosis is between acquired and constitutional hematopoietic failure, as the marrow appearance is the same. Physical anomalies, especially café au lait lesions, bony abnormalities of the hands, and unexpectedly short stature or peculiar facies, point to constitutional aplasia, which can be confirmed, or, in the absence of physical findings, diagnosed by stressed cytogenetic testing of peripheral blood (see Chapter 6).

PATHOPHYSIOLOGY

Hematopoiesis

By all measures, hematopoiesis is severely reduced in AA, including not only the morphologic and radiologic studies described earlier but also specific phenotypic and functional assays of blood cell progenitors.[54] By flow cytometry, the CD34+ cell population, containing most of the committed progenitor cells and stem cells, is greatly reduced in most patients; those with moderate disease or who have recovered may show higher CD34+ cell numbers, but levels may remain low despite improved blood counts.[55, 56] Hematopoietic progenitor cells that can be enumerated in semisolid medium and demonstrate lineage commitment are severely reduced in all studies: colonies formed by CFU_{GM} (granulocyte and macrophage progenitors), primitive erythroid progenitors (BFU-E) and CFU-E, and pluripotent progenitors measured as CFU-GEMM. Colony formation by bone marrow from patients with severe disease remains unresponsive even to very high levels of individual hematopoietic growth factors,[57, 58] although prolonged growth factor administration to patients may increase circulating colony-forming cells.[59] In general, however, low numbers of progenitors persist in patients long after successful treatment and hematologic recovery.[55, 60–62] Using stem cell surrogate assays, which assess cells capable of colony formation after more than a month in long-term bone marrow culture (long-term culture–initiating cells [LTC-IC]) or to produce "cobblestone" islands in long-term cultures, primitive progenitors also are virtually absent in every patient with severe aplasia[63, 64] and usually do not recover after either immunosuppressive or transplant therapies.[62] Combining the low LTC-IC number and the reduced marrow cellularity leads to an estimation that stem cells are reduced to 1% or less of normal in AA.

Qualitative abnormalities of hematopoiesis have also been documented. Least surprising is that the number of stem cell clones is reduced, as determined in assays based on X chromosome inactivation in heterozygous female patients.[65] Not only total numbers but also the yield of CFU_{GM} and BFU-E from a purified CD34+ population is diminished.[55] Telomere length is reduced in granulocytes and lymphocytes from patients with bone marrow failure syndromes and is correlated with disease duration[66]; however, telomere length is also shorter in patients who have received marrow transplants and may only reflect the highly proliferative status of the marrow compartment. In general, data from current assays do not allow a distinction between dysfunction of individual stem cells and abnormalities of the hematopoietic compartment as a whole.

Stroma and Hematopoietic Growth Factors

The survival and proliferation of hematopoietic cells is dependent on stromal cells, but the stroma is not usually defective in aplastic anemia (reviewed in Young and Maciejewski,[54] Kojima,[67] and Marsh[68]). For example, plastic-adherent cells from patients support hematopoiesis by normal CD34+ cells, while no hematopoietic colonies develop when patients' CD34+ cells are cultured in the presence of normal stroma.[69, 70] Stromal cells cultured from patients' bone marrow produce normal quantities of hematopoietic growth factors, measured as protein,[71] messenger RNA (mRNA),[72] or functionally.[73] A few studies have suggested deficiencies in some factors of uncertain pathophysiologic significance. Stroma isolated from a minority of patients may poorly manufacture granulocyte-macrophage colony-stimulating factor (GM-CSF),[74] interleukin-3 (IL-3), and granulocyte colony-stimulating factor (G-CSF)[75] or IL-1.[76] However, serum levels of erythropoietin (Epo),[77] thrombopoietin,[78] G-CSF,[79] and GM-CSF are usually much elevated. Cytokines that act at very early stages of hematopoiesis include Flt-3 ligand, for which blood levels are highly elevated in AA,[80] and stem cell factor (SCF), for which blood levels have been variable but at most only modestly decreased and stromal production normal.[81] Adequate stroma function is also implicit in the success of marrow transplantation in AA, because important stromal elements remain of host origin. Nor has treatment with hematopoietic growth factors—even those putatively deficient in patients—been very effective in restoring hematopoiesis in severely affected patients.

Mechanisms of Hematopoietic Cell Destruction

Direct Toxicity

The commonest form of AA is iatrogenic—the transient marrow failure that follows on cytotoxic chemotherapeutic drugs or irradiation therapy of cancer. Chemical or physical agents can act directly to injure both proliferating and quiescent hematopoietic cells; the introduction of sufficient damage to DNA leads to the process of apoptosis. As discussed later, among the drugs that are idiosyncratically associated with marrow failure may be a few that also directly cause marrow damage. However, patients with community-acquired AA rarely have a history of exposure to consistently toxic physicochemical agents.

Immune-mediated Marrow Failure

Mathé in the 1970s observed unexpected improvement of pancytopenia after failed marrow transplantation, and he speculated that the immunosuppressive conditioning regimen, intended to allow engraftment of the donor marrow, instead promoted the return of host marrow function.[82] Purposeful targeting of the immune system followed on these observations, and the effectiveness of diverse therapies to reduce lymphocyte number or to block T cell function strongly suggests that their success is due to an immunosuppressive mode of action.

Laboratory support for the immune hypothesis first came from coculture experiments, in which mononuclear cells from patients' blood or bone marrow suppressed colony formation by hematopoietic progenitor cells in vitro; removal of T cells from the patient samples sometimes improved their in vitro colony formation.[83] Peripheral blood and bone marrow from patients produced a soluble factor that inhibited hematopoiesis, and normal lymphocytes could be stimulated to release the same activity.[84] This soluble inhibitory activity was identified as interferon-γ (IFN-γ),[85] a product of lymphocytes and natural killer (NK) cells that inhibits hematopoiesis in vitro and in animals. AA patients' T cells overproduced IFN-γ[86] and also tumor necrosis factor (TNF),[87] another cytokine capable of suppressing hematopoietic cell proliferation.[88] IFN-γ mRNA, evidence of activity of the gene, was detectable in samples from most aplastic patients but not in normal persons or in control patients with other hematologic diseases.[89, 90] T cells infiltrated aplastic marrow,[91] and both blood and marrow of AA patients also contained elevated numbers of activated cytotoxic lymphocytes that could be assayed phenotypically (by expression of activation markers; Fig. 1–4A) or functionally (by their cytokine content, using intracellular staining for IFN-γ,[92] [Fig. 1–4B] or by suppression of colony formation[93]). The number and activity of these cells decreased appropriately with successful immunosuppressive therapy.[94, 95] Both activated cytotoxic lymphocytes and inhibitory lymphokines are specifically localized to the targeted bone marrow.

Late events in the immunosuppression of hematopoiesis are understood, at least in outline (Fig. 1–5A). In vitro, the lymphokines IFN-γ and TNF suppressed proliferation in tissue culture of early and late hematopoietic progenitor and stem cells.[88] These effects were far more potent when lymphokines were secreted into the marrow microenvironment than when they were simply added to culture,[96] consistent with their localization in the marrow of patients. While IFN-γ and

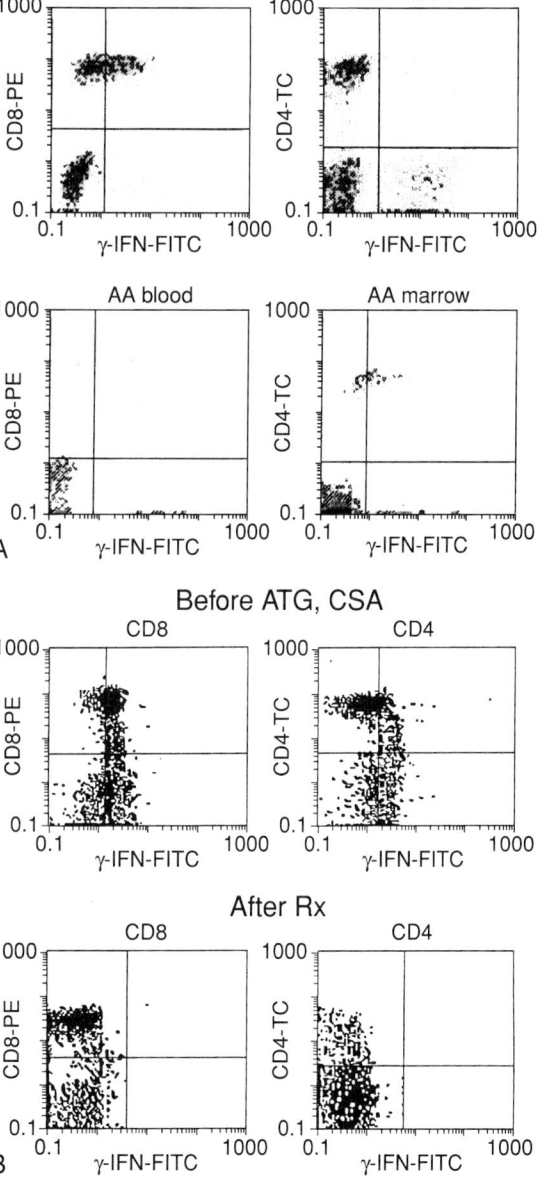

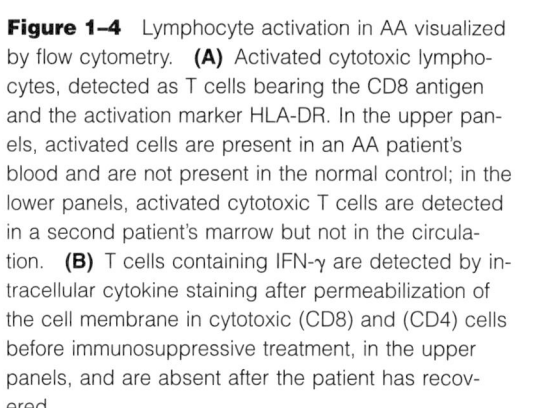

Figure 1–4 Lymphocyte activation in AA visualized by flow cytometry. **(A)** Activated cytotoxic lymphocytes, detected as T cells bearing the CD8 antigen and the activation marker HLA-DR. In the upper panels, activated cells are present in an AA patient's blood and are not present in the normal control; in the lower panels, activated cytotoxic T cells are detected in a second patient's marrow but not in the circulation. **(B)** T cells containing IFN-γ are detected by intracellular cytokine staining after permeabilization of the cell membrane in cytotoxic (CD8) and (CD4) cells before immunosuppressive treatment, in the upper panels, and are absent after the patient has recovered.

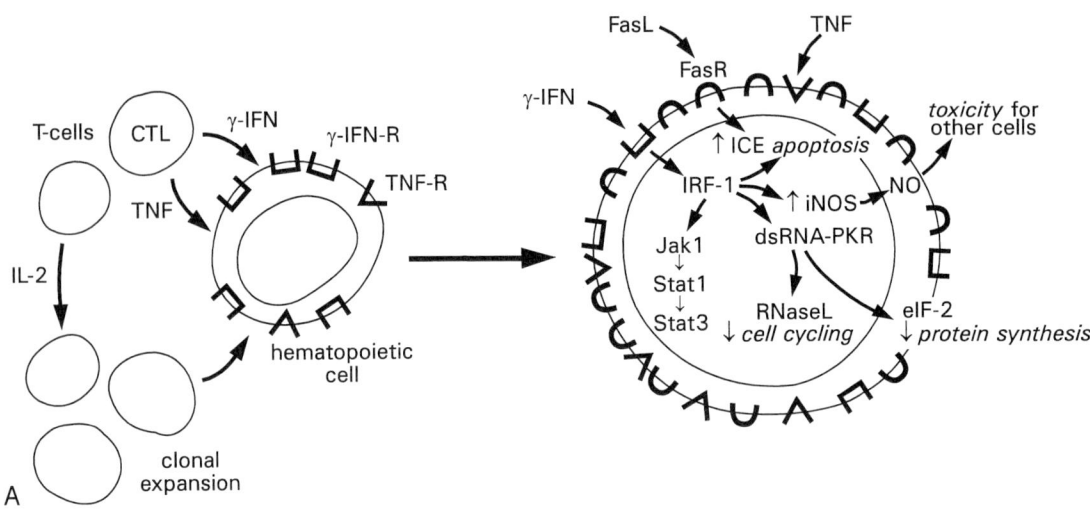
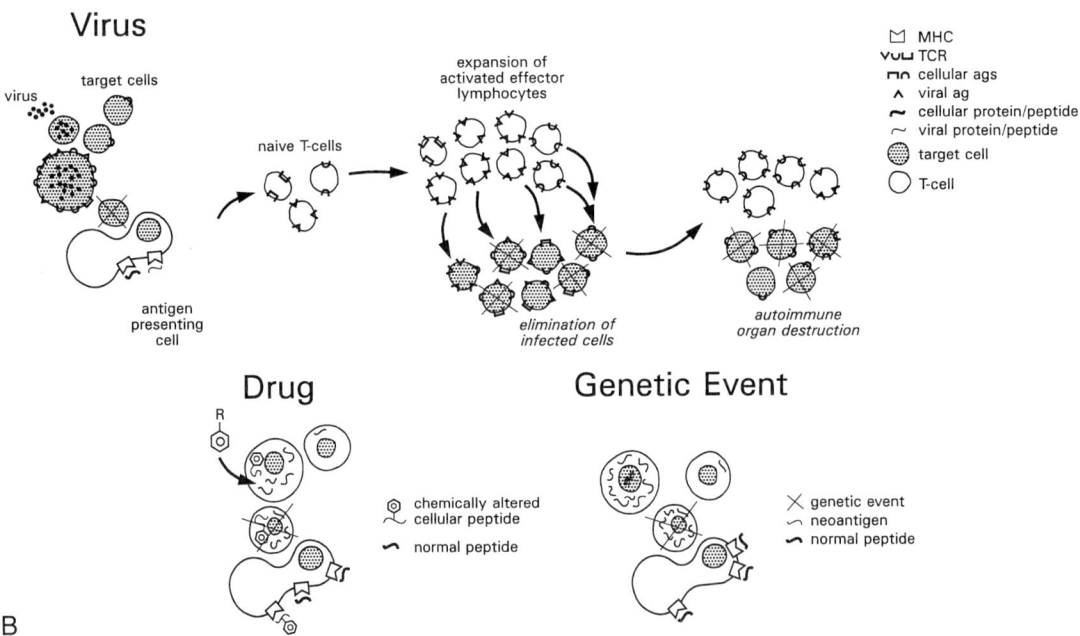

Figure 1–5 Immune-mediated marrow failure. **(A)** Proximal events, including cytotoxic T cell activation with production of inhibitory cytokines, IFN-γ, TNF, and IL-2 and recognition of CD34+ cell targets, with subsequent induction of Fas receptor expression and triggering of multiple signal transduction pathways leading to cell death.
(B) Early stages of autoimmunity in AA have been less well characterized. In theory, antigens derived from infection with a virus, exposure to drugs or chemicals, or neoantigens from a somatic genetic event would be processed by the immune system and lead to T cell activation that is both specific to the antigen and broadly reactive to normal cellular antigens, either aberrantly or excessively expressed in the affected tissue. In rare individuals, this physiologic, usually transient, process converts to a pathophysiologic, persisting, autoimmune response.

TNF can suppress hematopoiesis by effects on the mitotic cycle, an important and perhaps critical component of inhibition is cell killing through induction of programmed cell death. Both lymphokines induced expression of the Fas receptor on CD34+ progenitor cells; triggering of the Fas receptor by its ligand initiated apoptosis; both Fas receptor expression and the number of apoptotic cells were increased in patients' marrow.[97, 98] IFN and TNF also increased nitric oxide synthase and nitric oxide production by marrow cells,[99] which also would contribute to immune-mediated cytotoxicity and elimination of hematopoietic cells. Induction of interferon regulatory factor-1 (IRF-1), a transcription regulator experimentally associated with inhibition of cell proliferation, was required for the negative action of IFN-γ on hematopoiesis.[100]

The early immune system events that must precede the global destruction of hematopoietic cells are much less clearly elucidated. Involvement of CD4+ lymphocytes has been inferred from HLA typing of patients. As described earlier, HLA-DR2 is overrepresented in European and American patients with AA, and a more specific class II haplotype has been identified in Japanese patients. Several HLA antigens may be much more common in certain subsets of marrow failure, like B8 in posthepatitis aplasia. Clones of HLA-DR–restricted T helper cells derived from a few patients have been shown to proliferate in response to marrow cells.[101, 102] The initial antigen recognition event that leads to breached tolerance and the subsequent process of spreading autoimmunity are unknown. Chemicals, drugs, and viral infections that have been clinically associated with AA can be viewed as inciting complex, but ultimately similar immunologic attack on and destruction of hematopoietic cells (Fig. 1–5B). In outline, AA shares clinical, epidemiologic, and pathophysiologic features with other diseases of organ-specific autoimmunity, for which initiating antigens have been proposed from animal models and serologic studies: myelin basic protein for multiple sclerosis, islet cell proteins for type I diabetes mellitus, and keratin in uveitis.

Immune system destruction of the bone marrow is modeled in animals by runt disease, which is produced by infusion of donor lymphocytes that recognize host cells as foreign but are not themselves rejected; pancytopenia and death can be prevented by administration of monoclonal antibodies to IFN-γ.[103] In humans, transfusion-associated GvHD causes severe and almost invariably fatal marrow destruction by the same mechanism.[104] Very small numbers of effector cells can mediate disease under these conditions, which has been conveyed by residual lymphocytes contained in plasma or with solid organ transplants, and a single amino acid difference in an HLA molecule has sufficed to induce GvHD after marrow transplant between twins. AA is associated with peculiar rheumatic syndromes, particularly eosinophilic fasciitis,[105] and like systemic lupus erythematosus may appear or worsen with pregnancy.[106] Thus aberrant antigen presentation and recognition are suggested by some of the disease's clinical associations. While the antigens are unknown, the pathophysiology of the immune processes that operate in AA are broadly uniform, whatever the initial triggering event.

Specific Etiologic Associations

Radiation

Marrow aplasia is a major acute toxicity of radiation.[107–109] Stem and progenitor cells and the stroma may all be damaged. Bone marrow cells are most affected by high-energy gamma rays, and secondarily by alpha and beta particles. With the exception of lymphocytes, which are directly killed, a round of replication is required for radiation damage to become manifest. Mitotically active hematopoietic tissue is exquisitely sensitive to radiation with a rough correlation between cells' cycling status and their radiation sensitivity.[110] The dose-related occurrence of pancytopenia 2 to 4 weeks following exposure to radiation is due to injury to the actively replicating progenitor cell pool. Mortality from hematologic toxicity is a function of the marrow's ability to both tolerate depletion of hematopoietic cells and damage to the stem cell. The capacity for recovery of hematopoietic function following even massive single irradiation exposure is considerable, reflecting the resistance of the quiescent stem cell to damage and the enormous regenerative capacity of even a greatly reduced stem cell pool. At intermediate radiation doses around the median lethal dose (LD_{50}), where marrow toxicity limits survival, supportive efforts can drastically alter outcome. Autopsies of atom bomb victims in Japan showed acellular bone marrows in the first weeks of the explosion, but there frequently was regenerating bone marrow in those who survived longer.[111]

Bone marrow hypoplasia occurs with radiation doses above 1.5 to 2.0 Gy to the whole body. The histology of radiation-mediated aplasia includes necrosis, nuclear pyknosis and karyorrhexis, nuclear lysis, and ultimately cytolysis; the associated phagocytosis, marked congestion, and hemorrhage are rapidly followed by fatty replacement.[112] Precise LD_{50} figures for humans do not exist, and estimates are based on the limited direct human data and extrapolation from animal experiments. The LD_{50} is highly dependent on the quality of medical care: improved support may double the tolerated radiation dose.[113] From assessment of the outcome of radiation accidents and after high-dose therapeutic irradiation, the LD_{50} has been estimated at about 4.5 Gy,[114, 115] an almost mythical figure sometimes termed the Shields-Warren number.

In practice, the type and intensity of the source of radiation and the distance and shielding of the subject are the major determinants of radiation injury. Reconstruction methods are often used to estimate the received dose in an accidental exposure. The degree of pancytopenia also correlates well with the estimated radiation.[116] Because lymphocytes are particularly sensitive to radiation, their rate of fall can be used to estimate dose to a total body exposure of about 3 Gy[116]; at higher doses, the fall in granulocytes and the severity of thrombocytopenia and reticulocytopenia can be used as gauges.[108] After Chernobyl, measurement of dicentric chromosomes also provided an estimate of dose, which was better correlated with neutrophil than with lymphocyte kinetics.[117] The cytogenetic alterations in stem cells are dose-related, irreversible, and probably cumulative in increasing the probability of early leukemic transformation.[118, 119] The survival of some patients who received doses greater than 9 Gy suggests in retrospect that autologous marrow reconstitution can occur in many persons who survive the immediate consequences of radiation exposure.[120]

Pancytopenia may be a late consequence of a single radiation dose,[121] but AA is not well documented as a delayed sequela of radiation exposure. For example, out of 156 cases of AA in Japan in the 20 years following the atom bomb explosions, only 13 cases had received more than a 1 rad dose, and of the three patients who had been heavily irradiated, only one had typical AA.[122] In contrast, repeated low doses of radiation can damage bone marrow and have been associated with AA under very special circumstances, as for example, after thorium injection[123]; still, only a small proportion of exposed persons develop hematologic disease. Excessive numbers of deaths from AA were reported after therapeutic irradiation of the spine for ankylosing spondylitis, although the risk may have been overestimated.[124] Increased deaths from AA occurred among American radiologists who worked during the early part of the century with inadequate shielding.[125] Despite occasional instances in which marrow failure developed years after radiation and chemotherapy, AA was not found in unexpected numbers in a large population of cancer patients who had received therapeutic irradiation.[126] Marrow failure does not appear to be especially frequent among nuclear power plant or thorium processing factory workers or local residents,[127, 128] nor among persons exposed to higher natural background radiation.[129] With radiation, as with benzene exposure (see later), late marrow failure referred to in the older literature as "aplastic" might in fact be classified now as myelodysplasia, and its increased frequency therefore represents delayed manifestation of genetic damage rather than depletion of a limited stem cell reserve.

Drugs and Chemicals

Drugs are the most familiar clinical association with AA[130] (Table 1–5). Historically, drugs were linked to marrow failure after observations of benzene effects in workers at the end of the nineteenth century, establishment of a relationship of the analgesic amidopyrine to agranulocytosis in the early twentieth century, and description of an apparent epidemic of AA following the introduction of chloramphenicol in the 1960s. Initially suggested by the accumulation of case reports, specific drug associations have been established in formal case-control, population-based epidemiologic studies. In the IAAAS, conducted in Europe and Israel in the 1980s, relative risks were established for individual drugs and large classes of pharmaceutical agents, including NSAIDs, thyrostatics, certain cardiovascular agents, some psychotropics, and sulfa-based antibiotics[11] (see Table 1–4). Approximately 25% of the AA cases identified in this enormous study could be blamed on drug use. Drug use as a risk factor was also assessed by a similar methodology in Thailand, where the incidence of AA is higher than in the West.[19] Against expectations, chloramphenicol was not shown to be a risk factor; only sulfonamides reached statistical significance among medications, and the etiologic fraction blamed on drug use was only about 15%.[29]

Drug associations between chemicals and marrow aplasia are conveniently divided into two classes. Drugs used in cancer chemotherapy are selected for their cytotoxicity, and their regular, dose-dependent induction of marrow aplasia is expected. In contrast, most AA associated with medical drug use in the community is idiosyncratic, meaning that it occurs unexpectedly in rare individuals (although many of the drugs implicated in AA may more frequently be associated with milder and more restricted forms of marrow suppression such as neutropenia). While a difficult point to prove, some dose relationship probably does exist even for idiosyncratic reactions. In most case reports, patients have received normal or high

TABLE 1–5 Classification of Drugs and Chemicals Associated With Aplastic Anemia

I. Agents that regularly produce marrow depression as major toxicity in commonly employed doses or normal exposures:
  Cytotoxic drugs used in cancer chemotherapy
    Alkylating agents (busulfan, melphalan, cyclophosphamide)
    Antimetabolites (antifolic compounds, nucleotide analogues), antimitotics (vincristine, vinblastine), colchicine, some antibiotics, daunorubicin, doxorubicin
  Benzene (and less often benzene-containing chemicals: kerosene, carbon tetrachloride, Stoddard's solvent, chlorophenols)

II. Agents probably associated with aplastic anemia but with a relatively low probability relative to their use:
  Chloramphenicol
  Insecticides
  Antiprotozoals: quinacrine and chloroquine
  Nonsteroidal anti-inflammatory drugs, including phenylbutazone, indomethacin, ibuprofen, sulindac, diclofenac, naproxen, piroxicam, fenoprofen, fenbufen, mesalazine, aspirin (?)
  Anticonvulsants (hydantoins, carbamazepine, phenacemide, ethosuximide)
  Gold and arsenic (and other heavy metals, like bismuth, mercury)
  Sulfonamides as a class
  Some antibiotics
  Antithyroid drugs (methimazole, methylthiouracil, propylthiouracil)
  Antidiabetes drugs (tolbutamide, carbutamide, chlorpropamide)
  Carbonic anhydrase inhibitors (acetazolamide and methazolamide)
  D-Penicillamine
  2-Chlorodeoxyadenosine
  Estrogens (in pregnancy and in high doses in animals)

III. Agents more rarely associated with aplastic anemia:
  Antibiotics (streptomycin, tetracycline, methicillin, ampicillin, mebendazole and albendazole, sulfonamides [see above], flucytosine, mefloquine, dapsone)
  Antihistamines (cimetidine, ranitidine, chlorpheniramine)
  Sedatives and tranquilizers (chlorpromazine, prochlorperazine, piperacetazine, chlordiazepoxide, meprobamate, methyprylon, remoxipride)
  Antiarrhythmics (tocainide, amiodarone)
  Allopurinol (may potentiate marrow suppression by cytotoxic drugs)
  Ticlopidine
  Methyldopa
  Quinidine
  Lithium
  Guanidine
  Canthaxanin
  Potassium perchlorate
  Thiocyanate
  Carbimazole
  Cyanamide
  Desferrioxamine
  Amphetamines

doses of the agent and usually for a period of weeks to months. As for agranulocytosis (see Chapter 7), most marrow failure complications occur after a few weeks of therapy initiation and within the first 6 months of treatment.

The mechanisms that might lead to the very occasional development of AA after drug exposure include direct chemical toxicity and immune-mediated destruction. These pathophysiologic pathways have been better described for agranulocytosis, which is more commonly associated with prior medical drug use than is aplastic anemia (see Chapter 7). Unfortunately, drug-induced hematopoietic failure is difficult to study. AA is a rare rather than regular outcome, precluding an animal model, and the diversity of implicated drugs and the problem of confidently assigning causation in an individual case make clinical studies impractical. Drug-induced aplasia cannot be distinguished by history from idiopathic disease: the clinical course, including the favorable response to immunosuppressive therapy, of patients with histories of drug exposure is the same as in idiopathic disease[131]; serum assays are also unhelpful because antibodies to either drugs or cells have only occasionally been identified in AA.[132]

The low probability of developing AA from a drug exposure may be a reflection of the gene frequency for metabolic enzymes (for direct chemical effects) or immune response genes (for immune-mediated marrow failure) in the human population. The rarity of idiosyncratic drug reactions would then arise from the infrequent combination of unusual circumstances: exposure, genetic variations in drug metabolism, the physical properties of the agent, enzymatic pathways that chemically alter the drug, and the susceptibility of the host to the action of a toxic compound. Many drugs and chemicals, especially if they have limited water solubility, must be enzymatically degraded before conjugation and excretion. Degradative pathways for xenobiotics are complex, specific, redundant, and interrelated. Intermediate metabolites may be toxic, highly reactive, and responsible for some adverse effects of the primary agents. Examples of detoxifying enzyme systems directly applicable to bone marrow failure and also demonstrating genetic variability include arylhydrocarbon hydroxylase (relevant to benzene toxicity), epoxide hydrolases (for phenytoin toxicity), S-methylation (for 6-mercaptopurine, 6-thioguanine, and azathioprine) and N-acetylation (for sulfa drugs) (see Young[130] for a more detailed discussion). A nice example of the role of genetic background was provided by experiments using cells of a patient with carbamazapine-associated AA: only after generation of reactive metabolites from the incriminated agent by rat microsomes were the patient's lymphocytes killed in a dose-dependent, drug-specific pattern, while there was no toxicity for normal donors' cells, and intermediate killing of cells of the patient's mother.[133]

An immune basis for agranulocytosis was established early with the identification of leukoagglutinating antibodies and illustrated quite dramatically by the rapid reproduction of the syndrome on drug challenge of affected patients or with plasma infusions from patients into normal volunteers (see Chapter 7). Strong HLA class II linkage of clozapine[42, 134] and thiouracil[135] agranulocytosis in certain ethnic groups suggests involvement of CD4+ T cells in drug-induced marrow failure. The absence of serum antibodies in AA would suggest that drugs do not serve as simple haptens in the induction of this type of marrow failure. Other possible mechanisms include binding to cellular proteins leading to the loss of self-tolerance or disturbance of regulatory immune system networks with the same effect. The rarity of idiosyncratic drug reactions would be a function of genetic variation in drug metabolism systems, differences in major histocompatibility antigens and their peptide-binding properties, and the available repertoire of potentially self-reactive circulating lymphocytes during the period of drug exposure.

Benzene. Benzene is a ubiquitous chemical strongly linked to bone marrow failure and leukemia.[130, 136–139] Benzene myelotoxicity falls between the regular effects of chemotherapeutic agents and idiosyncratic drug reactions. Fugitive industrial emissions add greatly to the biologic sources of ambient benzene, and significant benzene exposure can also occur outside of industry. However, the concentrations of benzene to which consumers are exposed are orders of magnitude lower than those historically implicated in hematologic disease, and the effect on a population of chronic exposure to low doses of benzene, as with most "threshold" phenomena, is unknown.

Water-soluble products of benzene metabolism like phenols, hydroquinones, and catechols, rather than the parent compound, mediate marrow toxicity. Benzene's intermediate metabolites covalently and irreversibly bind to bone marrow DNA, inhibit DNA synthesis, and introduce DNA strand breaks. Benzene thus acts both as a "mitotic poison" and mutagen. Administration of benzene to animals produces bone marrow depression, but with variable marrow morphology, including often hyperplasia. Acutely, the more mature, actively cycling marrow precursor cells are preferentially damaged compared with primitive progenitors.[140] Intermittent is more damaging than continuous exposure as measured by impact on stem cell number.[141] The stroma can also be damaged by benzene.[142]

The range of hematologic effects attributable to benzene is broad, from relatively frequent but modest alterations in blood counts to marrow failure or leukemia. Studies of American workers earlier in this century suggested that the risk of AA was 3% to 4% in men exposed to concentrations higher than 300 ppm, and 50% of persons exposed to 100 ppm showed some blood count depression.[143, 144] The likelihood of some form of marrow suppression with heavy exposure can be high: over 10% of Chinese workers showed leukopenia; with improved hygiene the figure was lowered to 0.5%, a proportion which still resulted in a prevalence of 1 in 250.[145] Leukopenia, anemia, thrombocytopenia, and lymphocytopenia are common consequences of benzene; other manifestations include macrocytosis, acquired Pelger-Huët anomaly, eosinophilia, basophilia, and, more unusually, polycythemia, leukocytosis, thrombocytosis, or splenomegaly. The appearance of the marrow is usually normocellular but may be hypo- or hypercellular[146]; necrosis, fibrosis, edema, and hemorrhage have also been described.[147] Chronic benzene exposure clearly increases the risk of a variety of lymphohematopoietic malignancies. Aplasia and acute leukemia have occurred in the same person,[148] and pancytopenia not infrequently precedes acute leukemia.[149] Both marrow failure and leukemia in benzene workers can manifest decades after exposure, but malignancy may be the more frequent late consequence; the older literature seldom contains adequate histologic description of marrows to allow distinction between AA and myelodysplasia.

Aromatic Hydrocarbons. The common perception that other molecules resembling benzene or containing a benzene ring must also cause marrow suppression is not well supported by the facts. In contrast to benzene, neither closely related alkylbenzenes nor pure toluene and xylene are established marrow toxins. Often an aromatic hydrocarbon has been impugned by the clinician for lack of another apparent cause of disease. For some substances, toxicity may be due to the presence of benzene itself, either as a contaminant of the synthesis of the molecule or in the petroleum distillates used as solvent. Yet in total the number of AA cases reported is small considering the very large populations exposed to this heterogeneous group of chemicals. For example, surveys of AA patients found only 2%[150] to 6%[151] of cases associated with insecticide exposure, and the significance of a handful of case reports in the context of vast use of these compounds may be questioned. On the other hand, the very high prevalence of aromatic hydrocarbons in daily life would greatly amplify even a small individual risk. Pesticides and insecticides have been associated with AA for decades in almost 300 medical case reports[152]: most frequently cited are chlordane, lindane, and DDT. For the miscellaneous aromatic hydrocarbons, case reports also greatly outnumber series of patients and the results of systematic epidemiologic surveys are mixed. Significant excesses of AA have been reported for employment in certain industries with associated chemical exposures: printing (odds ratio [OR] = 6.2), lumber and wood products manufacture (OR = 3.7), agriculture (OR = 2.4), and construction (OR = 2.0).

Chloramphenicol. The structural similarity of chloramphenicol to amidopyrine, a drug earlier strongly associated with agranulocytosis, led to prescient prediction of possible hematotoxicity. During its time as a readily available and popular antibiotic, chloramphenicol was considered the commonest cause of AA in the United States,[153] blamed for 20% to 30% of total cases and 50% of drug-associated cases.[154, 155] Approximations of the numbers of cases of AA after a course of chloramphenicol ranged from 1 in 20,000[155] to 1 in 800,000,[156] or an estimated 13-fold increased risk. However, the assumption that the introduction of chloramphenicol into the American market had greatly increased the number of cases of AA[153, 157] was only weakly supported by epidemiologic data, and essentially the death rate from AA remained constant during the period of the drug's introduction, extensive use, and fall from favor in the prescription market. In recent series in the United States and Europe, of a total of 394 patients, only one was found who had ingested the drug.[26, 158] Nor has chloramphenicol appeared as a risk factor in Thailand, despite its high rate of use there, and in Hong Kong, where utilization of chloramphenicol is almost 100 times greater than in the West, drug-associated AA is infrequent.[159, 160] The early epidemiologic surveys stressed excessive dosage, high blood levels, repeated or intermittent courses, young age, and oral route of administration as particular risks for chloramphenicol marrow toxicity. However, in a later collection of 600 cases, most patients had received a dose of less than 10 g.[161] Even the small amounts of drug present in ophthalmic preparations were blamed for inducing fatal marrow aplasia, although this relationship too has not been supported by formal epidemiologic study.[162]

At ordinary doses, a stereotypic pattern of reversible alterations in erythropoiesis occurs in most patients treated with chloramphenicol.[163] In vitro, chloramphenicol can decrease hematopoietic colony number and size,[164] but usually at concentrations greater than those administered to patients; inhibition of marrow stromal cell proliferation and production of growth factors have also been reported.[165] There is no consistent evidence for abnormal marrow sensitivity to drug in affected patients. Chloramphenicol was claimed to produce marked chromosomal abnormalities in white blood cells.[166] Others have proposed that chloramphenicol toxicity is the result of covalent binding to cellular proteins of reactive oxidative metabolites, an oxalic acid derivative produced by cytochrome P-450–mediated oxidative dehalogenation to produce a chloramphenicol free radical and hydroxylamine intermediate, all capable of acylating proteins.[167] Ultimately, despite its fearsome reputation and extensive laboratory investigation, the mechanism of chloramphenicol-associated AA remains unknown.

Nonsteroidal Anti-inflammatory Drugs. In comparison to chloramphenicol, the association of phenylbutazone with AA was recognized more slowly. Estimates of mortality rates have ranged from 1 in 100,000 to 1 in 10^6 treatment courses.[168] Other, similar agents subsequently also were implicated by case reports, and the large case-control investigation in Europe not only confirmed the risk of phenylbutazone but identified even higher probabilities with other NSAIDs.[11] There was a suggestion of increased risk for drugs taken regularly for long periods at very high doses, and in some cases hematologic reactions were reproducible on reexposure.

Neuroleptics and Psychotropic Drugs. A variety of drugs with activity for the central nervous system (CNS) but extremely diverse chemical structures have been associated with AA: the hydantoins and carbamazepine, various antidepressants, tranquilizers, and, most recently, felbamate, the marketing of which was severely affected by the occurrence of aplasia in more than 30 patients.[169] Blood level and peripheral blood count monitoring of carbamazepine regimens were recommended despite fewer than two dozen aplastic anemia cases reported by 1982,[170] doubt about the validity of many cases in the literature, multiple large series of patients without hematologic toxicity, and an estimated marrow complication case rate of only about 1 in 200,000 treated patients.[171] "Bundling" of a monitoring system for blood counts with the marketing of clozapine, due to the occurrence of agranulocytosis, greatly increased the price of this drug (see Chapter 7, Agranulocytosis).

Gold and Other Heavy Metals. Gold salts have an extraordinarily high frequency of fatal adverse reactions, estimated at 1.6 per 10,000 prescriptions. Dose-dependent leukopenia is common, but several dozen cases of AA have been reported.[172] In the IAAAS, treatment with gold salts was the most significant drug exposure for general marrow failure, with an RR of 29 and an excess risk of 23 cases per 10^6 users in 1 week.[11] Spontaneous recovery rarely can occur; patients have been treated successfully by transplant or immunosuppression; chelation has not generally been helpful. High concentrations of gold salts inhibit hematopoietic colony formation in vitro,[173] and there is some evidence for a dose relationship in patients, as large doses have been associated with the development of blood dyscrasias in general and fatal pancytopenia, as opposed to transient neutropenia or thrombocytopenia.[174]

Arsenic poisoning can result in neutropenia, anemia, and thrombocytopenia,[175] with characteristic basophilic stippling, as in lead poisoning. Organic arsenicals, originally used in the treatment of syphilis (arsphenamine) and now as anthelmintics (arsenamide), historically were associated with AA,[176] but the quality of the older reports of both arsenic and other heavy metal effects do not allow myelodysplasia to be excluded as a more likely explanation for the marrow failure.

Viruses

Viral infections are frequently associated with limited marrow suppression, typically neutropenia and, less commonly, thrombocytopenia. Epidemiologic studies of AA have indirectly suggested an infectious agent: in Thailand, poverty,[27] grain farming (with attendant water and insect exposure),[177] and previous exposure to hepatitis A, an enteric agent,[178] support the hypothesis that a specific infectious exposure could trigger marrow failure in a susceptible individual. Viruses can damage the bone marrow directly, by cytolysis of hematopoietic cells, as exemplified by parvovirus B19 infection of erythroid progenitor cells and subsequent transient aplastic crisis (acute infection in a patient with underlying hemolysis) or pure red cell aplasia (chronic infection in a patient with underlying immunodeficiency) (see Chapter 6, Pure Red Cell Aplasia).[179] Viruses commonly produce pathologic changes indirectly by induction of secondary immune pathways; initiation of an autoimmune process in the marrow could lead to depletion of progenitor and stem cells or destruction of supporting stroma.

Known viruses under specific circumstances cause bone marrow failure. AA rarely complicates Epstein-Barr virus infection: pancytopenia may accompany or follow infectious mononucleosis,[180] or there may be evidence of new or reactivated viral infection in a patient with typical AA.[181] A genetic basis for an aberrant immune response to this virus is obvious from families of boys with X chromosome–linked lymphoproliferative disease syndrome, in which AA is often responsible for a fatal outcome,[182] or of the coexistence of nasopharyngeal carcinoma and AA in the same kindred.[183]

In the stereotypical posthepatitis aplasia syndrome, young males suffer an episode of acute, apparently viral hepatitis; in the convalescent phase, severe pancytopenia and marrow aplasia develop which, untreated, are uniformly fatal.[184] While this syndrome clinically seems to have a viral cause, it has not been linked to any known hepatitis virus, including hepatitis viruses A, B, C, E, and most recently G. There is a striking association between marrow failure, manifesting about the time of liver transplant, and fulminant hepatitis of childhood, which is also seronegative.[185] The same unknown etiologic agent is probably responsible for both these severe syndromes, as well as a proportion of non-A–G acute hepatitis, which, similar to AA, appears to be considerably more frequent in Asia than in the West. AA after either infectious mononucleosis or hepatitis is T cell–mediated and responsive to immunosuppressive therapy. Other viruses, including a variety of herpesviruses and retroviruses, have not been convincingly implicated in generalized bone marrow failure. Only a few cases of probably transient pancytopenia associated with marrow hypocellularity have been described following parvovirus B19 infection,[186, 187] which more usually causes only red blood cell aplasia.

An interesting parallel exists between AA and hemophagocytic syndrome, in which immune-mediated pancytopenia develops during convalescence from a wide variety of viral infections, especially herpesviruses such as Epstein-Barr virus but also parvovirus B19.[188–190] Cytotoxic T cell activation and circulating IFN-γ have been measured in patients, who can respond to immunosuppressive therapies. The morphologic finding of hemophagocytosis is an occasional feature of the bone marrow in typical AA.

DEFINITIVE TREATMENTS

Bone Marrow Transplantation

Allogeneic bone marrow transplantation (BMT) from a histocompatible matched sibling is curative therapy in the majority of aplastic patients who undergo the procedure[10, 191–195] (Table 1–6; see also Fig. 1–2B, C). Recently, cytokine-primed peripheral blood has also served as a regenerative source,[196, 197] and the convenience at least of this method likely will lead to its substitution for marrow harvesting as the major method of stem cell collection, but conclusions from marrow transplant should broadly hold for peripheral blood.

The first studies of allogeneic marrow transplants conclusively demonstrated their value in comparison to conventional supportive therapy; in a controlled trial of the International Aplastic Anemia Study Group, patients with severe disease who received transplants early had actuarial survival of greater than 60% compared with about 20% in patients who received androgens and blood transfusions only.[198] The results of marrow transplantation have steadily improved over time as the result of a combination of factors: progressive modification of conditioning regimens and lower procedure-related early mortality; improved transfusion support and antibiotic regimens; and the introduction of cyclosporine in graft-versus-host disease (GvHD) regimens. Some individual hospitals now report rates of survival of 80% to 90%[199–202] (see Table 1–5). Registry data, compilations of the collected experience of many units, also have shown generally better outcomes over the last several decades: in the International Bone Marrow Transplant Registry, rates had climbed from 48% in the years 1976 to 1980 to 66% for 1988 to 1992[203] and to 77% in the most recent cohort,[204] almost certainly creditable largely to the introduction of cyclosporine for GvHD prophylaxis as well as improved antibiotics and better blood product support.

Graft rejection and GvHD are the major complications of allogeneic transplantation in AA. Graft rejection has been more problematic for AA than for other diseases, perhaps due to the underlying immunopathophysiology in marrow failure, as well as the use of less intensive condi-

TABLE 1–6 Allogeneic Bone Marrow Transplantation in Aplastic Anemia

Study	Years of Study	N	Age (Median)	Rejection/ Failure (%)	Chronic Graft-versus-Host Disease (%)	Actuarial Survival (%)
Gluckman et al.[443]	1980–1989	107	5–46 (19) yr	3	35	68 ± 10 (at 5 yr)
Champlin et al.[444]	1984–1984	290	0.7–41 (19) yr	17	12	78 ± 10 (5 yr)
May et al.[200]	1984–1991	24	4–53 yr	29	0	79 ± 8
Storb et al.[199]	1988–1993	39	2–52 (25) yr	5	34	92 (3 yr)*
Passweg et al.[203]	1988–1992	471	1–51 (20) yr	16	32	66 + 6 (5 yr)
Reiter et al.[202]	1982–1996	20	17–37 (25) yr	0	53	95 (15 yr)

*In an update, a total of 55 patients treated by the same regimen (cyclophosphamide and antithymocyte globulin) were reported to have 89% survival at 8 years.[445]

tioning preparative chemotherapy than for malignant diseases like leukemia. Graft rejection is a major predictor of post-transplant survival. In transplants performed between 1981 and 1986, 29% of the deaths were secondary to graft rejection, the commonest single mortal event.[205] The rate of graft rejection has fallen with intensification of immunosuppressive conditioning, from 15% to 4% in Europe[205] and from 35% (1970s) to 9% (1982–1997) in Seattle.[206] The success of second transplants for the indication of graft rejection has also increased dramatically.[206]

That graft rejection might be intrinsic to the pathophysiology of AA has been suggested by the unexpectedly high proportion of failure in unprepared syngeneic transplants.[207–209] In a group of untransfused patients who received allogeneic stem cells, the incidence of graft rejection was 10%, indicating that AA patients may be especially sensitive to alloimmunization.[210] Nevertheless, the influence of transfusion on graft rejection is relative, and modest numbers of blood donations (less than 40 units in the International Registry experience[211] and less than 10 units of erythrocytes or 40 units of platelets among Seattle patients[212]) may not greatly increase the risk of graft rejection (see Fig. 1–6).

Intensification of immunosuppressive conditioning regimens, with use of total body[211] or lymphoid irradiation,[213] cyclosporine,[200, 211] or ATG[199] reduced the risk of graft rejection, but such measures often have not been shown to influence long-term survival (Table 1–6).[211, 214, 215] The effect of the conditioning program on graft rejection is probably through elimination of recipient lymphocytes and resulting mixed hematologic chimerism, which is highly associated with rejection.[216, 217] More rapid regeneration of bone marrow grafts has been observed in the presence of cyclosporine,[218] and second grafts have been successful when ATG has been added to the conditioning regimen.[219] The specific contribution of ATG to improved results post-transplant[199, 220, 221] is being tested in randomized studies.

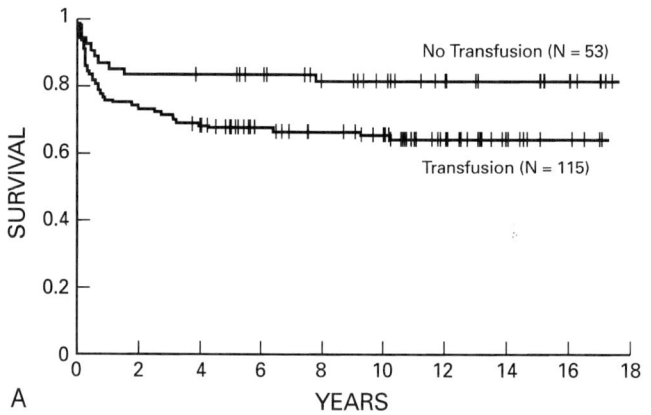

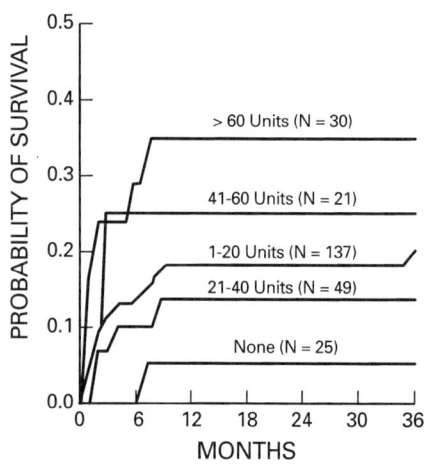

Figure 1–6 Two views of the influence of transfusion on transplantation success. **(A)** For procedures reported to the International Bone Marrow Transplant Registry between 1978 and 1986, there was little influence on the rate of graft failure for up to 40 units of transfused blood products (but radiation was used in conditioning more than half the patients).[211] **(B)** In contrast, at the University of Washington, the impact was favorable in the minority of patients who avoided transfusion until at least 3 days prior to infusion of donor cells.[325]

Rates of chronic GvHD vary, related to patient selection and treatment regimens. Age has been a major risk factor, with GvHD rates rising from 19% for patients 0 to 10 years old, to 46% at 11 to 30 years, and 90% in patients over 31 years old in a historical Seattle series.[222] With improved regimens, older patients have fared better, while children have a low probability of the occurrence of, and of death from, this complication.[223] Nevertheless, in the most recent analysis from Seattle, of 212 patients who survived for more than 2 years after transplant, 41% had developed chronic GvHD, with a mortality three times higher than in patients without this complication.[224] Age was a significant univariate risk factor for the development of chronic GvHD, with an increased probability of 1.04 per year (assuming that the median-age patient of 18 years had the average risk of 41%, the risk for infants would be about 20%; for adults, 30%; and for older patients, 70% to 98%). This analysis excluded patients who failed to survive 2 years post-transplant, many of whom presumably succumbed to GvHD as well.[224] The commonly cited boundary in survival figures at 20 to 30 years of age is almost certain due largely to chronic GvHD. In a European group analysis, a significant difference was observed in survival in those less than 20 years old (65%) compared with patients older than 20 years (56%), but there was no difference in survival for patients age 21 to 30 and those age 31 to 55 years.[214] Young adults have fared better in other series, but morbidity from severe GvHD was far more prevalent in them compared with children (43% vs. 10%).[225, 226]

Other very late complications also occur after transplantation, including effects on growth and development and endocrine, neurologic, and other organ systems.[224, 227] Deaths from pulmonary failure have been recorded years after transplantation.[224] A high rate of secondary malignancies has been registered after transplantation in general, as well as for AA. In a National Cancer Institute retrospective analysis of almost 20,000 marrow transplants, the risk of late cancer was eightfold higher at 10 years than anticipated for the general population and even higher—about 40-fold—for young patients.[228] The risk was greatest for the occurrence of malignant melanoma, buccal cavity tumors, and cancer of the liver, brain, thyroid, bone, and connective tissues. Multivariate analysis suggested that high-dose irradiation was an important factor. For AA, among 320 patients with aplasia receiving transplants in Seattle, four developed cancer, leading to a calculated risk seven times higher.[229] In a French survey, 4 of 147 aplastic patients developed solid tumors, an 8-year cumulative incidence rate of 22%, equivalent to an RR of 41.[230] Secondary solid tumors developed in the radiation field penumbra of 5 of 147 AA patients whose conditioning included thoracoabdominal irradiation.[231] Immune events have been implicated by associated risk factors: GvHD, treatment with ATG or monoclonal antibody, and total body irradiation.[229] Patients with second cancers do not fare well.[232] However, a significant risk of late malignancy exists in AA patients independent of transplant therapy and in a large registry of the European Bone Marrow Transplant Group was equivalent for immunosuppression and transplantation (compared with the general European population, the RR of malignancy was calculated at 5.15 for immunosuppression [confidence limits 3.26 to 7.94] and 6.67 [3.05 to 12.65] after transplantation[233]; see later).

In summary, excellent survival and low morbidity in younger patients make allogeneic BMT the treatment of choice for children and adolescents. Older patients have a higher risk of transplant-related morbidity and mortality. Young adults in the intermediate age group have a reasonable opportunity for cure with BMT but also face more complications than children. In addition to age, a prolonged interval between diagnosis and transplant, multiple transfusions, and serious infections before transplant are important risk factors.

Matched Unrelated and Nonhistocompatible Sibling Donors

Until recently, the lack of an HLA genotypically identical sibling donor precluded marrow transplantation, thus excluding this therapeutic option in about 70% of patients with AA. Alternative potential donors include either relatives who are phenotypically matched or partially matched and HLA phenotypically matched but unrelated volunteers.[234]

Phenotypically identical family donors are available in only 1% to 2% of cases, but haplotype sharing between parents occasionally has allowed identification and successful transplantation between such matched relatives.[235] Long-term survival after family donations of even one locus mismatched has been inferior to genotypically matched transplants, due mainly to the familiar problems of graft rejection and GvHD. In the large European experience, for phenotypically identical family matches actuarial survival was 45%; for patients with a single locus mismatch, 25%; and for two or three loci mismatched, 11%.[236, 237] In a recent Seattle report, while all patients who received such transplants that were fully HLA-matched survived, those with mismatches of one or more loci had much poorer outcomes, and even with total body irradiation added to the conditioning regimen, survival was only 50%.[235] In Minneapolis, only two of seven children survived mismatched donation from their fathers, one with chronic GvHD (four failed engraftment entirely).[238] Satisfactory engraftment and low incidence of GvHD have been achieved in partially matched related donors with conditioning that included total body irradiation and multiple and high doses of cytotoxic drugs in combination with T cell depletion.[239]

Many more donors histocompatible at the major HLA loci are available outside the family, but in comparison to standard HLA-matched sibling transplantation, most large studies have shown inferior long-term survival and higher rates of complications of graft rejection,[240] GvHD,[241, 242] and delayed immune system reconstitution.[243] Age, even more than in matched sibling transplants, is a crucial factor and probably more important even than the level of match, conditioning regimen, or use of T cell depletion.[234, 237, 244, 245] For AA patients who received unrelated transplants reported to the National Marrow Donor Program, survival at 2 years was 29%.[246] In the European group registry 1994 report, survival for 110 recipients of marrow other than from a matched sibling was 34%, about half the rate with standard transplantation.[247] At the University of Minnesota seven children with AA were prepared with cyclophosphamide and total body irradiation; all eventually were engrafted, most developed severe GvHD, but three have survived with restored hematopoiesis (one with profound leukoencephalopathy but the others free of major complications).[248] Superior results have been obtained at Children's Hospital in Milwaukee, where T cell depletion of the donor graft is combined with a rigorous conditioning program of cytosine arabinoside, cyclophosphamide, and total body irradiation: for 28 transfused and previously treated children with severe AA, survival was 54% with no chronic GvHD (median follow-up of almost 3 years).[245, 249]

Thus, alternative donor transplantation is feasible; the rare phenotypic match from within the family may be equivalent to a sibling donation, but for other family members or unrelated donors, there are greatly increased risks of transplant-related mortality and morbidity. As the logistics of unrelated donor transplantation require months to arrange the procedure, it should be considered early. At the best centers, alternative donor transplantation represents an option, especially for the young patient with very severe pancytopenia who has failed immunosuppression. Poor results at most institutions, as well as the likelihood of increased late complications due to the severe preparation regimen, temper enthusiasm for the procedure.

Autologous Transplantation

Circulating hematopoietic progenitor cells can be mobilized by prolonged G-CSF administration to AA patients,[250] although increased CD34 cell counts or the yield of colony-forming cells may not reflect true stem cell content. In one patient reportedly rescued by infusion of peripheral blood cells collected during remission,[251] interpretation of any benefit is obscured by the concurrent use of high-dose cyclophosphamide as conditioning (see later).

Immunosuppression

Antithymocyte and Antilymphocyte Globulins

Immunosuppression is an effective alternative treatment for patients who are not candidates for BMT. Immunoglobulin preparations made from the sera of horses and rabbits immunized against human lymphocytes are the mainstays of current regimens.[10, 252, 253] In Europe, thoracic duct lymphocytes are the antigens for antilymphocyte globulin (ALG) and in the United States thymocytes (from children undergoing cardiac surgery) are the immunogen for ATG. ALG dosages are often expressed in lytic units for lymphocytes in vitro, and ATG in milligrams. Both horse ATG and rabbit ALG are currently licensed for use in the United States.

The efficacy of ALG in marrow failure was discovered serendipitously in the late 1960s, when Mathé observed recovery of autologous hematopoietic function in a patient who had received antilymphocyte serum as conditioning for marrow transplantation.[82] In an early collection of European cases from Basel, Paris, and Leiden, treated with different serum preparations and in a variety of dose regimens, sustained hematologic improvement occurred in 12 of 29 severe AA patients (41%) and 1-year survival of the entire group was 55%.[254] Outcome of treatment has improved with time, and in the most recent analysis of European data a Kaplan-Meier survival of 64% was estimated for patients treated with ALG alone between 1974 and 1997.[255] Two important controlled trials were performed in the United States. In a combined center study, Swiss ALG was clearly superior to androgen treatment with significantly better response (70% vs. 18%) and 1-year survival rates (76% vs. 22%).[256] Similar results were also obtained in a small randomized study of ATG vs. supportive care (52% vs. 0% response rate).[257] In a big multicenter American trial, 47% of patients improved.[258] Review of published results from Europe and America suggested that overall about half the patients treated with either ATG or ALG would show hematologic improvement, broadly defined as an end to transfusion-dependence and increase in the neutrophil number adequate to protect from serious infection; response rates vary with centers from 20% to 85%.[259] Putative etiology does not predict response: virus-associated[181, 184] and drug-induced aplasia[131, 260, 261] behave similarly to idiopathic disease; nor do cytogenetic abnormalities preclude improvement, as both AA with chromosomal abnormalities,[262–264] as well as frank myelodysplasia (see Chapter 3), may respond. The response rate to ATG or ALG was not increased by addition of androgens[265] or very high doses of corticosteroids[266]; intensification of immunosuppression with cyclosporine is discussed later.

A hematologic response to ATG is usually apparent within several months of therapy (Fig. 1–7); in some cases, all blood counts rise dramatically, while in others, increases in platelets or red blood cells may be gradual or delayed. The average time to improvement in neutrophil number shows a normal distribution around 1 to 2 months,[258] and transfusion-independence occurs about 2 to 3 months after initiating treatment. Continued improvement without further therapy not uncommonly occurs after 3 months, but it is clinical status at 3 months that is strongly correlated with long-term survival.[258, 267] Patient selection is important, as the likelihood of response to ALG has been inversely correlated with disease severity,[268] and, in particular, with low neutrophil count.[214, 269]

Antilymphocyte sera have three major toxicities: immediate allergic phenomena, serum sickness (Plate 3), and transient blood count depression. Fever, rigors, and an urticarial cutaneous eruption are common on the first day or two of ATG or ALG therapy, and these symptoms respond to antihistamines and meperidine. Anaphylaxis is rare, but its occurrence has been fatal even in the prepared medical setting.[270] A positive immediate wheal and flare reaction to the epicutaneous application of the 50 mg/mL stock solution

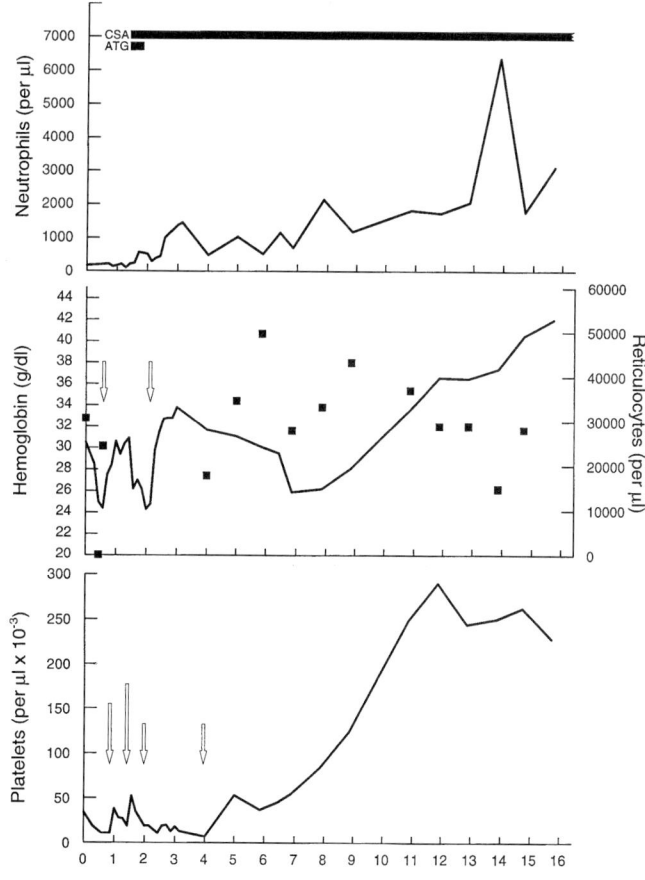

Figure 1–7 A typical hematologic response to ATG and cyclosporine in a 16-year-old with posthepatitis severe aplastic anemia.

of ATG may be predictive of massive histamine release on systemic infusion, and desensitization with gradually increasing doses of ATG administered intradermally, subcutaneously, and then intravenously has permitted ATG use in allergic patients.[270] Corticosteroids are usually administered in moderate doses (1 mg/kg of prednisone or methylprednisolone) during the first 2 weeks to ameliorate serum sickness. Doses and regimens of ATG and ALG have varied widely, from 5 to 50 mg/kg and from 4 to 28 days. It is more rational to administer equivalent doses of ATG or ALG by the schedule originally employed in Europe, 40 mg/kg/day for 4 days; antiserum will then have reached low levels in the circulation by the time host antibody appears.[271] A shorter course is easier to administer and associated with less serum sickness and is equally effective as the same dose given over more prolonged time periods.

Antilymphocyte sera are immunosuppressive. ATG and ALG contain a heterogeneous mix of antibody specificities for lymphocytes, including reactivity to antigens such as CD2, CD3, CD4, CD8, CD25 (the receptor for IL-2), and HLA-DR.[272-274] Horse sera fix human complement efficiently, and all preparations are cytotoxic to T cells in vitro, with little difference between ATG and ALG or among lots for lymphocyte killing in vitro.[273] In vitro, ALG efficiently inhibited T cell proliferation and blocked IL-2 and IFN-γ production and IL-2 receptor expression[275]; ATG induced Fas-mediated apoptosis in T cells, especially after activation.[276] In monkeys, ATG and ALG suppressed cutaneous allograft rejection.[274] In studies of rabbit ATG in rhesus monkeys undergoing kidney transplant, persisting specific antibodies may have been responsible for the chronic anergic state and tolerance induced in this animal model.[277] In patients, administration of ATG and ALG results in rapid reduction in the number of circulating lymphocytes, usually to less than 10% of starting values, and lymphocytopenia persists for several days after discontinuing the last infusion. When lymphocyte numbers have returned to pretreatment values at 3 months, reductions in activated lymphocyte numbers in recovered patients persist.[94, 278-280]

While it is highly probable that such negative effects on T cells are responsible for their clinical efficacy, the ability of ATG and ALG to also stimulate lymphocyte function by acting as a mitogen might also have a role in treatment. ATG and ALG provoked both IL-2 and hematopoietic growth factor production by peripheral blood mononuclear cells,[281] later identified as GM-CSF[87, 282, 283] and IL-3.[282] T cells cloned after ALG stimulation produced GM-CSF or IL-3, or both, and less frequently, IL-2 and IFN-γ.[284] Acutely, ALG administration reduced serum GM-CSF levels in one study.[285] In a mouse model, ATG has increased circulating levels of colony-stimulating activity,[286] and administration of ATG post human marrow transplantation was associated with increased serum levels of IL-3.[287] ATG also binds to bone marrow precursor[288] and progenitor[289] cells and might modestly have a direct enhancement of hematopoiesis, possibly through binding to CD45RO, a molecule capable of tyrosine phosphatase signaling activity.[290]

Reliable methods to predict which patients will respond to ATG are lacking. In some cases, lymphocyte inhibitory activity for hematopoietic progenitors disappeared after successful ATG therapy[291]; in one recent study, CD8 cells obtained from patients before treatment inhibited autologous hematopoietic colony formation, whereas CD8 lymphocytes from the same patients after they had recovered were no longer inhibitory (CD4 cells had no effect on hematopoietic progenitors in vitro).[292] Good correlations were reported between clinical response to immunosuppression and pretreatment improvement in hematopoietic colony formation after T cell depletion,[293, 294] incubation of marrow with ALG[295] or in coculture assays,[296] but these promising findings have not been confirmed in other studies. We recently have detected IFN-γ in circulating and marrow lymphocytes using intracellular staining followed by flow cytometric analysis, and the presence in patients before treatment of such cytokine-containing cells, especially in marrow specimens, has been predictive of responsiveness to immunosuppressive therapy.[92] The lymphocyte stimulatory effects of ATG and ALG have been correlated with clinical outcomes in some[297, 298] but not other[282] studies.

Cyclosporine

Shahidi and others had success with cyclosporine, usually combined with androgens, in individual patients with AA, many of whom had failed other therapies.[299] Subsequently, several groups reported efficacy of cyclosporine in patients refractory to ALG or ATG treatment, with salvage rates of about 50%.[300, 301] Efficacy of cyclosporine as initial therapy was promoted in a large French cooperative randomized study, in which low but equivalent response rates were observed in comparison with standard ALG.[302] However, in a more recent randomized European trial in patients with severe AA, cyclosporine was clearly inferior to the combination of ALG with cyclosporine as measured by response rates (46% vs. 74%) and short-term survival (at 180 days, 67% vs. 90%), and a second course of immunosuppression was more frequently required in the patients treated with cyclosporine alone.[303]

The optimal regimen has not been determined. In the United States, cyclosporine has usually been employed at 12 mg/kg/day for adults and 15 mg/kg/day for children, with adjustment of doses to plasma drug concentrations, serum creatinine levels, or other toxicities. In Europe, lower doses, 3 to 7 mg/kg/day, have appeared to be sufficient.[304] Hematologic improvement may occur in a few weeks or months; a 6-month trial is reasonable. When achieved, remissions usually have been durable, but some proportion of patients relapse when cyclosporine is discontinued; although most will then respond to its reinstitution,[304, 305] some require maintenance treatment.[300, 306]

Cyclosporine toxicity is not minor. Hypertension and azotemia are the most common serious side effects; hirsutism and gingival hypertrophy are also frequent complaints. Increasing serum creatinine levels are an indication to lower the dose. Chronic nephropathy, characterized by interstitial fibrosis and tubular atrophy, can be irreversible and must be avoided; the risk of nephropathy is increased by high doses and long-duration therapy, and occurs more commonly in older than younger patients. Cyclosporine, especially in combination with corticosteroids, converts patients with AA to temporary immunodeficiency and new susceptibility to unusual infectious agents; monthly aerosolized pentamidine prophylaxis will prevent *Pneumocystis* infection in patients receiving cyclosporine. Convulsions, possibly related to hypomagnesemia, are also a potential serious complication of therapy.

Combined or Intensive Immunosuppressive Therapy

The combination of an agent that lyses lymphocytes (ATG or ALG) with a drug to block T cell function is rational. In a German randomized trial in which patients were treated initially with a combination of ALG and cyclosporine or with ALG only, the addition of cyclosporine led to higher hematologic response rates and more complete responses than with ALG alone: 65% vs. 39% and 70% vs. 46% at 3 and 6 months, respectively[307] (Table 1–7). In a single-center study at the National Institutes of Health (NIH) that combined cyclosporine with ATG,[308] and in a multicenter European study of ALG and cyclosporine,[309] the hematologic response rates at 1 year were about 80%, and in all the trials 5-year survival rates for responding patients have been high: 80% to 90%.

Intensive immunosuppression has been beneficial, especially for patients with extreme neutropenia (fewer than 200 absolute neutrophils per microliter), and in children, both of whom fared poorly with ALG alone but have good response and survival rates with combined treatment.

Immunosuppression has been intensified in other regimens. In Europe, repeated courses of ALG are commonly given in an effort to induce hematologic improvement.[268, 310–312] A longer course of ATG (28 days vs. 10 days) appeared to produce more complete responses in an American multicenter trial[258] (but with much more serum sickness toxicity). The addition of high-dose methylprednisolone to ALG has been associated with very high response rates in some trials,[310, 313] but no benefit was apparent in a randomized trial.[266] Most recently, the experience with 11 patients who received high doses of cyclophosphamide, 45 mg/kg/day for 4 days without stem cell rescue, were reported, with an overall response rate similar to that with ATG; blood counts normalized.[314] Cyclophosphamide appears to offer the promise of eliminating relapse or late hematologic complications[315] at the cost of more acute toxicity, especially a prolonged period of profound neutropenia.

Corticosteroids

Methylprednisolone in modest doses is usually administered during ATG and ALG therapy to ameliorate serum sickness. Otherwise, low-dose corticosteroids are not effective treatment for aplastic anemia. Very high ("industrial") doses have been administered, as boluses of 6-methylprednisolone given intravenously and starting at 20 mg/kg/day may be effective, especially in recently diagnosed cases,[312, 316, 317] and, as mentioned earlier, high-dose methylprednisolone has also been added to antilymphocyte globulin therapy but with inconsistent results. Because antilymphocyte globulins have better response rates and many fewer toxicities, they are generally preferable as initial therapy. Modest doses of corticosteroids do not have a role in the treatment of AA except in combination with antilymphocyte globulins: not only is there little evidence of their effectiveness in either reversing marrow failure or improving hemostasis but even limited courses may contribute to aseptic vascular necrosis of bones, a troubling complication in the pancytopenic patient.[318]

Relapse. Recurrence of pancytopenia is common. In 719 European patients treated with immunosuppression, the actuarial rate of relapse among 358 responders was 35% at 14 years; relapse occurred more commonly among patients who had shown

TABLE 1–7 Intensive Immunosuppression in Severe Aplastic Anemia

Study (Year)	Regimen	N	Median Age (Range)	Median ANC per µL/<0.2/ µL	Response	Survival	Relapse	Median Follow-Up (Days)
German multicenter, (1992)[307]	ALG + CSA	43	32 (7–80) yr	0.48/19%	70% at 6 mo	64% at 41 mo	11%	516 (183–1295)
EGBMT (1995)[308]	ALG + CSA + G-CSF	40	16 (2–72) yr	0.19/50%	82% at 1 yr	92% at 34 mo	3%	428 (122–1005)
NIH (1995)[309]	ATG + CSA	51	28 (3–79) yr	0.34/42%	78% at 1 yr	86% at 1 yr, 72% at 2 yr	18% at 1 yr, 36% at 2 yr	912 (218–1714)

ANC, absolute neutrophil count; ALG, antilymphocyte globulin; ATG, antithymocyte globulin; CSA, cyclosporine; G-CSF, granulocyte colony-stimulating factor; EGMBT, European Group for Bone Marrow Transplantation; NIH, National Institutes of Health.

initial rapid responses to treatment.[319] About half the relapsed patients could be induced to respond to a second course of immunosuppression, but survival was lower in patients who suffered a relapse compared with those who had not. In our NIH cohort of 112 patients, relapse, which was defined as a need for further treatment, was even more common, with a risk estimated at 87% at 7 years; however, survival was unaffected by the occurrence of relapse, and most patients responded to further therapy, usually reinstitution of cyclosporine alone.[320] These observations are consistent with a view of AA as a chronic immunologic disease that is not cured by a single course of immunosuppressive therapy.

The much more serious complication of late clonal hematologic disease is discussed later.

Immunosuppression vs. Bone Marrow Transplantation

Combined immunosuppressive therapy and BMT are alternative effective therapies for AA[10] (see Fig. 1–2B). Lack of a matched sibling donor, the cost and availability of transplant, and risk factors such as active infection, older age, or a heavy transfusion burden mean that most patients will automatically undergo treatment with ATG or ALG and cyclosporine.[321] For a few patients with AA and their physicians, a choice does exist between the two different therapies. Marrow transplant offers the opportunity of permanent cure of hematopoietic failure; its disadvantages are cost, the risk of procedure-related morbidity and mortality, especially GvHD in older patients, and an increased rate of late solid organ malignancies. Immunosuppression is easier and, at least initially, less costly. However, many patients do not achieve normal blood counts, remain at high risk of relapse and a need for additional therapy, and some proportion will develop the serious complication of late clonal hematologic disease, especially myelodysplasia.

Retrospective analyses of the large number of European patients reported to the European Bone Marrow Transplantation Group show consistently improved results with both therapies but have repeatedly failed to demonstrate a survival advantage for transplantation over immunosuppression[9, 214, 322, 323]: the most recent 5-year survival figures were 75% for immunosuppression and 77% for transplant.[204] Results of single-center studies are similar: whether immunosuppression is equivalent to transplant or superior[310, 324] or inferior,[322, 325] the observed differences usually do not reach statistical significance. Certain categories of patients, defined by neutrophil number and age, likely benefit from choosing one therapy over the other. In the European Group analysis, marrow transplantation yielded superior results in children age 10 years and younger with neutrophil counts of less than 400/µL, whereas immunosuppression was better for adults 40 years and older, and for patients in the intermediate age category, a neutrophil count below 300/µL favored transplant.[204, 205] Better results for matched sibling transplant in children have been reported by other groups.[269, 326–328] In contrast, older persons do less well than children with this therapy. In a compilation of early results in transplantation for AA from 1970 to 1989 in Seattle, long-term survival in patients over 40 years old was about 10%, and in patients 30 to 39 years old, only 35%[329]; for patients transplanted between 1978 and 1991, the survival figures had improved to about 70% at 16 years for those age 20 to 39 years and about 40% for those 40 years and older.[325] While the results of transplant clearly have improved in adults over the subsequent decade, the most recent report from the same institution still describes age as a major risk factor for GvHD, which in turn has a marked influence on survival.[224] Even its enthusiasts do not recommend transplantation as first-line therapy in patients over 50 years old[330]; 40 years was adopted as a boundary in one review.[331]

In some cases, an unsuccessful trial of immunosuppression has been followed by marrow sibling donor transplant rescue.[332] Delayed transplant could be employed not only for aplasia refractory to standard immunosuppression but also for relapse and the development of late clonal disease.[321]

Androgens

Testosterone and synthetic anabolic steroids seemed a major advance in the treatment of AA when they were introduced in the 1960s.[333, 334] High response rates that were reported in early series may be retrospectively reinterpreted as influenced by the inclusion of patients with only moderate acquired AA or Fanconi's anemia. For severe acquired disease, modern studies generally have failed to demonstrate efficacy, measured as survival[335] or hematologic improvement.[258] As adjuncts to immunosuppression, a controlled trial in the United States did not show an increase in the response rate,[265] and in a randomized study in Europe a modest survival advantage was observed only in women with severe neutropenia.[336]

Certain androgen regimens have their advocates, who have reported response rates similar to those observed after ATG[337] and long survivals.[338] Androgens are helpful in some patients when used as second-line therapy, and most hematologists have observed patients who appeared to respond or even to develop hematologic dependence on continued administration of hormone.[339, 340] Androgens are popular in the Orient[341, 342] and Mexico[343] because they are inexpensive and thought effective. Diverse androgens in various doses have given indistinguishable response rates of 35% to 60% at 6 months.[344] Nevertheless, transplantation or immunosuppression must be the strongly preferred options in newly diagnosed severe AA.

Popular commercial preparations include nandrolone decanoate, oxymetholone, and danazol. The hemoglobin response is usually more impressive than either increases in granulocytes or platelets. An adequate trial is at least 3 months and possibly as long as 6 months at full doses. Despite multiple toxic effects, among long-term survivors after androgen treatment complications are infrequent and the patients' quality of life is good. Some rare complications are more serious and may limit effective therapy, especially in the elderly. The cholestatic pattern of liver function test abnormalities is usually reversible. Hepatotoxicity (bile duct proliferation, peliosis, atypical hepatocyte hyperplasia, and tumors) can occur with all preparations but less frequently with parenteral formulations.[345] Children appear to tolerate high doses of androgens without lasting effects on growth or maturation.[346]

The mechanism of action of the male hormones on improving failed hematopoiesis remains unclear.[347, 348] Increased secretion of erythropoietin, the most definite effect, is probably not very important in the setting of AA, given the excessive growth factor production intrinsic to the disease. Modest direct effects on progenitor cells in colony cultures[349] or in animals[350] are of uncertain clinical significance. In in vitro and in animal models of autoimmune disease, androgens appear to act as immunomodulators, perhaps acting specifically to downregulate the TH1 response.[351]

Hematopoietic Growth Factors

Even if hematopoietic growth factor production is normal or increased in most patients with aplasia, pharmacologic stimulation with very high doses of cytokines might be effective, either through a direct effect on residual stem cells, promoting marrow recovery, or by increasing progenitor cell activity and allowing patients to survive long enough to respond to other, more definitive therapy; G-CSF may also modulate the immune response (for reviews, see references 67, 68).[352, 353]

Neutropenia most often leads to serious and life-threatening complications, and both G-CSF and GM-CSF can increase neutrophil counts in patients with AA.[354–358] Controlled trials have not been performed, so there is no formal demonstration that growth factor administration, even when granulocyte counts are beneficially affected, ultimately either decreases serious infections or improves survival. Unfortunately, neutrophil responses to growth factors usually have been transient, dependent on their continuous administration, and, most important, restricted to patients with quantitatively less depressed granulocyte levels. Nevertheless, occasional bilineage and trilineage responses have been observed.[359] Children may be more sensitive to the effects of prolonged administration of G-CSF.[357]

G-CSF and GM-CSF have some immediate toxicities, including bone pain and "cytokine flu." GM-CSF may increase eosinophil and monocyte counts, and G-CSF can cause a concurrent reduction in platelet numbers. Of greatest concern has been the possibility that prolonged administration of G-CSF increases the probability of late clonal disease, especially monosomy 7; in retrospective analyses of Japanese children[360–362] and adults[363] with severe AA, this serious syndrome appeared to occur only among patients who had received growth factor. However, this experience has yet to be confirmed in Europe or the United States (where the practice of long-term use of growth factors may be less frequent) or in prospective studies. Additionally, growth factors often are inappropriately employed as first therapy in AA, where they have not been shown to be useful, potentially leading to delay in the institution of definitive treatments of proven efficacy.[10, 364]

IL-1, IL-3, IL-6, and SCF have been tested in small pilot trials, usually in patients with refractory AA. IL-1, the monocyte production of which is deficient in severe AA, is not effective and highly toxic.[365, 366] IL-3 can increase neutrophil numbers but less frequently platelet levels, with significant side effects.[367–370] A trial of IL-6 in AA was discontinued prematurely due to increased bleeding and worsening of anemia.[371] Anemia[372, 373] and pancytopenia[374] have responded in occasional patients to prolonged administration of high doses of erythropoietin.

Clinically meaningful hematologic responses to single cytokines have been limited in marrow failure syndromes, but combinations of growth factors might be more effective due to physiologic or pharmacologic synergism. Some complete remissions have been reported to GM-CSF and erythropoietin,[375–377] and in a large randomized protocol, the combination of G-CSF and high doses of erythropoietin improved hemoglobin values, mainly in patients with moderate disease.[378] The combination of stem cell factor and G-CSF has led to increased blood counts, including trilineage recovery, in some refractory patients, including patients who had failed each administered individually.[379]

Growth factors have also been combined with definitive medical therapy with the purpose of improving neutrophil counts in granulocytopenic patients during the early phase of immunosuppression. Often, G-CSF or GM-CSF is instituted because the neutropenic patient is febrile and unresponsive to antibiotics; its value in this circumstance is unknown. A brief course of GM-CSF before or concurrent with ALG has not added appreciable benefit in two small trials.[380, 381] A few case reports suggested that the combination of a growth factor with cyclosporine might rescue refractory patients.[382, 383] However, a randomized trial showed G-CSF and cyclosporine to be much inferior to ALG and cyclosporine as first therapy for AA.[384] Prolonged G-CSF in the European group's trial of intensive immunosuppression was credited with the very high hematologic response and survival rates[309] (as opposed to the use of sequential courses of immunosuppression), and G-CSF also appeared to greatly improve the hematologic response to ALG administered to Chinese patients.[385] However, a recently completed randomized trial failed to confirm the value of G-CSF as an adjunct to initial immunosuppressive therapy.[386]

In the absence of definitive evidence of benefit, either in the short or long term, the use of growth factor in AA continues to be dictated by the physician's judgment. Most severely neutropenic patients who are persistently or seriously infected will undergo a therapeutic trial in the hope of clinical benefit. G-CSF may be preferred to GM-CSF because of a more favorable toxicity profile. Some patients who are refractory to other forms of treatment may also receive prolonged courses of factors in the hope of inducing either improvement in a low neutrophil count or a reduction in transfusion requirements. Preferably, the use of growth factors over long treatment periods, especially in patients who are not severely neutropenic, should be in the context of a formal study, especially until the most recent data concerning usefulness and risk are reported and assessed.

SUPPORTIVE TREATMENT

The ultimate benefit of definitive therapies like transplantation or immunosuppression will be unrealized if the patient succumbs to an early clinical catastrophe or suffers unnecessary bleeding or infectious complications. A haphazard transfusion policy increases the risk of graft rejection after a marrow transplant; too frugal an approach to providing blood products can jeopardize the patient's life and increase morbidity. Supportive management therefore requires both meticulous attention to the daily problems presented by pancytopenia and appreciation of their impact on the ultimate possibilities for cure or amelioration of the disease.

Principles of supportive care of AA apply to other chronic pancytopenias. Further details and references can be obtained from hematology textbooks and monographs (see, in particular, Young[387]).

Bleeding

Bleeding is a common symptom in AA, and death due to hemorrhage was frequent in the premodern era. The effective use of platelet transfusions has been credited with a substantial improvement in survival in this disease. Measurable correction of the platelet count by transfusion almost always alleviates the minor mucocutaneous bleeding common in thrombocytopenic patients. Major bleeding from the gastrointestinal and genitourinary tracts is usually not due to thrombocytopenia alone, and ancillary explanations for massive hemorrhage should always be sought. The bleeding time improves after erythrocyte transfusion in patients with anemia, and there is a strong inverse correlation between the hematocrit and bleeding; the treatment of serious hemorrhage should include correction of severe anemia as red blood cell transfusions may lessen bleeding symptoms.

Modern transfusion medicine practice has made platelets readily available and safe to administer. Other than cost and convenience, the major problem related to platelet transfusions is the development of the refractory state in the recipient.[388] The life span of the transfused platelet in the circulation is dramatically shortened by host antibodies, almost always directed to HLA class I antigens. Alloimmunization is suggested by poor recovery at the 1 hour post-transfusion platelet count and confirmed by finding specific HLA antibodies in serum. Refractoriness often can be overcome by selection of HLA-matched donors; nevertheless, 6% to 39% of perfectly HLA-matched transfusions fail.[389] Alloimmunization can be prevented by the use of single-donor platelets rather than pooled platelets.[390] Apparently of equal utility are physical methods of leukocyte depletion by filtration or ultraviolet treatment[391]; such techniques have been successfully piloted in AA patients.[392] Avoidance of platelet transfusions except when there is active bleeding is another alternative to prevent alloimmunization. However, the dose relationship between exposure to different donors' platelets and the probability of developing refractoriness is not clearly established, and in one study, only transfusion of more than 40 units increased the risk of alloimmunization.[393]

Prophylactic platelet transfusion is controversial.[394, 395] The primary indication for platelet prophylaxis is to avoid intracranial hemorrhage, but the risk of this complication in the chronically thrombocytopenic patient, while real, is low. Prophylactic platelet transfusions have not been shown to alter patient survival,[395, 396] but the beneficial effects on minor bleeding complications and improvement in the quality of life have been considered sufficient justification.[394] Maintenance of platelet counts above 20,000/μL will reduce bleeding episodes,[397] but this numerical threshold is based only on a single study published in 1962 showing reduction in bleeding days and serious hemorrhage among children with acute leukemia.[398] If some reports have suggested little difference in the risk of bleeding over a wide range of platelet counts between 5000 and 100,000/μL,[399] tradition until recently has led to resistance to attempts to lower the threshold.[400] In one study, a rigorous, defined transfusion policy during induction therapy was proposed: platelet transfusions for every patient with a count less than 5000/μL; for counts of 6000 to 10,000/μL if fresh minor hemorrhage or fever was present; for 11,000 to 20,000/μL if a coagulation disorder was present or before a minor procedure; and platelets for more than 20,000/μL only for major bleeding complications or surgery.[401] Fatal or severe bleeding episodes were rare and did not occur in patients with platelet counts higher than 10,000/μL. The worst episodes in these cases were associated with refractoriness to platelet transfusions. In a recent randomized trial in acute myeloid leukemia patients, the risk of major bleeding was no different when 10,000 or 20,000/μL was chosen as a threshold, while the lower value led to a 20% reduction in platelet use.[402] Any prophylaxis program must be modified to the individual patient, but the goal of maintaining platelet counts above 5000/μL is reasonable.

Bone marrow sampling can be performed without prior platelet transfusions. Major surgery can be accomplished in the setting of thrombocytopenia: in one study, blood loss and morbidity were low, even at platelet levels less than 30,000/μL.[403]

Anemia

Complete replacement of erythrocytes requires transfusion of about 2 units of packed red blood cells every 2 weeks. Other than in expectation of an imminent stem cell transplant, there is no rationale for allowing a patient to suffer symptoms of chronic anemia; once equilibrium is achieved, a constant amount of blood will be required to maintain any hemoglobin concentration. With acclimation, fit patients are usually not symptomatic at hemoglobin concentrations of more than 7 g/dL; patients with underlying cardiovascular disease should be maintained at a higher level, above 9 g/dL. Perhaps in contrast to alloimmunization by platelet transfusions, AA patients show a relatively low frequency (about 11%) of alloimmunization due to packed red blood cell transfusions.[404] Iron chelation is indicated for patients with unresponsive chronic anemia who have a reasonable expectation of survival.

Transfusions and Transplantation

Alloimmunization as a result of blood product administration increases the probability of graft rejection and of a fatal outcome after marrow transplantation. Blood products from a potential marrow donor, almost always a sibling, or from another family member, such as a parent who shares histocompatibility antigens, should be avoided. Small numbers of transfusions from unrelated donors do not have a major deleterious effect on survival after allogeneic transplantation. The risk of rejection of about 5% in entirely untransfused patients was increased to 15% with receipt of 1 to 40 units and to greater than 25% only in heavily transfused patients, according to a survey by the IBMTR[211]; in Seattle, increased graft rejection was observed in patients who had received more than 10 units of erythrocytes or 40 units or more of platelets.[212] Speed in arranging histocompatibility typing and transfer to an appropriate center have a greater impact on the survival of the patient than the judicious transfusion of a few units of red blood cells to a severely anemic patient or platelets to a bleeding patient. Of course, transfusions need not be withheld in an older patient in whom immunosuppression will be first therapy.

Infection

There are very few specific investigations of infections and their therapy in patients with AA.[405] Duration is the major difference between the neutropenia of bone marrow failure and that induced by cytotoxic chemotherapy; with longer periods of neutropenia, the probability of serious bacterial or fungal infection increases. A second major difference is that neutropenia is part of a complex of problems in malignant disease and its therapy. In AA, in contrast, the immune system is activated and, with the exception of intravenous catheter placement, the integument is preserved. Studies of cancer patients have usually identified a "low-risk" category, determined by the relatively brief period of neutropenia; by this criterion, almost all unresponsive AA patients are "high-risk."

In classic observations in leukemic children, neutropenia was shown to increase susceptibility to bacterial infections and the number of infectious episodes was quantitatively correlated with the degree and duration of neutropenia: 9% to 10% of days at granulocyte levels above 1500/μL were associated with proven infection, but this number rose to 20% with granulocyte counts of 500 to 1000/μL; to 36% with 100 to 500/μL, and to 53% with neutrophil counts of less than 100/μL; levels of extreme neutropenia, less than 100/μL, were associated with the most serious infections and very high mortality.[407] Susceptibility to serious infection is so extreme at an absolute neutrophil count below 200/μL that this value has been used to define a category of "supersevere" AA. As severe granulocytopenia becomes prolonged, infection is inevitable.

Similar recommendations for initiation of empirical antibiotic therapy apply to AA patients as to other patients with neutropenia. The cardinal rule is: if the absolute neutrophil count is less than 500/μL and infection is suspected, immediately begin broad-spectrum, parenteral antibacterial therapy. Any regimen may require modification based on results of cultures, new symptoms or signs, or a deteriorating clinical course.[408] In general, bacteremia is present in only 20% of febrile neutropenic episodes, and in only about 40% can a microbiologic cause or localizing physical findings be identified.[409] ATG itself is a frequent cause of fever.[410] Nevertheless, early discontinuation of antibiotics, because cultures are unrevealing, in persistently neutropenic patients can be dangerous. Sometimes patients remain febrile despite antibacterial antibiotics; fever may also recrudesce after a few days or weeks. In the absence of additional microbiologic data or clinical clues from the patient's complaints or physical examination, antifungal therapy like amphotericin B should be instituted in patients who remain febrile despite adequate antibacterial therapy for more than 3 days. Fungemia during an initial febrile episode is rare, but fungal infection becomes more likely with repeated courses of antibiotics and ultimately the major cause of death in AA refractory to definitive therapy.[411] *Candida* and *Aspergillus* species account for almost all fungal disease in AA.[411] Early aggressive treatment of neutropenic patients can reverse fungal disease.[412] Unfortunately, attempts to avoid fungal infections in neutropenic patients using prophylactic regimens have neither consistently prevented aspergillosis nor produced survival benefits.[413, 414]

Polymorphonuclear cells have a relatively brief life in the circulation, their major activity is in infected tissue, and there are no simple measures of therapeutic efficacy. Harvesting of granulocytes from the peripheral blood was feasible in the 1970s, but controlled trails failed to demonstrate significant improvement in survival in patients who received such transfusions; these negative studies were criticized because of the relatively low numbers of granulocytes transfused (less than $10^{10}/m^2/day$), which were usually insufficient to increase neutrophil levels in recipients.[415] As granulocyte transfusions fell from favor, they tended to be used in more desperate clinical circumstances, making them appear even less efficacious. In addition, this type of transfusion is expensive and associated with serious toxicities: severe febrile reactions, pulmonary capillary leak syndrome, increased risk of cytomegalovirus transmission, and inevitable alloimmunization. However, a meta-analysis of the published studies suggested that granulocyte transfusions were beneficial in patients with sepsis unresponsive to antibiotics if (1) adequate cell numbers were administered cells (2 to 3×10^{10} cells daily), (2) donor and recipient were compatible, and (3) the patients treated were unlikely to have imminent improvement in marrow function.[416]

Cytokines offer a new strategy for increasing the efficiency of donor harvests. Administration of G-CSF to normal donors can greatly increase the yield of leukapheresis without adverse effects on the volunteers. Such large numbers of neutrophils can be obtained as to allow dramatic increases in the blood levels of absolute granulocytes in neutropenic recipients, and case reports have suggested that G-CSF–mobilized granulocyte transfusions were of clinical benefit in the treatment of life-threatening fungal infections in severely neutropenic patients.[417, 418] A randomized trial to test the efficacy of these preparations is needed.

Some infections in neutropenic patients can be prevented. Most important are simple but often neglected measures directed at increasing general hygiene. A hospital ward's physical surroundings should be well maintained to reduce nosocomial infection. Dental hygiene should be sustained and sources of infection removed with antibiotic and platelet prophylaxis. Nystatin oral rinses prevent thrush. "Routine" rectal examinations are more likely to be harmful than helpful. Blood should not be taken from fingertips and ear lobes. Early attention to the signs of infection, especially after discharge from hospital, can avert many of the catastrophic complications of initially minor infectious episodes.

Total protection environments, often in combination with nonabsorbable antibiotics or selective gut decontamination to preserve some anaerobic bacteria, have had their strong advocates. However, laminar flow rooms with gut sterilization are not obviously superior to simpler methods of isolation,[419] and simple reverse isolation accomplishes little more than compulsive handwashing.[420] Sterile diets, avoidance of fresh fruits and vegetables, and no flowers in the room are simple proscriptions of similarly unproven practical value.

PROGNOSIS

Blood counts are the most important indicators of prognosis in AA. The most popular criteria define severe disease as the presence of two of three greatly diminished blood counts: neutrophils, less than $500/\mu L$; platelets, less than $20,000/\mu L$; corrected reticulocytes, less than 1% (less than $40,000/\mu L$).[198] More complicated formulas are less easy to use and often only quantitate the obvious: patients who tolerate low blood counts without symptoms do better than those who bleed or become infected quickly; patients who do well will continue to do well, at least for a time; and those who do not "go steadily down from bad to worse," in Cabot's phrase.[421] In a comparative study of prognostic factors, decreasing blood counts during the first 3 months of therapy was uniformly associated with death before 5 years, while stable or increased counts correctly predicted long-term survival in 75% of patients, and of the prognostic indices, the simple Camitta criteria were most accurate at 6 months, correctly predicting poor survival in 85% of patients with 100% sensitivity.[422] One modification to the standard criteria is useful. While bleeding was a major cause of death in the early large series, infection kills the overwhelming proportion of modern cases. Accordingly, in the large European cooperative trials the category of supersevere AA has recently been defined as an extremely low absolute neutrophil count of less than $200/\mu L$.[269]

In contrast to blood counts, bone marrow examination is subject to sampling error and cellularity is not usually quantitated, and it is not surprising that gross marrow appearance has not correlated with survival. Predominance of lymphoid cells has been claimed as a bad prognostic factor,[423] the presence of residual hematopoiesis, particularly erythropoiesis, as favorable.[424] The permanence of marrow depression after an insult may also be predicted by continued low marrow cellularity despite blood count recovery,[425] but discordance between correction of pancytopenia and marrow histology in recovered patients is frequent.

The rate of spontaneous recovery is difficult to estimate, and most current observers believe it to be low. Collections of published cases of AA from the era when diagnosis was made at autopsy described a disease with a mortal outcome in days to months and truly untreated severe disease must be almost invariably fatal. In contrast, moderate AA has a good prognosis, and some patients with minimal blood count depression will recover normal blood counts with little or no therapy.[426] Nevertheless, in an older series of pediatric patients treated mainly with transfusions, only 3% of 334 were judged to be cured,[157] and among more recently reported African patients who were treated with transfusions, corticosteroids, and androgens, mortality at 1 year was 56% and at 18 months, 72%.[24] Interpretation of older publications is complicated by uncertainties in diagnosis, both of AA as distinct from other marrow failure syndromes and because of the inclusion of a large proportion of moderate disease. In a randomized study from our own era, none of 21 patients assigned to supportive care only improved during 3 months of observation.[257]

Late Clonal Hematologic Disease

Improved survival after effective treatment has brought its own considerations relevant to prognosis, especially late clonal hematologic diseases, when bone marrow failure is reversed without stem cell replacement, and late malignancies following aggressive conditioning regimens used in BMT (see earlier). When pancytopenia recurs in the patient who has received immunosuppression, a satisfactory response usually will be obtained with reinstitution of cyclosporine. Less frequently but more ominously, recurrent marrow failure is secondary to a new pathologic process, associated with abnormal marrow morphology or cytogenetic abnormalities. The delayed syndromes—which can occur years after apparently successful immunosuppressive therapy—include PNH, myelodysplasia, and AML.[427, 428] Late clonal disease may represent part of the natural history of AA now manifest due to improved survival. Prior to the recent dramatic improvements in treatment, leukemia was considered an unusual complication,[429, 430] but late clonal disease does not appear to be a simple result of the introduction of immunosuppressive therapy. In a series of 156 patients treated with androgens, there was a 10% actuarial probability of developing PNH as well as 5 cases of late-onset myelodysplasia and one of non-Hodgkins lymphoma.[338] For patients in the modern era who undergo immunosuppression, the most accurate figures derive from retrospective analysis of reports to European Group for Bone Marrow Transplantation: of 223 long-term survivors after immunosuppression, 19 developed PNH (13% risk at 7 years) and 11 had myelodysplasia, 5 of whom later manifested AML (combined risk of 15% at 7 years).[431] In a later and larger analysis from the same group, of 860 patients treated by immunosuppression, 19 developed myelodysplasia, 15 acute leukemia, and there was also a case of lymphoma and 7 solid tumors; the cumulative incidence of all malignant tumors at 10 years was almost 19%.[432] In our series of 122 NIH patients treated with intensive immunosuppression, the actuarial risk of a clonal hematologic disease was 33% at about 10 years.[432] Using the Ham test, PNH appeared early, usually in responding patients; with the more sensitive flow cytometric assays, PNH is recognized at diagnosis in about a quarter of patients and may not be a late development at all[433] (see Chapter 4). PNH may be solely a laboratory diagnosis; the patient is often without symptoms and the hemolysis may be mild or well compensated. In contrast, myelodysplasia occurred late and usually in patients who had failed treatment and remained pancytopenic. Myelodysplasia after aplasia has had a particularly high risk of leukemic transformation[427] but may also be surprisingly indolent.[434]

REFERENCES

1. Ehrlich P: Ueber einem Fall von Anämie mit Bemerkungen über regenerative Veränderungen des Knochenmarks. Charite Ann 1888; 13:300–309.
2. Vaquez MH, Aubertin C: L'anémie pernicieuse d'après les conceptions actuelles. Bull Mem Soc Hop Med Paris 1904; 21:288–297.
3. Cabot RC: Pernicious anaemia. In Osler W (ed): A System of Medicine. London, Frowde, 1908, pp 637–639.
4. Minot GR: Diminished blood platelets and marrow insufficiency. Arch Intern Med 1917; 19: 1062–1084.
5. Santesson CG: Über chronische Vergiftung mit Steinkohlentheerbenzin; vier Todesfälle. Arch Hyg Berl 1897; 31:336–376.
6. Kracke RR, Parker FP: The etiology of granulopenia (agranulocytosis) with particular reference to the drugs containing the benzene ring. J Lab Clin Med 1934; 19:799–818.
7. Welch H, Lewis CN, Kerlan I: Blood dyscrasias. A nationwide survey. Antibiot Chemother 1954; 4:607–623.
8. Storb R, Anasetti C, Appelbaum F, et al: Marrow transplantation for severe aplastic anemia and thalassemia major. Semin Hematol 1991; 28:235–239.
9. Gluckman E, Marmont A, Speck B, et al: Immunosuppressive treatment of aplastic anemia as an alternative treatment for bone marrow transplantation. Semin Hematol 1984; 21:11–19.
10. Young NS, Barrett AJ: The treatment of severe acquired aplastic anemia. Blood 1992; 85:3367–3377.
11. Kaufman DW, Kelly JP, Levy M, et al: The Drug Etiology of Agranulocytosis and Aplastic Anemia. New York, Oxford University Press, 1991.
12. Vital Statistics of the United States, ed 2. Washington, DC, US Dept of Health and Human Services, 1986, p 122.
13. Aul C, Gattermann N, Schneider W: Age-related incidence and other epidemiological aspects of myelodysplastic syndromes. Br J Haematol 1992; 82:358–367.
14. Kaufman D, Young NS: Epidemiology of acquired aplastic anemia. Blood 2000, In Press.
15. Shima S, Kato Y: Incidence of aplastic anemia among workers in major industries in Japan and suspected causal factors. In Aoki K, Hosoda Y,

Yanagawa H, et al (eds): Epidemiology of Intractable Diseases in Japan. Nagoya, Japan, Department of Preventive Medicine, Nagoya University School of Medicine, 1986, pp 53–63.
16. Yin D, Wu Y, Lin Z, et al: Epidemiological and etiological studies on aplastic anemia in the Mudanjiang area. Chin J Hematol 1980; 1:33–34.
17. Corrigan GE: An autopsy survey of aplastic anemia. Am J Clin Pathol 1974; 62:488–490.
18. Aoki K, Fujiki N, Shimizu H, et al: Geographic and ethnic differences of aplastic anemia in humans. *In* Najean Y (ed): Medullary Aplasia. New York, Masson, 1980, pp 79–88.
19. Issaragrisil S, Sriratanasatavorn C, Piankijagum A, et al: The incidence of aplastic anemia in Bangkok. Blood 1991; 77:2166–2168.
20. Chongli Y, Xiaobo Z: Incidence survey of aplastic anemia in China. Chin Med Sci J 1991; 6:203–207.
21. Yong ASM, Goh M, Rahman J, et al: Epidemiology of aplastic anemia in the state of Sabah, Malaysia (abstract). Cell Immunol 1996; 1,284:S75.
22. Sánchez-Medal L, Castanedo JP, Garcia-Rojas F: Insecticides and aplastic anemia. N Engl J Med 1963; 269:1365–1367.
23. Mukiibi J, Paul B, Nkrumah F: Aplastic anaemia in Zimbabweans. Cent Afr J Med 1987; 33:1–8.
24. Aken'ova YA, Okunade MA: Aplastic anaemia: A review of cases at the University College Hospital, Ibadan, Nigeria. Cent Afr J Med 1992; 38:362–367.
25. Szklo M, Sensenbrenner L, Markowitz J, et al: Incidence of aplastic anemia in metropolitan Baltimore: A population-based study. Blood 1985; 66:115–119.
26. Linet MS, Markowitz JA, Sensenbrenner LL, et al: A case-control study of aplastic anemia. Leuk Res 1989; 13:3–11.
27. Issaragrisil S, Kaufman D, Anderson T, et al: An association of aplastic anaemia in Thailand with low socioeconomic status. Br J Haematol 1995; 91:80–84.
28. Issaragrisil S, Chansung K, Kaufman DW, et al: Aplastic anemia in rural Thailand: Its association with grain farming and agricultural pesticide use. Am J Public Health 1997; 87:1551–1554.
29. Issaragrisil S, Kaufman DW, Anderson TE, et al: Low drug attributability of aplastic anemia in Thailand. Blood 1997; 89:4034–4039.
30. Linet MS, McCaffrey LD, Morgan WF, et al: Incidence of aplastic anemia in a three county area in South Carolina. Cancer Res 1986; 46:426–429.
31. Custer RP: Aplastic anemia in soldiers treated with atabrine. Am J Med Sci 1946; 212:211–224.
32. Qazilbash M, Liu J, Vlachos A, et al: A new syndrome of familial aplastic anemia and chronic liver disease. Acta Haematol 1997; 97:164–167.
33. Nimer SD, Ireland P, Meshkinpour A, et al: An increased HLA DR2 frequency is seen in aplastic anemia patients. Blood 1994; 84:923–927.
34. Dausset J, Gluckman E, Lemarchand F, et al: Excès d'HLA-A2 et d'homozygotes HLA-A2 parmi les malades atteints d'aplasie medullaire et maladie de Fanconi. Nouv Rev Fr Hematol 1977; 18:315–324.
35. D'Amaro J, van Rood JJ, Rimm AA, et al: HLA associations in Italian and non-Italian Caucasoid aplastic anaemia patients. Tissue Antigens 1983; 21:184–191.
36. Brown KE, Tisdale J, Dunbar CE, et al: Hepatitis/aplastic anemia: an immune-mediated disease of unknown viral (?) etiology. (abstract). Blood 1996; 88(Suppl 1):309.
37. Aaron S, Davis P, Bertouch J: HLA-DR antigens in gold-induced neutropenia. Arthr Rheum 1986; 29:1515–1517.
38. Odum N, Platz P, Morling N, et al: Increased frequency of HLA-DPw3 in severe aplastic anemia (AA). Tissue Antigens 1987; 29:184–185.
39. Nakao S, Yamaguchi M, Saito M, et al: HLA-DR2 predicts a favorable response to cyclosporine therapy in patients with bone marrow failure (letter). Am J Hematol 1992; 40:239–240.
40. Nakao S, Takamatsu H, Shiobara S, et al: Susceptibility to relapse of aplastic anemia after successful immunosuppresive therapy is closely associated with an HLA class II haplotype (abstract). Blood 1994; 84(suppl 1):215a.
41. Nakao S, Takamatsu H, Chuhjo T, et al: Identification of specific HLA class II haplotype strongly associated with susceptibility to cyclosporine-dependent aplastic anemia. Blood 1994; 84:4257–4261.
42. Corzo D, Yunis JJ, Salazar M, et al: The major histocompatibility complex region marked by HSP70-1 and HSP70-2 variants is associated with clozapine-induced agranulocytosis in two different ethnic groups. Blood 1995; 86:3835–3840.
43. Gordon-Smith EC: Clinical features of aplastic anemia. *In* Heimpel H, Gordon-Smith EC, Heit W, ct al (eds): Aplastic Anemia—Pathophysiology and Approaches to Therapy. Berlin, Springer-Verlag, 1979, pp 10–13.
44. Hall SE, Rosse WF: The use of monoclonal antibodies and flow cytometry in the diagnosis of paroxysmal nocturnal hemoglobinuria. Blood 1996; 87:5332–5340.
45. Morely AA, Brisco MJ, Rice M, et al: Leukaemia presenting as marrow hypoplasia: Molecular detection of the leukaemic clone at the time of initial presentation. Br J Haematol 1997; 98:940–944.
46. Young NS: The problem of clonality in aplastic anemia. Dr. Dameshek's riddle, restated. Blood 1992; 79:1385–1392.
47. Tuzuner N, Cox C, Rowe JM, et al: Hypocellular myelodysplastic syndromes (MDS): New proposals. Br J Haematol 1995; 91:612–617.
48. Geary CG, Marsh JCW, Gordon-Smith EC: Hypoplastic myelodysplasia (MDS). Br J Haematol 1996; 94:582–583.
49. Elghetany MT, Vyas S, Yuoh G: Significance of p53 overexpression in bone marrow biopsies from patients with bone marrow failure; aplastic anemia, hypocellular refractory anemia, and hypercel-

lular refractory anemia. Ann Hematol 1998; 77:261–264.
50. Maulopoulos L, Dimopoulos M: Magnetic resonance imaging of the bone marrow in hematologic malignancies. Blood 1997; 90:2127–2147.
51. Molldrem J, Caples M, Mavroudis D, et al: Antithymocyte globulin (ATG) abrogates cytopenias in patients with myelodysplastic syndrome. Br J Haematol 1997; 99:669–705.
52. Jonasova A, Neuwirtova R, Cermak J, et al: Cyclosporin A therapy in hypoplastic MDS patients and certain refractory anaemias without hypoplastic bone marrow. Br J Haematol 1998; 200:304–309.
53. Molldrem JJ, Jiang YZ, Stetler-Stevenson M, et al: Haematological response of patients with myelodysplastic syndrome to antithymocyte globulin is associated with a loss of lymphocyte-medicated inhibition of CFU-GM and alterations in T-cell receptor Vβ profiles. Br J Haematol 1998; 102:1314–1322.
54. Young NS, Maciejewski J: The pathophysiology of acquired aplastic anemia. N Engl J Med 1997; 336:1365–1372.
55. Maciejewski JP, Anderson S, Katevas P, et al: Phenotypic and functional analysis of bone marrow progenitor cell compartment in bone marrow failure. Br J Haematol 1994; 87:227–234.
56. Manz CY, Nissen C, Wodnar-Fillipowicz A: Deficiency of CD34+ c-kit+ and CD34+38− hematopoietic precursors in aplastic anemia after immunosuppressive treatment. Am J Hematol 1996; 52:264–274.
57. Bacigalupo A, Piaggio G, Figari O, et al: Response of CFU-GM to increasing doses of rhGM-CSF in patients with aplastic anemia. Exp Hematol 1991; 19:829–832.
58. Aoki I, Higashi K, Homori M, et al: Responsiveness of bone marrow erythropoietic stem cells (CFU-E and BFU-E) to recombinant human erythropoietin (rh-Ep) in vitro in aplastic anemia and myelodysplastic syndrome. Am J Hematol 1990; 35:6–12.
59. Bacigalupo A, Piaggio G, Podestà M, et al: Early hemopoietic progenitors in the peripheral blood of patients with severe aplastic anemia (SAA) after treatment with antilymphocyte globulin (ALG), cyclosporin-A and G-CSF. Haematologica 1997; 82:133–137.
60. Li S, Champlin R, Fitchen JH, et al: Abnormalities of myeloid progenitor cells after "successful" bone marrow transplantation. J Clin Invest 1985; 75:234–241.
61. Yoshida K, Miura I, Takahashi T, et al: Quantitative and qualitative analysis of stem cells of patients with aplastic anemia. Scand J Haematol 1983; 30:317–323.
62. Podestà M, Piaggio G, Frassoni F, et al: The assessment of the hematopoietic reservoir after immunosuppressive therapy or bone marrow transplantation in severe aplastic anemia. Blood 1988; 91:1959–1965.
63. Maciejewski JP, Selleri C, Sato T, et al: A severe and consistent deficit in marrow and circulating primitive hematopoietic cells (long term culture-initiating cells) in acquired aplastic anemia. Blood 1996; 88:1983–1991.
64. Schrezenmeier H, Jenal M, Herrmann F, et al: Quantitative analysis of cobblestone area–forming cells in bone marrow of patients with aplastic anemia by limiting dilution assay. Blood 1996; 88:4474–4480.
65. Raghavachar A, Janssen JWG, Schrezenmeier H, et al: Clonal hematopoiesis as defined by polymorphic-X-linked loci occurs infrequently in aplastic anemia. Blood 1995; 86:2938–2974.
66. Ball SE, Gibson FM, Rizzo S, et al: Progressive telomere shortening in aplastic anemia. Blood 1998; 91:3582–3592.
67. Kojima S: Hematopoietic growth factors and marrow stroma in aplastic anemia. Int J Hematol 1998; 68:19–28.
68. Marsh JCW: Hematopoietic growth factors in the pathogenesis and for the treatment of aplastic anemia. Semin Hematol 2000; 37:81–90.
69. Marsh JCW, Chang J, Testa NG, et al: In vitro assessment of marrow "stem cell" and stromal cell function in aplastic anaemia. Br J Haematol 1991; 78:258–267.
70. Novitzky N, Jacobs P: Immunosuppressive therapy in bone marrow aplasia: The stroma functions normally to support hematopoiesis. Exp Hematol 1995; 23:1472–1477.
71. Kojima S, Matsuyama T, Kodera Y: Hematopoietic growth factors released by marrow stromal cells from patients with aplastic anemia. Blood 1992; 79:2256–2261.
72. Gibson FM, Scopes J, Daly S, et al: Haemopoietic growth factor production by normal and aplastic anaemia stroma in long-term bone marrow culture. Br J Haematol 1995; 91:551–561.
73. Stark R, Andre C, Thierry D, et al: The expression of cytokine and cytokine receptor genes in long-term bone marrow culture in congenital and acquired bone marrow hypoplasias. Br J Haematol 1993; 83:560–566.
74. Migliaccio AR, Migliaccio G, Adamson JW, et al: Production of granulocyte colony–stimulating factor and granulocyte/macrophage-colony–stimulating factor after interleukin-1 stimulation of marrow stromal cell cultures from normal or aplastic anemia donors. J Cell Physiol 1992; 152:199–206.
75. Tani K, Ozawa K, Ogura H, et al: The production of granulocyte colony–stimulating factor and interleukin 6 by human bone marrow stromal cells in aplastic anemia. Tohoku J Exp Med 1993; 169:325–334.
76. Nakao S, Matsushima K, Young N: Deficient interleukin 1 production by aplastic anemia monocytes. Br J Haematol 1989; 71:431–436.
77. Das Gaines RE, Milne A, Rowley M, et al: Serum immunoreactive erythropoietin in patients with idiopathic aplastic and Fanconi's anaemias. Br J Haematol 1992; 82:601–607.
78. Emmons RVB, Reid D, Cohen RL, et al: Human

thrombopoietin levels are high when thrombocytopenia is due to megakaryocyte deficiency and low when due to increased platelet destruction. Blood 1996; 87:4068–4071.
79. Watari K, Asano S, Shirafuji N, et al: Serum granulocyte colony–stimulating factor levels in healthy volunteers and patients with various disorders as estimated by enzyme immunoassay. Blood 1989; 73:117–122.
80. Lyman SD, Seaberg M, Hanna R, et al: Plasma/serum levels of flt3 ligand are low in normal individuals and highly elevated in patient with Fanconi anemia and acquired aplastic anemia. Blood 1995; 86:4091–4096.
81. Kojima S, Matsuyama T, Kodera Y: Plasma levels and production of soluble stem cell factor by marrow stromal cells in patients with aplastic anaemia. Br J Haematol 1997; 99:440–446.
82. Mathé G, Amiel JL, Schwarzenberg L, et al: Bone marrow graft in man after conditioning by antilymphocytic serum. BMJ 1970; 2:131–136.
83. Kagan WA, Ascensao JA, Pahwa RN, et al: Aplastic anemia: Presence in human bone marrow of cells that suppress myelopoiesis. Proc Natl Acad Sci U S A 1976; 73:2890–2894.
84. Bacigalupo A, Podestà M, Frassoni F, et al: Generation of CFU-C suppressor T cells in vitro V. A multistep process. Br J Haematol 1982; 52:421–427.
85. Zoumbos N, Djeu J, Young N: Interferon is the suppressor of lymphocytes generated by stimulated lymphocytes in vitro. J Immunol 1984; 133:769–774.
86. Zoumbos N, Gascon P, Djeu J, et al: Interferon is a mediator of hematopoietic suppression in aplastic anemia in vitro and possibly in vivo. Proc Natl Acad Sci U S A 1985; 82:188–192.
87. Tong J, Bacigalupo A, Piaggio G, et al: In vitro response of T cells from aplastic anemia patients to antilymphocyte globulin and phytohemagglutinin: Colony-stimulating activity and lymphokine production. Exp Hematol 1991; 19:312–316.
88. Selleri C, Sato T, Anderson S, et al: Interferon-γ and tumor necrosis factor-α suppress both early and late stages of hematopoiesis and induce programmed cell death. J Cell Physiol 1995; 165:538–546.
89. Nakao S, Yamaguchi M, Shiobara S: Interferon gamma gene expression in unstimulated bone marrow mononuclear cells predicts a response to cyclosporine therapy in aplastic anemia. Blood 1992; 79:2532–2535.
90. Nisticò A, Young NS: Gamma-interferon gene expression in the bone marrow of patients with acquired aplastic anemia. Ann Intern Med 1994; 120:463–469.
91. Melenhorst JJ, van Krieken JHJM, Dreef E, et al: T cells selectively infiltrate bone marrow areas with residual haemopoiesis of patients with acquired aplastic anaemia. Brit J Haematol 1997; 99:517–519.
92. Sloand E, Kim S, Maciejewski JP, et al: Presence of intracellular interferon-gamma (IFN-gamma) in circulating lymphocytes and response to immunosuppressive therapy in patients with aplastic anemia (abstract). Blood 1998; 10(suppl 1):158a.
93. Maciejewski JP, Hibbs JR, Anderson S, et al: Bone marrow and peripheral blood lymphocyte phenotype in patients with bone marrow failure. Exp Hematol 1994; 22:1102–1110.
94. Platanias L, Gascon P, Bielory L, et al: Lymphocyte subsets and lymphokines following anti-thymocyte globulin therapy in patients with aplastic anaemia. Br J Haematol 1987; 66:433–443.
95. Laver J, Castro-Malaspina H, Kernan NA, et al: In vitro interferon-gamma production by cultured T-cells in severed aplastic anemia: Correlation with granulomonopoietic inhibition in patients who respond to anti-thymocyte globulin. Br J Haematol 1988; 69:545–550.
96. Selleri C, Maciejewski JP, Sato T, et al: Interferon-γ constitutively expressed in the stromal microenvironment of human marrow cultures mediates potent hematopoietic inhibition. Blood 1996; 87:4149–4157.
97. Maciejewski JP, Selleri C, Sato T, et al: Increased expression of Fas antigen on bone marrow CD34+ cells of patients with aplastic anemia. Br J Haematol 1995; 91:245–252.
98. Philpott NJ, Scopes J, Marsh JCW, et al: Increased apoptosis in aplastic anemia bone marrow progenitor cells: Possible pathophysiologic significance. Exp Hematol 1995; 23:1642–1648.
99. Maciejewski JP, Selleri C, Sato T, et al: Nitric oxide suppression of human hematopoiesis in vitro: Contribution to inhibitory action of interferon-γ and tumor necrosis factor-α. J Clin Invest 1995; 96:1085–1092.
100. Sato T, Selleri C, Young NS, et al: Inhibition of interferon regulatory factor-1 expression results in predominance of cell growth stimulatory effects of interfcron-gamma due to phosphorylation of Stat1 and Stat3. Blood 1997; 90:4749–4758.
101. Moebius U, Hermann F, Hercent T, et al: Clonal analysis of CD4+/CD8+ T cells in a patient with aplastic anemia. J Clin Invest 1991; 87:1567–1574.
102. Nakao S, Takamatsu H, Yachie A, et al: Establishment of a CD4+ T cell clone recognizing autologous hematopoietic progenitor cells from a patient with immune-mediated aplastic anemia. Exp Hematol 1995; 23:433–438.
103. Wolk A, Simon-Stoos K, Nami I, et al: A mouse model of immune-mediated aplastic anemia (abstract). Blood 1998; 10(suppl 1):158a–159a.
104. Anderson KC, Weinstin HJ: Transfusion-associated graft-versus-host disease. N Engl J Med 1990; 323:315–321.
105. Debusscher L, Bitar N, De Maubeuge J, et al: Eosinophilic fasciitis and severe aplastic anemia: Favorable response to either antithymocyte globulin or cyclosporine A in blood and skin disorders. Transplant Proc 1988; 10:310–313.
106. Aitchison RGM, Marsh JCW, Hows JM, et al: Pregnancy associated aplastic anaemia: A report

of five cases and review of current management. Br J Haematol 1989; 73:541–545.
107. Champlin R: Bone marrow aplasia due to radiation accidents: Pathophysiology, assessment and treatment. Baillière's Clin Haematol 1989; 2:69:–82.
108. Wald N, Thoma GE, Broun GJ: Hematological manifestations of radiation exposure in man. Prog Hematol 1962; 3:1–52.
109. Young NS: Bone marrow failure secondary to genetic injury: Radiation; myelodysplasia and related syndromes. In Young NS, Alter BP (eds): Aplastic Anemia, Acquired and Inherited. Philadelphia, WB Saunders, 1994, pp 465–467.
110. Meijne EIM, Van der Winden-von Groenewegen RJM, Ploemacher RE, et al: The effects of x-irradiation of hematopoietic stem cell compartments in the mouse. Exp Hematol 1991; 19:617–623.
111. Liebow AA, Warren S, DeCoursey E: Pathology of atomic bomb casualties. Am J Pathol 1949; 25:853–1027.
112. Congdon CC, Fliedner TM: Morphological aspects of radiation injury. In Manual on Radiation Hematology. Vienna, International Atomic Energy Agency, 1971, pp 85–87.
113. Morris MD, Jones TD: Hematopoietic death of unprotected man from photon irradiations: Statistical modeling from animal experiments. Int J Radiat Biol 1989; 55:445–461.
114. Baverstock KF, Ash PJND: A review of radiation accidents involving whole body exposure and the relevance to LD50/60 for man. Br J Radiol 1983; 56:837–849.
115. Mole RH: The LD50 for uniform low LET irradiation of man. Br J Radiol 1984; 57:355–369.
116. LeRoy GV: Hematology of atomic bomb casualties. Arch Intern Med 1950; 86:691–710.
117. Baranov A, Gale RP, Guskova A, et al: Bone marrow transplantation after the Chernobyl nuclear accident. N Engl J Med 1989; 321:205–212.
118. Krishbaum JD, Matsuo T, Sato K, et al: A study of aplastic anemia in an autopsy series with special reference to atomic bomb survivors in Hiroshima and Nagasaki. Blood 1971; 38:17–26.
119. Kato H, Schull WJ: Studies of the mortality of A-bomb survivors. 7. Mortality, 1950–1978: Part 1. Cancer morality. Radiat Res 1982; 90:395–432.
120. Mathé G, Jammet H, Pendic B, et al: Transfusions et greffes de moelle osseuse homologue chez des humains irradiés à haute dose accidentellement. Rev Fr Études Clin Biol 1959; 4:226–238.
121. Betz EA: Late effects on haemopoiesis and life-shortening. In Manual on Radiation Hematology. Vienna, International Atomic Energy Agency, 1971, pp 181–190.
122. Ichimaru M, Ichimaru T, Tsuchimoto T, et al: Clinical aspects and survival of aplastic anemia cases in Hiroshima and Nagasaki, 1946–67. J Kyushu Hematol 1973; 22:91–98.
123. Parreira F, Carneiro de Moura M: Morphological study of the bone marrow in patients injected with ThO2. Environ Res 1979; 1861:614–664.
124. Darby SC, Doll R, Gill SK, et al: Long term mortality after a single treatment course with X-rays in patients treated for ankylosing spondylitis. Br J Cancer 1987; 55:179–190.
125. Matanoski GM, Seltser R, Sartwell PE, et al: The current mortality rates of radiologists and other physician specialists: Specific causes of death. J Epidemiol 1975; 101:199–210.
126. Kitabatake T, Sakai K, Saito A: Expectation of aplastic anemia following radiotherapy for malignancy. Radiology 1978; 129:169–171.
127. Gilbert ES, Fry A, Wiggs LD, et al: Analyses of combined mortality data on workers at the Hanford Site, Oak Ridge National Laboratory, and Rocky Flats Nuclear Weapons Plant. Radiat Res 1989; 120:19–35.
128. Wiggs LD, Cox-DeVore CA, Wilkinson GS, et al: Mortality among workers exposed to external ionizing radiation at a nuclear facility in Ohio. J Occup Med 1991; 33:632–637.
129. Hickey RJ, Bowers EJ, Spence DE, et al: Low level ionizing radiation and human mortality: Multi-regional epidemiological studies. Health Phys 1981; 40:625–641.
130. Young NS: Drugs and chemicals. In Young NS, Alter BP (eds): Aplastic Anemia, Acquired and Inherited. Philadelphia, WB Saunders, 1994, pp 100–132.
131. Bacigalupo A: Aetiology of severe aplastic anaemia and outcome after allogeneic bone marrow transplantation or immunosuppression. Eur J Haematol 1996; 57(suppl 60):16–19.
132. Kelton HG, Huang AT, Mold N, et al: The use of in vitro technics to study drug-induced pancytopenia. N Engl J Med 1979; 301:621–624.
133. Gerson WT, Fine DG, Spielberg SP, et al: Anticonvulsant-induced aplastic anemia: Increased susceptibility to toxic drug metabolites in vitro. Blood 1983; 61:889–893.
134. Yunis JJ, Corzo D, Salazar M, et al: HLA associations in clozapine-induced agranulocytosis. Blood 1995; 86:1177–1183.
135. Tamai H, Sudo T, Kimura A, et al: Association between the DRB1*08032 histocompatibilty antigen and methimazole-induced agranulocytosis in Japanese patients with Graves disease. Ann Intern Med 1996; 124:490–494.
136. Marcus WL: Chemical of current interest—benzene. Toxicol Ind Health 1987; 3:205–266.
137. Kalf GF: Recent advances in the metabolism and toxicity of benzene. Crit Rev Toxicol 1987; 18:141–159.
138. Smith MT: Overview of benzene-induced aplastic anaemia. Eur J Haematol 1996; 57(suppl):107–110.
139. Ross D. Metabolic basis of benzene toxicity. Eur J Haematol 1996; 57(suppl):111–118.
140. Gill DP, Jenkins VK, Kempen RR, et al: The importance of pluripotential stem cells in benzene toxicity. Toxicology 1980; 16:163–171.
141. Green JD, Snyder CA, LoBue J, et al: Acute and chronic dose/response effects of inhaled benzene on multipotential hematopoietic stem (CFU-S) and

141. granulocyte/macrophage progenitor. Toxicol Appl Pharmacol 1981; 58:492–503.
142. Chertkov JL, Lutton JD, Jiang S, et al: Hematopoietic effects of benzene inhalation assessed by murine long-term bone marrow culture. J Lab Clin Med 1992; 119:412–419.
143. Hamilton A: Benzene (benzol) poisoning. Arch Pathol 1931; 11:434–454, 631–637.
144. Oldfeldt CO: Benzene poisoning; clinical considerations. Acta Med Scand 1944; 119:380–425.
145. Yin S-N, Li Q, Liu Y, et al: Occupational exposure to benzene in China. Br J Ind Med 1987; 44:192–195.
146. Aksoy M, Koray D, Akgun T, et al: Haematological effects of chronic benzene poisoning in 217 workers. Br J Ind Med 1971; 28:296–302.
147. Ruiz MA, Vassallo J, de Souza CA: Hematological abnormalities in patients chronically exposed to benezene. An update. Rev Saude Publica 1993; 27:145–151.
148. DeGowin RL: Benzene exposure and aplastic anemia followed by leukemia 15 years later. JAMA 1963; 185:748–751.
149. Aksoy M. Benzene as a leukemogenic and carcinogenic agent. Am J Ind Med 1985; 8:9–20.
150. Aksoy M, Erdem S, Dincol G, et al: Aplastic anemia due to chemicals and drugs: A study of 108 patients. Sex Transm Dis 1984; 11:347–350.
151. Williams DM, Lynch RE, Cartwright GE: Drug-induced aplastic anemia. Semin Hematol 1973; 10:195–223.
152. Fleming LE, Timmeny W: Aplastic anemia and pesticides. An etiologic association? J Occup Med 1993; 35:1106–1116.
153. Scott JL, Cartwright GE, Wintrobe MM: Acquired aplastic anemia: An analysis of thirty-nine cases and review of the pertinent literature. Medicine (Baltimore) 1958; 38:119–172.
154. Smick KM, Condit PK, Proctor RL, et al: Fatal aplastic anemia: An epidemiological study of its relationship to the drug chloramphenicol. J Chronic Dis 1964; 17:899–914.
155. Wallerstein RO, Condit PK, Kasper CK, et al: Statewide study of chloramphenicol therapy and fatal aplastic anemia. JAMA 1969; 208:2045–2050.
156. Leikin SL, Welch H: Aplastic anemia due to chloramphenicol. Clin Proc Child Hosp D C 1961; 17:171–181.
157. Wolff JA: Anemias caused by infections and toxins, idiopathic aplastic anemia and anemia caused by renal disease. Pediatr Clin North Am 1957; 469–480.
158. Kelly JP, Kaufman DW: Anti-infective drug use in relation to the risk of agranulocytosis and aplastic anemia. Arch Intern Med 1989; 149:1036–1040.
159. Kumana CR, Li KY, Chau PY: Worldwide variation in chloramphenicol utilization: Should it cause concern? J Clin Pharmacol 1988; 28:1071–1075.
160. Kumana CR, Li KY, Kou M: Do chloramphenicol blood dyscrasias occur in Hong Kong? Adverse Drug React Toxicol Rev 1993; 12:97–106.
161. Polak BCP, Wesseling H, Schut D, et al: Blood dyscrasias attributed to chloramphenicol. Acta Med Scand 1972; 192:409–414.
162. Laporte JR, Vidal X, Ballarin E, et al: Possible association between ocular chloramphenicol and aplastic anaemia—the absolute risk is very low. Br J Clin Pharmacol 1998; 46:181–184.
163. Gussoff BD, Lee SL: Chloramphenicol-induced hematopoietic depression: A controlled comparison with tetracycline. Am J Med Sci 1966; 251:46–53.
164. Hara H, Kohsaki M, Noguchi K, et al: Effect of chloramphenicol on colony formation from erythrocytic precursors. Am J Hematol 1978; 5:123–130.
165. Sawada H, Tezuka H, Kamamoto T, et al: Effects of chloramphenicol on hemopoietic cells and their microenvironment in vitro. Acta Haematol Jpn 1985; 48:1323–1331.
166. Mitus WJ, Coleman N: In vitro effect of chloramphenicol on chromosomes. Blood 1970; 35:689–694.
167. Pohl LR, Reddy GB, Krishna G: A new pathway of metabolism of chloramphenicol which influences the interpretation of its irreversible binding to protein in vivo. Biochem Pharmacol 1979; 28:2433–2440.
168. Chaplin S: Bone marrow depression due to mianserin, phenylbutazone, oxyphenbutazone, and chloramphenicol. Part I. Adverse Drug React Toxicol Rev 1986; 5:97–101.
169. Brodie MJ, Pellock JM: Taming the brain storms: Felbamate updated. Lancet 1995; 346:918–919.
170. Joffe RT, Post RM, Roy-Byrne PP, et al: Hematological effects of carbamazepine in patients with affective illness. Am J Psychiatry 1985; 142:1196–1199.
171. Pellock JM: Carbamazepine side effects in children and adults. Epilepsia 1987; 28(suppl 3):S64–S70.
172. MacCarty DJ, Brill JM, Harrop DH: Aplastic anemia secondary to gold-salt therapy. Report of fatal case and a review of literature. JAMA 1962; 179:655–657.
173. Howell A, Gumpel JM, Watts RWE: Depression of bone marrow colony formation in gold-induced neutropenia. BMJ 1975; 1:432–434.
174. Kay AGL: Myelotoxicity of gold. BMJ 1976; 1:1266–1268.
175. Kyle RA, Prase GL: Hematologic aspects of arsenic intoxication. N Engl J Med 1965; 273:18–23.
176. Loveman AB: Toxic granulocytopenia, purpura hemorrhagica and aplastic anemia following the arsphenamines. Ann Intern Med 1932; 5:1238–1256.
177. Kaufman DW, Issaragrisil S, Anderson T, et al: Use of household pesticides and the risk of aplastic anaemia in Thailand. Int J Epidemiol 1997; 26:643–650.
178. Issaragrisil S, Kaufman D, Anderson T, et al: Association of seropositivity for hepatitis viruses and aplastic anemia in Thailand. Hepatology 1997; 25:1255–1257.

179. Anderson LJ, Young NS (eds): Human parvovirus B19. Basel, Karger, 1997.
180. Sullivan JL: Hematologic consequences of Epstein-Barr virus infection. Hematol Oncol Clin North Am 1987; 1:397–417.
181. Baranski B, Armstrong G, Truman JT, et al: Epstein-Barr virus in the bone marrow of patients with aplastic anemia. Ann Intern Med 1988; 109:695–704.
182. Purtilo DT, Sakamoto K, Barnabei V, et al: Epstein-Barr virus–induced diseases in boys with the X-linked lymphoproliferative syndrome (XLP). Update on studies of the registry. Am J Med 1982; 73:49–56.
183. Schimke RN, Collins D, Cross D: Nasopharyngeal carcinoma, aplastic anemia, and various malignancies in a family. Possible role of Epstein-Barr virus. Am J Med Genet 1987; 27:195–202.
184. Brown KE, Tisdale J, Dunbar CE, et al: Hepatitis-associated aplastic anemia. N Engl J Med 1997; 336:1059–1064.
185. Tzakis AG, Arditi M, Whitington PF, et al: Aplastic anemia complicating orthotopic liver transplantation for non-A, non-B hepatitis. N Engl J Med 1988; 319:393–396.
186. Frickhofen N, Raghavachar A, Heit W, et al: Human parvovirus infection (letter). N Engl J Med 1986; 314:646.
187. Osaki M, Matsubara K, Iwasaki T, et al: Severe aplastic anemia associated with human parvovirus B19 infection in a patient without underlying disease. Ann Hematol 1999; 78:83–86.
188. Akashi K, Hayashi S, Gondo H, et al: Involvement of interferon-gamma and macrophage colony–stimulating factor in pathogenesis of hemophagocytic lymphohistiocytosis in adults. Br J Haematol 1994; 87:243–250.
189. Imashuku S. Differential diagnosis of hemophagocytic syndrome: Underlying disorders and selection of the most effective treatment. Int J Hematol 1997; 66:135–151.
190. Tsuda H: Hemophagocytic syndrome (HPS) in children and adults. Int J Hematol 1997; 65:215–226.
191. Storb R, Longton G, Anasetti C, et al: Changing trends in marrow transplantation for aplastic anemia. Bone Marrow Transplant 1992; 10:45–52.
192. Horowitz MM: Current status of allogeneic bone marrow transplantation in acquired aplastic anemia. Semin Hematol 2000; 37:30–42.
193. Young NS: Definitive treatment of acquired aplastic anemia. In Young NS, Alter BP (eds): Aplastic Anemia, Acquired and Inherited. Philadelphia, WB Saunders, 1994, pp 159–200.
194. Tsai TW, Freytes CO: Allogeneic bone marrow transplantation for leukemias and aplastic anemia. Adv Intern Med 1997; 42:423–451.
195. Margolis DA, Cammita BM: Hematopoietic stem cell transplantation for severe aplastic anemia. Curr Opin Hematol 1998; 5:441–444.
196. Hsu HC, Tsai WH, Lin JS, et al: Primary transplantation of allogeneic peripheral blood stem cell for severe aplastic anemia. Ann Hematol 1997; 74:191–192.
197. Redei I, Waller EK, Holland HK, et al: Successful engraftment after primary graft failure in aplastic anemia using G-CSF mobilized peripheral stem cell transfusions. Bone Marrow Transplant 1997; 19:175–177.
198. Camitta BM, Thomas ED, Nathan DG, et al: Severe aplastic anemia: A prospective study of the effect of early marrow transplantation on acute mortality. Blood 1976; 48:63–69.
199. Storb R, Etzioni R, Anasetti C, et al: Cyclophosphamide combined with antithymocyte globulin in preparation for allogeneic marrow transplants in patients with aplastic anemia. Blood 1994; 84:941–949.
200. May WS, Sensenbrenner LL, Burns WH, et al: BMT for severe aplastic anemia using cyclosporine. Bone Marrow Transplant 1993; 11:459–464.
201. Ladenstein R, Peters C, Minkov M, et al: A single centre experience with allogeneic stem cell transplantation for severe aplastic anaemia in childhood. Klin Padiatr 1997; 209:201–208.
202. Reiter E, Keil F, Brugger S, et al: Excellent long-term survival after allogeneic marrow transplantation in patients with severe aplastic anemia. Bone Marrow Transplant 1997; 19:1191–1196.
203. Passweg J, Socie G, Hinterberger W, et al: Bone marrow transplantation for severe aplastic anemia: Has outcome improved? Blood 1997; 90:858–864.
204. Bacigalupo A, Brand R, Obeto R, et al: Treatment of acquired aplastic anemia: Bone marrow transplantation compared with immunosuppressive therapy—The European Group for Blood and Marrow Transplantation Experience. Semin Hematol 2000; 37:69–80.
205. Bacigalupo A, Hows J, Gluckman E, et al: Bone marrow transplantation (BMT) versus immunosuppression for the treatment of severe aplastic anaemia (SAA): A report of the EBMT SAA working party. Br J Haematol 1988; 70:177–182.
206. Stucki A, Leisenring W, Sandmaier BM, et al: Decreased rejection and improved survival of first and second marrow transplants for severe aplastic anemia (a 26-year retrospective analysis). Blood 1998; 92:2742–2749.
207. Champlin RE, Feig SA, Sparkes RS, et al: Bone marrow transplantation from identical twins in the treatment of aplastic anaemia: Implication for the pathogenesis of the disease. Br J Haematol 1984; 56:455–463.
208. Lu DP: Syngeneic bone marrow transplantation for treatment of aplastic anemia: Report of a case and review of the literature. Exp Hematol 1981; 9:257–263.
209. Hinterberger W, Rowlings PA, Hinterberger-Fischer M, et al: Results of transplanting bone marrow from genetically identical twins into patients with aplastic anemia. Ann Intern Med 1997; 126:116–122.
210. Anasetti C, Doney KC, Storb R, et al: Marrow

211. Champlin RE, Horowitz MM, vanBekkum DW, et al: Graft failure following bone marrow transplantation for severe aplastic anemia: Risk factors and treatment results. Blood 1989; 73:606–613.
212. Deeg HJ, Self S, Storb R, et al: Decreased incidence of marrow graft rejection in patients with severe aplastic anemia: Changing impact of risk factors. Blood 1986; 68:1363–1368.
213. Ramsay NKC, Kim TH, McGlave P, et al: Total lymphoid irradiation and cyclophosphamide conditioning prior to bone marrow transplantation for patients with severe aplastic anemia. Blood 1983; 62:622–626.
214. Bacigalupo A. Treatment of severe aplastic anaemia. In Gordon-Smith EC (ed): Aplastic Anaemia. Clinical Haematology, vol 2. London, Bailliere Tindall, 1989, pp 19–36.
215. Sullivan KM, Witherspoon RP, Storb R, et al: Long-term results of allogeneic bone marrow transplantation. Transplant Proc 1988; 21:2926–2928.
216. Hill RS, Petersen FB, Storb R, et al: Mixed hematologic chimerism after allogeneic marrow transplantation for severe aplastic anemia is associated with a higher risk of graft rejection and a lessened incidence of acute graft-versus-host disease. Blood 1986; 67:811–816.
217. Weitzel JN, Hows JM, Jeffreys AJ, et al: Use of a hypervariable minisatellite DNA probe (33.15) for evaluating engraftment two or more years after bone marrow transplantation for aplastic anaemia. Br J Haematol 1988; 70:91–97.
218. Hows JM, Kaffaf S, Palmer S, et al: Regeneration of peripheral blood cells following allogeneic bone marrow transplantation for severe aplastic anaemia. Br J Haematol 1982; 52:551–558.
219. Storb R, Weiden PL, Sullivan KM, et al: Second marrow transplants in patients with aplastic anemia rejecting the first graft: Use of a conditioning regimen including cyclophosphamide and antithymocyte globulin. Blood 1987; 70:116–121.
220. Hortsmann M, Stockschlader M, Kruger W, et al: Cyclophosphamide/antithymocyte globulin conditioning of patients with severe aplastic anemia for marrow transplantation from HLA-matched siblings: Preliminary results. Ann Hematol 1995; 71:77–81.
221. Azuma E, Kojima S, Kato K, et al: Conditioning with cyclophosphamide/antithymocyte globulin for allogeneic bone marrow transplantation from HLA-matched siblings in children with severe aplastic anemia. Bone Marrow Transplant 1997; 19:1085–1087.
222. Storb R, Prentice RL, Sullivan KM, et al: Predictive factors in chronic graft-versus-host disease in patients with aplastic anemia treated by marrow transplantation from HLA-identical siblings. Ann Intern Med 1983; 98:461–466.
223. Sanders JE, Whitehead J, Storb R, et al: Bone marrow transplantation experience for children with aplastic anemia. Pediatrics 1986; 77:179–186.
224. Deeg HJ, Leisenring W, Storb R, et al: Long-term outcome after marrow transplantation for severe aplastic anemia. Blood 1998; 91:3637–3645.
225. Champlin R, Ho W, Bayever E, et al: Treatment of aplastic anemia: Results with bone marrow transplantation, antithymocyte globulin, and a monoclonal anti-T cell antibody. In Young NS, Levine AS, Humphries RK (eds): Aplastic Anemia: Stem Cell Biology and Advances in Treatment. New York, Alan R Liss, 1984, pp 227–238.
226. McGlave PB, Haake R, Miller W, et al: Therapy of severe aplastic anemia in young adults and children with allogeneic bone marrow transplantation. Blood 1987; 70:1325–1330.
227. Sklar C: Growth and endocrine disturbances after bone marrow transplantation in childhood. Acta Paediatr 1995; 411:57–61.
228. Curtis ER, Rowlings PA, Deeg J, et al: Solid cancers after bone marrow transplantation. N Engl J Med 1997; 336:897–904.
229. Witherspoon RP, Fisher LD, Schock G, et al: Secondary cancers after bone marrow transplantation for leukemia or aplastic anemia. N Engl J Med 1989; 321:784–789.
230. Socié G, Henry-Amar M, Cosset JM, et al: Increased incidence of solid malignant tumors after bone marrow transplantation for severe aplastic anemia. Blood 1991; 78:277–279.
231. Pierga J, Socié G, Gluckman E, et al: Secondary solid malignant tumors occurring after bone marrow transplantation for severe aplastic anemia given thoraco-abdominal irradiation. Radiother Oncol 1994; 30:55–58.
232. Socié G, Henry-Amar M, Devergie A, et al: Poor clinical outcome of patients developing malignant solid tumors after bone marrow transplantation for severe aplastic anemia. Leuk Lymphoma 1992; 7:419–423.
233. Socié G, Henry-Amar M, Bacigalupo A, et al for the European Bone Marrow Transplantation-Severe Aplastic Anaemia Working Party: Malignant tumors occurring after treatment of aplastic anemia. N Engl J Med 1993; 329:1152–1157.
234. Anasetti C, Etzioni R, Petersdorf EW, et al: Marrow transplantation from unrelated volunteer donors. Annu Rev Med 1995; 46:169–179.
235. Wagner JL, Deeg HJ, Seidel K, et al: Bone marrow transplantation for severe aplastic anemia from genotypically HLA-nonidentical relatives. Transplantation 1996; 61:54–61.
236. Bacigalupo A, Hows J, Gordon-Smith EC, et al: Bone marrow transplantation for severe aplastic anemia from donors than HLA identical siblings: A report of the BMT working party. Bone Marrow Transplant 1988; 3:531–535.
237. Hows JM: Severe aplastic anaemia: The patient without a HLA-identical sibling. Br J Haematol 1991; 77:1–4.
238. Filipovich AH, Ramsay NKC, Arthur DC, et al: Allogeneic bone marrow transplantation with related donors other than HLA MLC-matched

siblings, and the use of antithymocyte globulin, prednisone, and methotrexate for prophylaxis of graft-versus-host disease. Transplantation 1985; 39:282–285.
239. Henslee-Downey PJ, Abhyankar SH, Parrish RS, et al: Use of partially mismatched related donors extends access to allogeneic marrow transplant. Blood 1997; 89:3864–3872.
240. Davies SM, Ramsay NKC, Haake RJ, et al: Comparison of engraftment in recipients of matched sibling or unrelated donor marrow allografts. Bone Marrow Transplant 1994; 13:51–57.
241. Hows J, Bradley BA, Gore S, et al: Prospective evaluation of unrelated donor bone marrow transplantation. Bone Marrow Transplant 1993; 12: 371–380.
242. Vowels MR, Lam PT, Mameghan H, et al: Bone marrow transplantation in children using closely matched related and unrelated donors. Bone Marrow Transplant 1991; 8:87–92.
243. Ochs L, Shu XO, Miller J, et al: Late infections after allogeneic bone marrow transplantation: Comparison of incidence in related and unrelated donor transplant recipients. Blood 1995; 86:3979–3986.
244. Hows JM, Szydlo R, Anasetti C, et al: Unrelated donor transplants for severe aplastic anemia. Bone Marrow Transplant 1992; 10(suppl 1):102–106.
245. Margolis DA, Casper JT: Alternative donor hematopoietic stem-cell transplantation for severe aplastic anemia. Semin Hematol 2000; 37:43–55.
246. Kernan NA, Bartsch G, Ash RC, et al: Analysis of 462 transplantations from unrelated donors facilitated by the National Marrow Donor Program. N Engl J Med 1993; 328:593–602.
247. Bacigalupo A: Severe Aplastic Anaemia Working Party. *In* EBMT Working Parties Reports. Harrogate, UK, European Group for Bone Marrow Transplantation, 1994, pp 49–62.
248. Davies SM, Wagner JE, Defor T, et al: Unrelated donor bone marrow transplantation for children and adolescents with aplastic anaemia or myelodysplasia. Br J Haematol 1997; 96:749–756.
249. Margolis D, Camitta B, Pietryga D, et al: Unrelated donor bone marrow transplantation to treat severe aplastic anaemia in children and young adults. Br J Haematol 1996; 94:65–72.
250. Bacigalupo A, Piaggio G, Podestà M, et al: Collection of peripheral blood hematopoietic progenitors (PBHP) from patients with severe aplastic anemia (SAA) after prolonged administration of granulocyte colony–stimulating factor. Blood 1993; 82:1410–1414.
251. Koza V, Jindra P, Svojgrová M, et al: Successful autologous transplantation in a patient with severe aplastic anemia (SAA). Bone Marrow Transplant 1998; 21:957–959.
252. Camitta BM, Doney K: Immunosuppressive therapy for aplastic anemia: Indications, agents, mechanisms, and results. Am J Pediatr Hematol Oncol 1990; 12:411–424.
253. Marsh JC, Gordon-Smith EC: Treatment of aplastic anaemia with antilymphocyte globulin and cyclosporin. Int J Hematol 1995; 62:133–144.
254. Speck B, Gluckman E, Haak HL, et al: Treatment of aplastic anaemia by antilymphocyte globulin with and without allogeneic bone-marrow infusions. Lancet 1977; 2:1145–1148.
255. Tichelli A, Socié G, Henry-Amar M, et al: Effectiveness of immunosuppressive therapy in older patients with aplastic anemia. The European Group for Blood and Marrow Transplantation Severe Aplastic Anaemia Working Party. Ann Intern Med 1999; 130:193–201.
256. Camitta B, Sensenbrenner L, O'Reilly RJ, et al: Antithoracic duct lymphocyte globulin therapy of severe aplastic anemia. Blood 1983; 62:883–888.
257. Champlin R, Ho W, Gale RP: Antithymocyte globulin treatment in patients with aplastic anemia. N Engl J Med 1983; 308:113–118.
258. Young N, Griffith P, Brittain E, et al: A multicenter trial of anti-thymocyte globulin in aplastic anemia and related diseases. Blood 1988; 72:1861–1869.
259. Young N, Speck B: Antithymocyte and antilymphocyte globulins: Clinical trials and mechanism of action. *In* Young NS, Levine AS, Humphries RK (eds): Aplastic Anemia. Stem Cell Biology and Advances in Treatment. New York, Alan R Liss, 1984, 221–226.
260. Doney K, Storb R, Buckner CD, et al: Treatment of gold-induced aplastic anaemia with immunosuppressive therapy. Br J Haematol 1988; 68:469–472.
261. Frickhofen N, Rosenfeld SJ: Immunosuppressive treatment of aplastic anemia with antithymocyte globulin and cyclosporine. Semin Hematol 2000; 37:56–68.
262. Van Kamp H, Landegent JE, Jansen RPM, et al: Clonal hematopoiesis in patients with acquired aplastic anemia. Blood 1991; 78:3209–3214.
263. Wun T, Lewis JP: Clonal remission in aplastic anemia after treatment with antithymocyte globulin. Am J Hematol 1992; 40:229–231.
264. Geary CG, Harrison CJ, Philpott NJ, et al: Abnormal cytogenetic clones in patients with aplastic anaemia: Response to immunosuppressive therapy. Br J Haematol 1999; 104:271–274.
265. Champlin RE, Ho WG, Feig SA, et al: Do androgens enhance the response to antithymocyte globulin in patients with aplastic anemia? A prospective randomized trial. Blood 1985; 66:184–188.
266. Doney K, Pepe M, Storb R, et al: Immunosuppressive therapy of aplastic anemia: Results of a prospective, randomized trial of antithymocyte globulin (ATG), methylprednisolone, and oxymetholone to ATG, very high-dose methylprednisolone, and oxymetholone. Blood 1992; 79:2566–2571.
267. Doney KC, Weiden PL, Buckner CD, et al: Treatment of severe aplastic anemia using antithymocyte globulin with or without an infusion of HLA haploidentical marrow. Exp Hematol 1981; 9:829–834.
268. Marsh JCW, Hows JM, Bryett KA, et al: Survival after antilymphocyte globulin therapy for aplastic

anemia depends on disease severity. Blood 1987; 70:1046–1052.
269. Locasciulli A, van't Veer L, Bacigalupo A, et al: Treatment with marrow transplantation or immunosuppression of childhood acquired severe aplastic anemia: A report from the EBMT SAA working party. Bone Marrow Transplant 1990; 6: 211–217.
270. Bielory L, Wright R, Nienhuis AW, et al: Antithymocyte globulin hypersensitivity in bone marrow failure patients. JAMA 1988; 260:3164–3167.
271. Heyworth MF: Effects of anti-lymphocytic globulin in human subjects. J Immunol 1981; 43:793–802.
272. Smith AG, O'Reilly RJ, Hansen JA, et al: Specific antibody-blocking activities in antilymphocyte globulin as correlates of efficacy for the treatment of aplastic anemia. Blood 1985; 66:721–723.
273. Raefsky E, Gascon P, Gratwohl A, et al: Biological and biochemical characterization of anti-thymocyte globulins (ATG) and anti-lymphocyte globulins (ALG). Blood 1986; 68:712–719.
274. Bonnefoy-Bérard N, Vincent C, Revillard J-P: Antibodies against functional leukocyte surface molecules in polyclonal antilymphocyte and antithymocyte globulins. Transplantation 1991; 51: 669–673.
275. Bonnefoy-Berard N, Verrier V, Vincent C, et al: Inhibition of CD25 (IL-2Rα) expression and T-cell proliferation by polyclonal anti-thymocyte globulins. Immunology 1992; 77:61–67.
276. Genestier L, Fournel S, Flacher M, et al: Induction of Fas (Apo-, CD95)-mediated apoptosis of activated lymphocytes by polyclonal antithymocyte globulin. Blood 1998; 91:2360–2368.
277. Rebellato LM, Gross U, Verbanac KM, et al: A comprehensive definition of the major antibody specificities in polyclonal rabbit antithymocyte globulin. Transplantation 1994; 57:685–694.
278. López-Karpovitch X, Zarzosa ME, et al: Changes in peripheral blood mononuclear cell subpopulations during antithymocyte globulin therapy for severe aplastic anemia. Acta Haematol 1989; 81:176–180.
279. Pawelski S, Rokicka-Milewska R, Oblakowski P, et al: ALG/ATG treatment—a useful alternative for BMT in selected aplastic anaemia patients. Folia Haematol 1989; 116:377–381.
280. Nikitin DO, Gavrilova LV: Influence of antilymphocytic globulin on immunologic parameters in children with aplastic anemia. Gematol Transfuziol 1992; 37:15–17.
281. Gascon P, Zoumbos N, Djeu J, et al: Lymphokine abnormalities in aplastic anemia. Implications for the mechanism of action of ATG. Blood 1985; 65:407–413.
282. Nimer SD, Golde DW, Kwan K, et al: In vitro production of granulocyte-macrophage colony stimulating factor in aplastic anemia: Possible mechanisms of action of antithymocyte globulin. Blood 1991; 78:163–168.
283. Kojima S, Matsuyama T, Kodera Y: In vitro granulocyte-macrophage colony–stimulating factor production by peripheral blood mononuclear cells in aplastic anemia. Acta Haematol 1994; 91:175–180.
284. Barbano GC, Schenone A, Roncella S, et al: Antilymphocyte globulin stimulates normal human T cells to proliferate and to release lymphokines in vitro. A study at the clonal level. Blood 1988; 72:956–963.
285. Schrezenmeier H, Raghavachar A, Heimpel H: Granulocyte-macrophage colony–stimualting factor in the sera of patients with aplastic anemia. Clin Invest 1993; 71:102–108.
286. Mookerjee BK, Azzolina L, Poultar L: Interaction of anti-thymocyte serum with hematopoietic stem cells. I. Effects in vitro and in vivo. J Immunol 1974; 112:822–829.
287. Mangan KF, Mullaney MT, Barrientos TD, et al: Serum interleukin-3 levels following autologous or allogeneic bone marrow transplantation: Effects of T-cell depletion, blood stem cell infusion, and hematopoietic growth factor treatment. Blood 1993; 81:1915–1922.
288. Greco B, Bielory L, Stephany D, et al: Antithymocyte globulin reacts with many normal human cell types. Blood 1983; 62:1047–1054.
289. Barrett AJ, Longhurst P, Rosengurt N, et al: Cross-reaction of antilymphocyte globulin with human granulocyte colony forming cells. J Clin Pathol 1978; 31:129–135.
290. Huang AT, Mold NG: The role of CD45RO in antithymocyte globulin's stimulation of primitive haemopoietic cells. Br J Haematol 1994; 88:643–646.
291. Hanada T, Abe T, Fukao K, et al: Severe aplastic anaemia treated with anti-lymphocyte globulin. Scand J Haematol 1982; 29:128–134.
292. Teramura M, Kobayashi S, Iwabe K, et al: Mechanism of action of antithymocyte globulin in the treatment of aplastic anaemia: In vitro evidence for the presence of immunosuppressive mechanism. Br J Haematol 1997; 96:80–84.
293. Bacigalupo A, Podestà M, van Lint MT, et al: Severe aplastic anaemia: Correlation of in vitro tests with clinical response to immunosuppression in 20 patients. Br J Haematol 1981; 47:423–433.
294. Amare M, Abdou NL, Robinson MG, et al: Aplastic anemia associated with bone marrow suppressor T-cell hyperactivity: Successful treatment with antithymocyte globulin. Am J Hematol 1978; 5:25–32.
295. Faille A, Barrett AJ, Balitrand N, et al: Effect of antilymphocyte globulin on granulocyte precursors in aplastic anemia. Br J Haematol 1979; 42:371–380.
296. Blasetti A, Faille A, Balitrand N, et al: Inhibitory effects of peripheral blood cells on in vitro colony formation by autologous bone marrow in aplastic anemia: Relation with response to immunosuppressive therapy. J Clin Pathol 1982; 35:1316–1319.
297. Abe T, Matsuoka H, Kojima S, et al: Correlation of response of aplastic anemia patients to antilymphocyte globulin with in vitro lymphocyte stimu-

latory effect: Predictive value of in vitro test for clinical response. Blood 1991; 77:2225–2230.
298. Killick S, Marsh JCW, Gordon-Smith EC, et al: In vitro antithymocyte globulin (ATG) stimulation of hemopoietic stem cells: Correlation with clinical response in patients with aplastic anemia (AA) and myelodysplastic syndromes (MDS) (abstract). Blood 1998; 92(suppl 1):693a.
299. Finlay JL, Toretsky J, Hoffman R, et al: Cyclosporine A (CyA) in refractory severe aplastic anemia (AA) (abstract). Blood 1984; 64(suppl 1):104a.
300. Leonard EM, Raefsky E, Griffith P, et al: Cyclosporine therapy of aplastic anaemia, congenital and acquired red cell aplasia. Br J Haematol 1989; 72:278–284.
301. Hinterberger-Fischer M, Hocker P, Lechner K, et al: Oral cyclosporin-A is effective treatment for untreated and also for previously immunosuppressed patients with severe bone marrow failure. Eur J Haematol 1989; 43:136–142.
302. Gluckman E, Esperou-Bourdeau H, Baruchel A, et al: A multicenter randomized study comparing cyclosporin-A alone and antithymocyte globulin with prednisone for treatment of severe aplastic anemia. J Autoimmun 1992; 5:271–275.
303. Marsh J, Schrezenmeier H, Marin P, et al: Prospective randomized multicenter study comparing cyclosporin alone versus the combination of antithymocyte globulin and cyclosporin for treatment of patients with nonsevere aplastic anemia: A report from the European Blood and Marrow Transplant (EMBT) Severe Aplastic Anemia Working Party. Blood 1991; 93:2191–2195.
304. Leeksma OC, Thomas LLM, Van der Leslie J, et al: Effectiveness of low dose cyclosporine in acquired aplastic anaemia with severe neutropenia. Neth J Med 1992; 41:143–148.
305. Schrezenmeier H, Schlander M, Raghavachar A: Cyclosporin A in aplastic anemia—report of a workshop. Ann Hematol 1992; 65:33–36.
306. Bridges R, Pineo G, Blahey W: Cyclosporin A for the treatment of aplastic anemia refractory to antithymocyte globulin. Am J Hematol 1987; 26:83–87.
307. Frickhofen N, Kaltwasser JP, Schrezenmeier H, et al: Treatment of aplastic anaemia with antilymphocyte globulin and methylprednisolone with or without cyclosporine. N Engl J Med 1991; 324:1297–1304.
308. Rosenfeld SJ, Kimball J, Vining D, et al: Intensive immunosuppression with antithymocyte globulin and cyclosporine as treatment for severe acquired aplastic anemia. Blood 1995; 85:3058–3065.
309. Bacigalupo A, Broccia G, Corda G, et al: Antilymphocyte globulin, cyclosporin, and granulocyte colony–stimulating factor in patients with acquired severe aplastic anaemia (SAA): A pilot study of the EBMT SAA working party. Blood 1995; 85:1348–1353.
310. Speck B, Gratwohl A, Nissen C, et al: Treatment of severe aplastic anemia. Exp Hematol 1986; 14:126–132.
311. Means RT, Krantz SB, Dessypris EN, et al: Retreatment of aplastic anemia with antithymocyte globulin or antilymphocyte serum. Am J Med 1988; 84:678–682.
312. Marmont AM, Bacigalupo A, van Lint MT, et al: Treatment of severe aplastic anemia with sequential immunosuppression. Exp Hematol 1983; 11:856–865.
313. Novitzky N, Wood L, Jacobs P: The treatment of aplastic anaemia with antilymphocyte globulin and high dose methylprednisolone. Am J Hematol 1991; 36:227–234.
314. Brodsky RA, Sensenbrenner LL, Jones RJ: Complete remission in severe aplastic anemia after high-dose cyclophosphamide without bone marrow transplantation. Blood 1996; 87:491–494.
315. Tisdale JF, Dunn DE, Rosenfeld SE, et al: Report of a randomized trial comparing cyclophosphamide and cyclosporine vs antithymocyte globulin and cyclosporine as initial treatment for severe aplastic anemia. (abstract). Blood 1999; 94(suppl 1):407a.
316. Bacigalupo A, van Lint MT, Cerri R, et al: Treatment of severe aplastic anemia with bolus 6-methylprednisolone and antilymphocytic globulin. Blut 1980; 41:168–171.
317. Marmont AM, Bacigalupo A, van Lint MT, et al: Treatment of severe aplastic anemia with high-dose methylprednisolone and antilymphocyte globulin. In Young NS, Levine AS, Humphries RK (eds): Aplastic Anemia: Stem Cell Biology and Advances in Treatment. New York, Alan R Liss, 1984, pp 271–287.
318. Marsh JCW, Zomas A, Hows JM, et al: Avascular necrosis after treatment of aplastic anaemia with antilymphocyte globulin and high-dose methylprednisolone. Br J Haematol 1993; 84:731–735.
319. Schrezenmeier H, Marin P, Raghavachar A, et al: Relapse of aplastic anaemia after immunosuppressive treatment: A report from the European Bone Marrow Transplantation Group SAA Working Party. Br J Haematol 1993; 85:371–377.
320. Rosenfeld SJ, Young NS: Aplastic anemia treated by immunosuppression is a chronic relapsing illness but prognosis is unaffected by relapse. Blood 1997; 90(suppl 1):435a.
321. Young NS: Autoimmunity and its treatment in aplastic anemia. Ann Intern Med 1997; 126:166–168.
322. Paquette RL, Tebyani N, Frane M, et al: Long-term outcome of aplastic anemia in adults treated with antithymocyte globulin: Comparison with bone marrow transplantation. Blood 1995; 85:283–290.
323. Arranz R, Otero MJ, Ramos R, et al: Clinical results in 50 multiply transfused patients with severe aplastic anemia treated with bone marrow transplantation or immunosuppressive therapy. Bone Marrow Transplant 1994; 13:383–387.
324. Speck B, Gratwohl A, Nissen C, et al: Treatment of severe aplastic anaemia with antilymphocyte globulin or bone-marrow transplantation. BMJ 1981; 282:860–863.

325. Doney K, Leisenring W, Storb R, et al: Primary treatment of acquired aplastic anemia: Outcomes with bone marrow transplantation and immunosuppressive therapy. Ann Intern Med 1997; 126:107–115.
326. Bayever E, Champlin R, Ho W, et al: Comparison between bone marrow transplantation and antithymocyte globulin in treatment of young patients with severe aplastic anemia. J Pediatr 1984; 105:920–925.
327. Kojima S, Fukuda M, Horibe K, et al: Comparison between bone marrow transplantation and immunosuppressive therapy in treatment of patients younger than 20 years with severe aplastic anemia. Acta Haematol Jpn 1988; 51:28–35.
328. Halperin DS, Grisaru D, Freedman MH, et al: Severe acquired aplastic anemia in children: 11-year experience with bone marrow transplantation and immunosuppressive therapy. Am J Pediatr Hematol Oncol 1989; 11:304–309.
329. Loughran TP Jr, Storb R: Treatment of aplastic anemia. Bone Marrow Transplant 1990; 4:559–575.
330. Klingemann H-G, Storb R, Fefer A, et al: Bone marrow transplantation in patients aged 45 years and older. Blood 1986; 67:770–776.
331. Gordon-Smith E, Marsh JC: Bone marrow transplantation in the management of acquired aplastic anemia. J Hematother 1994; 3:238–243.
332. Crump M, Larratt LM, Maki E, et al: Treatment of adults with severe aplastic anemia: Primary therapy with antithymocyte globulin (ATG) and rescue of ATG failures with bone marrow transplantation. Am J Med 1992; 92:596–602.
333. Shahidi NT, Diamond LK: Testosterone-induced remission in aplastic anemia of both acquired and congenital types. Further observations in 24 cases. N Engl J Med 1961; 264:953–967.
334. Sanchez-Medal L, Gomez-Leal A, Duarte L, et al: Anabolic androgenic steroids in the treatment of acquired aplastic anemia. Blood 1969; 34:283–295.
335. Camitta BM, Thomas D, Nathan DG, et al: A prospective study of androgens and bone marrow transplantation for treatment of severe aplastic anemia. Blood 1979; 53:504–514.
336. Bacigalupo A, Chaple M, Hows J, et al: Treatment of aplastic anemia (AA) with antilymphocyte globulin (ALG) and methylprednisolone (MPred) with or without androgens: A randomized trial from the EBMT SAA working party. Br J Haematol 1993; 83:145–151.
337. Gardner FH, Juneja HS: Androstane therapy to treat aplastic anaemia in adults: An uncontrolled pilot study. Br J Haematol 1987; 65:295–300.
338. Najean Y, Haguenauer O: Long-term (5 to 20 years) evolution of nongrafted aplastic anemia. Blood 1990; 76:2222–2228.
339. Azen EA, Shahidi NT: Androgen dependency in acquired aplastic anemia. Am J Med 1977; 63:320–324.
340. Yoshida Y, Yamagishi M, Uchino H: Problems in androgen treatment in aplastic anemia with reference to androgen dependency and acquisition of refractoriness. Acta Haematol Jpn 1981; 44:1360–1372.
341. Urabe A, Takaku F, Akatsuka J, et al: Immunosuppression or androgen therapy for aplastic anemia: A cooperative study. Jpn J Clin Hematol 1984; 25:554–560.
342. Israngkura P, Hathirat P, Ratanabanangkoon K, et al: The prognosis of acquired aplastic anemia in Thai children. J Med Assoc Thail 1976; 59:479–489.
343. Pizzuto J, Conte G, Sinco A, et al: Use of androgens in acquired aplastic anaemia. Relation of response to aetiology and severity. Acta Haematol 1980; 64:18–24.
344. Hirota Y: Effects of androstanes on aplastic anemia—A prospective study. Acta Haematol Jpn 1981; 44:1341–1359.
345. Turani H, Levi J, Zevin D, et al: Hepatic lesions in patients on anabolic androgenic therapy. Isr J Med Sci 1983; 19:332–337.
346. Bourliere B, Najean Y: Influence of long-term androgen therapy on growth: An analysis of 18 cases of aplastic anemia in children. Pediatr Forum 1987; 141:718–719.
347. Ammus SS: The role of androgens in the treatment of hematologic disorders. Adv Intern Med 1989; 34:191–208.
348. Besa EC: Hematologic effects of androgens revisited: An alternative therapy in various hematologic conditions. Semin Hematol 1994; 31:134–145.
349. Selleri C, Catalano L, De Rosa G, et al: Danazol: In vitro effects on human hemopoiesis and in vivo activity in hypoplastic and myelodysplastic disorders. Eur J Haematol 1991; 47:197–203.
350. Udupa KB, Reissmann KR: Stimulation of granulopoiesis by androgens without concomitant increase in the serum level of colony stimulating factor. Exp Hematol 1975; 3:26–31.
351. Dalal M, Kim S, Voskuhl RR: Testosterone therapy ameliorates experimental autoimmune encephalomyelitis and induces a T helper 2 bias in the autoantigen-specific T lymphocyte response. J Immunol 1997; 159:3–6.
352. Kumar M, Alter BP: Hematopoietic growth factors for the treatment of aplastic anemia. Curr Opin Hematol 1998; 5:226–234.
353. Devetten MP, Young NS: Hematopoietic growth factors in the pathophysiology and treatment of aplastic anemia. In Hoelzer D, Ganser A (eds): Cytokines in the Treatment of Hematopoietic Failure. New York, Marcel Dekker, 1998.
354. Vadhan-Raj S, Buescher S, Broxmeyer HE, et al: Stimulation of myelopoiesis in patients with aplastic anemia by recombinant human granulocyte-macrophage colony-stimulating factor. N Engl J Med 1988; 319:1628–1634.
355. Antin JH, Smith BR, Holmes W, et al: Phase I/II study of recombinant human granulocyte-macrophage colony–stimulating factor in aplastic anemia and myelodysplastic syndrome. Blood 1988; 72:705–713.
356. Champlin RE, Nimer SD, Ireland P, et al: Treat-

ment of refractory aplastic anemia with recombinant human granulocyte-macrophage-colony–stimulating factor. Blood 1989; 73:694–699.
357. Kojima S, Matsuyama T: Stimulation of granulopoiesis by high-dose recombinant human granulocyte colony–stimulating factor in children with aplastic anemia and very severe neutropenia. Blood 1994; 83:1474–1478.
358. Sonoda Y, Ohno Y, Fujii H, et al: Multilineage response in aplastic anemia patients following long-term administration of filgrastim (recombinant human granulocyte colony stimulating factor). Stem Cells 1993; 11:543–554.
359. Higuchi T, Shimizu T, Okada S, et al: Delayed granulocyte response to G-CSF in aplastic anemia. Am J Hematol 1994; 46:164–165.
360. Imashuku S, Hibi S, Mitsui T, et al: A review of 125 cases to determine the risk of myelodysplasia and leukemia in pediatric neutropenic patients after treatment with recombinant human granulocyte colony–stimulating factor. Blood 1996; 84:2380–2381.
361. Ohsaka A, Sugahara Y, Imai Y, et al: Evolution of severe aplastic anemia to myelodysplasia with monosomy 7 following granulocyte colony–stimulating factor; erythropoietin and high-dose methylprednisolone combination therapy. Intern Med 1995; 34:892–895.
362. Yamazaki E, Kanamori H, Taguchi J, et al: The evidence of clonal evolution with monosomy 7 in aplastic anemia following granulocyte colony–stimulating factor using the polymerase chain reaction. Blood Cells Mol Dis 1997; 23:213–218.
363. Kaito K, Kobayashi M, Katayama T, et al: Long-term administration of G-CSF for aplastic anaemia is closely related to the early evolution of monosomy 7 MDS in adults. Br J Haematol 1998; 103:297–303.
364. Marsh JCW, Socié G, Schrezenmeier H, et al: Haemopoietic growth factors in aplastic anaemia: A cautionary note. Lancet 1994; 344:172–173.
365. Walsh CE, Liu JM, Anderson SM, et al: A trial of recombinant human interleukin-1 in patients with severe, refractory aplastic anemia. Br J Haematol 1991; 80:106–110.
366. Nemunaitis J, Ross M, Meisenberg B, et al: Phase I study of recombinant human interleukin-1β (rhIL-1β) in patients with bone marrow failure. Bone Marrow Transplant 1994; 14:583–588.
367. Falk S, Seipelt G, Ganser A, et al: Bone marrow findings after treatment with recombinant human interleukin-3. Am J Clin Pathol 1991; 95:355–362.
368. Ganser A, Lindemann A, Seipelt G, et al: Effects of recombinant human interleukin-3 in aplastic anemia. Blood 1990; 76:1287–1292.
369. Nimer SD, Paquette RL, Ireland P, et al: A phase I/II study of interleukin-3 in patients with aplastic anemia and myelodysplasia. Exp Hematol 1994; 22:875–880.
370. Bargetzi MJ, Gluckman E, Tichelli A, et al: Recombinant human interleukin-3 in refractory severe aplastic anaemia: a phase I/II trial. Br J Haematol 1995; 91:306–312.
371. Schrezenmeier H, Marsh JCW, Stromeyer P, et al: A phase I/II trial of recombinant human interleukin-6 in patients with aplastic anaemia. Br J Haematol 1995; 90:283–292.
372. Rodriguez JN, Martino ML, Dieguez JC, Prados D: Sustained trilineage response to erythropoietin therapy in a case of aplastic anaemia (letter). J Intern Med 1997; 242:437–439.
373. Stebler C, Tichelli A, Dazzi H, et al: High-dose recombinant human erythropoietin for treatment of anemia in myelodysplastic syndromes and paroxysmal nocturnal hemoglobinuria: A pilot study. Exp Hematol 1990; 18:1204–1208.
374. Bernell P: Aplastic anemia with a trilineage response to erythropoietin therapy. J Intern Med 1996; 239:79–81.
375. Takahashi M, Aoki A, Mito M, et al: Combination therapy with rhGM-CSF and rhEpo for two patients with refractory anemia and aplastic anemia. Hematol Pathol 1993; 7:153–158.
376. Nawata J, Toyoda Y, Nisihira H, et al: Haematological improvement by long-term administration of recombinant human granulocyte-colony stimulating factor and recombinant human erythropoietin in a patient with severe aplastic anaemia. Eur J Pediatr 1994; 153:325–327.
377. Kurzrock R, Talpaz M, Gutterman JU: Very low doses of GM-CSF administered alone or with erythropoietin in aplastic anemia. Am J Med 1992; 93:41–48.
378. Bessho M, Hirashima K, Asano S, et al: Treatment of the anemia of aplastic anemia patients with recombinant human erythropoietin in combination with granulocyte colony–stimulating factor: A multicenter randomized controlled study. Eur J Haematol 1997; 58:265–272.
379. Kurzrock R, Paquette R, Gratwohl A, et al: Use of stem cell factor (Stemgen, SCF) and filgrastimm (GCSF) in aplastic anemia (AA) patients who have failed ATG/ALG therapy (abstract). Blood 1997; 90(suppl 1):173a.
380. Doney K, Storb R, Applebaum FR, et al: Recombinant granulocyte-macrophage colony stimulating factor followed by immunosuppressive therapy for aplastic anaemia. Br J Haematol 1993; 85:182–184.
381. Gordon-Smith EC, Yandle A, Milne A, et al: Randomized placebo-controlled study of RH-GM-CSF following ALG in the treatment of aplastic anaemia (abstract). Bone Marrow Transplant 1991; 7(suppl 2):78–80.
382. Bertrand Y, Amri F, Capdeville R, et al: Successful treatment of two cases of severe aplastic anemia with granulocyte-colony stimulating factor and cyclosporin A. Br J Haematol 1991; 79:648–652.
383. Weide R, Lyttelton M, Samson D, et al: Sustained trilineage response in a patient with ALG-resistant severe aplastic anaemia after treatment with G-CSF, erythropoietin and cyclosporin A: Association of recovery with marked elevation of serum alkaline phosphatase. Br J Haematol 1993; 85:608–610.

384. Raghavachar A, Kolbe K, Höffken K, et al: A randomized trial of standard immunosuppression versus cyclosporine and filgastrim in severe aplastic anemia (abstract). Blood 1997; 90(suppl 1):439a.
385. Shao Z, Chu Y, Zhang Y, et al: Treatment of severe aplastic anemia with an immunosuppressive agent plus recombinant human granulocyte-macrophage colony–stimulating factor and erythropoietin. Am J Hematol 1998; 59:185–191.
386. Gluckman E, Rokicka-Milewska R, Gordon-Smith EC, et al: Results of a randomized study of glycosylated rHuG-CSF Lenogastrim in severe aplastic anemia (abstract). Blood 1998; 92(suppl 1):376a.
387. Young NS: Supportive treatment of aplastic anemia. In Young NS, Alter BP (eds): Aplastic Anemia, Acquired and Inherited. Philadelphia, WB Saunders, 1994, pp. 201–215.
388. Sandler SG: Alloimmune refractoriness to platelet transfusions. Curr Opin Hematol 1998; 4:470–473.
389. Menitove JE: Platelet transfusion for alloimmunized patients. Clin Oncol 1983; 2:587–609.
390. Sintnicolaas K, Vriesendorf HM, Sizoo W, et al: Delayed alloimmunisation by random single donor platelet transfusions. A randomised study to compare single donor and multiple donor platelet transfusions in cancer patients with severe thrombocytopenia. Lancet 1981; 1:750–753.
391. The Trial to Reduce Alloimmunization to Platelets Study Group: Leukocyte reduction and ultraviolet B irradiation of platelets to prevent alloimmunization and refractoriness to platelet transfusions. N Engl J Med 1997; 337:1861–1869.
392. Killick SB, Win N, Marsh JC, et al: Pilot study of HLA alloimmunization after transfusion with pre-storage leucodepleted blood products in aplastic anaemia. Br J Haematol 1997; 97:677–684.
393. Klingemann HG, Self S, Banaji M, et al: Refractoriness to random donor platelet transfusions in patients with aplastic anaemia: A multivariate analysis of data from 264 cases. Br J Haematol 1987; 66:115–121.
394. Baer MR, Bloomfield CD: Controversies in transfusion medicine. Prophylactic platelet transfusion therapy: Pro. Transfusion 1992; 32:337–380.
395. Patten E: Controversies in transfusion medicine. Prophylactic platelet transfusion revisited after 25 years: Con. Transfusion 1992; 32:381–385.
396. Platelet transfusion therapy. JAMA 1987; 257:1775–1780.
397. Heckman K, Weiner GJ, Strauss RG, et al: Randomized evaluation of the optimal platelet count for prophylactic platelet transfusions in patients undergoing induction therapy for acute leukemia (abstract). Blood 1993; 82(suppl 1):192a.
398. Gaydos LA, Freireich EJ, Mantel N: The quantitative relation between platelet count and hemorrhage in patients with acute leukemia. N Engl J Med 1962; 266:905–909.
399. Kelton JG, Ali AM: Platelet transfusions—a critical appraisal. Clin Oncol 1983; 2:549–585.
400. Shulkin DJ, Fox KR, Stadtmauer EA: Guidelines for prophylactic platelet transfusions: Need for a concurrent outcomes management system. Qual Rev Bull 1992; 12:477–479.
401. Gmür J, Burger J, Schanz U, et al: Safety of stringent prophylactic platelet transfusion policy for patients with acute leukaemia. Lancet 1991; 338:1223–1226.
402. Rebulla P, Finazzi G, Marangoni F, et al: The threshold for prophylactic platelet transfusions in adults with acute myeloid leukemia. N Engl J Med 1997; 337:1870–1875.
403. Bishop JF, Schiffer CA, Aisner J, et al: Surgery in acute leukemia: A review of 167 operations in thrombocytopenic patients. Am J Hematol 1987; 26:147–155.
404. Blumberg N, Peck K, Ross K, et al: Immune response to chronic red blood cell transfusion. Vox Sang 1983; 44:212–217.
405. Keidan AJ, Tsatalas C, Cohen J, et al: Infective complications of aplastic anaemia. Br J Haematol 1986; 63:503–508.
406. Bodey GP, Buckley M, Sathe YS, et al: Quantitative relationships between circulating leukocytes and infection in patients with acute leukemia. Ann Intern Med 1966; 64:328–340.
407. van der Meer JWM, Alleman M, Boekhout M: Infectious episodes in severely granulocytopenic patients. Infection 1979; 7:171–175.
408. Pizzo PA: Fever in immunocompromised patients. N Engl J Med 1999; 341:893–900.
409. Klastersky J, Zinner SH, Calandra T, et al: EORTC: Empiric antimicrobial therapy for febrile granulocytopenic cancer patients: Lessons from four EORTC trials. Eur J Cancer Clin Oncol 1988; 24:S35–S45.
410. Dearden C, Foukaneli T, Lee P, et al: The incidence and significance of fevers during treatment with antithymocyte globulin for aplastic anemia. Br J Haematol 1998; 103:846–848.
411. Weinberger M, Elatta I, Marshall D, et al: Patterns of infection in patients with aplastic anemia: The emergence of *Aspergillus* as a major cause of death. Medicine (Baltimore) 1992; 71:24–43.
412. Rahemtulla A, Durrant STS, Coonar HS, et al: Zygomycosis in aplastic anaemia: Response to a combined regimen of amphotericin B and antilymphocyte globulin. Eur J Haematol 1988; 40:315–317.
413. Menichetti F, Del Favero A, Martino P, et al: Itraconazole oral solution as prophylaxis for fungal infections in neutropenic patients with hematologic malignancies: A randomized, placebo-controlled, double-blind, multicenter trial. GIMEMA Infection Program. Gruppo Italiano Malattie Ematologiche dell' Adulto. Clin Infect Dis 1999; 28:250–255.
414. Kelsey SM, Goldman JM, McCann S, et al: Liposomal amphotericin (AmBisome) in the prophylaxis of fungal infections in neutropenic patients: A randomised, double-blind, placebo-controlled study. Bone Marrow Transplant 1999; 23:163–168.
415. Menitove JE, Abrams RA: Granulocyte transfu-

sions in neutropenic patients. Crit Rev Oncol Hematol 1987; 7:89–113.
416. Strauss RG: Therapeutic granulocyte transfusions in 1993. Blood 1993; 81:1675–1678.
417. Leitman SF, Oblitas JM, Emmons R, et al: Clinical efficacy of daily G-CSF–recruited granulocyte transfusions in patients with severe neutropenia and life-threatening infections (abstract). Blood 1996; 88(suppl 1):331a.
418. DiMario A, Sica S, Salutari P, et al: Granulocyte colony-stimulating factor–primed leukocyte transfusions in *Candida tropicalis* fungemia in neutropenic patients. Haematologica 1997; 82:362–363.
419. Dietrich M, Gaus W, Vossen J, et al: Protective isolation and antimicrobial decontamination in patients with high susceptibility to infection. A prospective cooperative study of gnotobiotic care in acute leukemia patients. I: Clinical results. Infection 1977; 5:107–114.
420. Nauseef WM, Maki DG: A study of the value of simple protective isolation in patients with granulocytopenia. N Engl J Med 1981; 304:448–453.
421. Cabot RC: Case 13321. Bleeding from the gums. Boston Med Surg J 1927; 197:236–239.
422. Najean Y, Pecking A: Prognostic factors in acquired aplastic anemia. A study of 352 cases. Am J Med 1979; 67:564–571.
423. Frisch B, Lewis SM: The bone marrow in aplastic anaemia: Diagnostic and prognostic features. J Clin Pathol 1974; 27:231–241.
424. Nakao S, Yamaguchi M, Takamatsu H, et al: Relative erythroid hyperplasia in the bone marrow at diagnosis of aplastic anemia: A predictive marker for a favourable response to cyclosporine therapy. Br J Haematol 1996; 92:318–323.
425. Keisu M, Heit W, Lambertenghi-Deliliers G, et al: Transient pancytopenia. A report from the International Agranulocytosis and Aplastic Study. Blut 1990; 61:240–244.
426. Khatib Z, Wilimas J, Wang W: Outcome of moderate aplastic anemia in children. Am J Pediatr Hematol Oncol 1994; 16:80–85.
427. de Planque MM, Kluin-Nelemans HC, van Krieken HJM, et al: Evolution of acquired severe aplastic anaemia to myelodysplasia and subsequent leukaemia in adults. Br J Haematol 1988; 70:55–62.
428. Tichelli A, Gratwohl A, Würsch A, et al: Secondary leukemia after severe aplastic anemia. Blut 1988; 56:79–81.
429. Marsh JC, Geary CG: Annotation—Is aplastic anaemia a pre-leukaemic disorder? Br J Haematol 1991; 77:447–442.
430. Orlandi E, Alessandrino EP, Caldera D, et al: Adult leukemia developing after aplastic anemia: Report of 8 cases. Acta Haematol 1988; 79:174–177.
431. de Planque MM, Bacigalupo A, Würsch A, et al: Long-term follow-up of severe aplastic anaemia patients treated with antithymocyte globulin. Br J Haematol 1989; 73:121–126.
432. Socié G, Rosenfeld S, Frickhofen N, et al: Late clonal disease of treated aplastic anemia. Semin Hematol 2000; 37:91–101.
433. Dunn DE, Tanawattanacharoen P, Boccuni P, et al: Paroxysmal nocturnal hemoglobinuria cells in patients with bone marrow failure syndromes. Ann Intern Med 1999; 131:401–408.
434. Narayanan MN, Geary CG, Freemont AJ, et al: Long-term follow-up of aplastic anaemia. Br J Haematol 1994; 86:837–843.
435. Cartwright RA, McKinney PA, Williams L, et al: Aplastic anaemic incidence in parts of the United Kingdom in 1985. Leuk Res 1988; 12:459–463.
436. Clausen N: A population study of severe aplastic anemia in children: Incidence, etiology and course. Acta Paediatr Scand 1986; 75:58–63.
437. The International Agranulocytosis and Aplastic Anemia Study: Risks of agranulocytosis and aplastic anemia: A first report of their relation to drug use with special reference to analgesics. JAMA 1986; 256:1749–1788.
438. Aggio MC, Alvarez RV, Bartomioli MA, et al: Incidence and etiology of aplastic anemia in a defined population of Argentina (1966–1977). Medicina (B Aires) 1988; 48:231–233.
439. Mary JY, Baumelou E, Guiguet M: Epidemiology of aplastic anemia in France: A prospective multicenter study. Blood 1990; 75:1646–1653.
440. Clausen N, Kreuger A, Salmi T, et al: Severe aplastic anemia in the Nordic countries: A population based study of incidence, presentation, course, and outcome. Arch Dis Child 1996; 74:319–322.
441. Tweddle DA, Reid MM: Aplastic anaemia in the Northern Region of England (letter). Acta Paediatr 1996; 85:1388–1389.
442. Rawson NS, Harding SR, Malcolm E, et al: Hospitalization for aplastic anemia and agranulocytosis in Saskatchewan: Incidence and associations with antecedent prescription drug use. J Clin Epidemiol 1988; 51:1343–1355.
443. Gluckman E, Socié G, Devergie A, et al: Bone marrow transplantation in 107 patients with severe aplastic anemia using cyclophosphamide and thoraco-abdominal irradiation for conditioning: Long-term follow-up. Blood 1991; 78:2451–2455.
444. Champlin RE, Ho WG, Nimer SD, et al: Bone marrow transplantation for severe aplastic anemia. Transplantation 1990; 49:720–724.
445. Storb R, Leisenring W, Anasetti C, et al: Long-term follow-up of allogeneic marrow transplants in patients with aplastic anemia conditioned by cyclophosphamide combined with antithymocyte globulin (letter). Blood 1997; 89:3890–3891.
446. Lynch RE, Williams DM, Reading JC, et al: The prognosis in aplastic anemia. Blood 1975; 45:517–528.
447. Bielory L, Gascon P, Lawley TJ, et al: Human serum sickness: A prospective analysis of 35 patients treated with equine anti-thymocyte globulin for bone marrow failure. Medicine (Baltimore) 1988; 67:40–57.

2

Fanconi's Anemia

Johnson M. Liu, M.D.

Fanconi's anemia (FA), the best-defined inherited bone marrow failure disorder, was first described by the Swiss pediatrician Guido Fanconi in three brothers with a syndrome of aplastic anemia and congenital physical anomalies.[1] In addition to the chief criteria of pancytopenia, hyperpigmentation, malformation of the skeleton, small stature, and hypogonadism noted by Fanconi, diverse malformations of the eye, ear, genitourinary and gastrointestinal tracts, and cardiopulmonary and central nervous systems can occur. FA is notoriously heterogeneous in the degree and number of clinical manifestations,[2] and patients presenting solely with either congenital malformations or hematologic abnormalities may either be misdiagnosed or go unrecognized entirely. Fanconi himself was sufficiently puzzled by the number and variability of the manifestations of the disease that as late as 1967 he questioned the autosomal recessive inheritance pattern.[3]

Since the original clinical description, FA has drawn from the scientific and medical community an attention that is disproportionate to the small number of patients. A breakthrough in the conceptualization of the FA phenotype was the recognition that patients' cells and chromosomes are sensitive to certain chromosome-damaging (clastogenic) agents such as diepoxybutane (DEB) or mitomycin C (MMC). In the last decade, this disease-defining property was successfully used, first to segregate FA into different complementation groups and then to identify the FA genes in (now) three such groups. From a clinical perspective, FA was the first disease to be treated by umbilical cord blood stem cell transplantation and has ushered in new approaches to cell and gene therapy, which are described in detail below.

The modern diagnosis of FA no longer rests upon the constellation of abnormalities described by Fanconi but depends instead upon finding chromosomal breakage after incubation of the patient's cells with DEB or MMC[4,5] (Fig. 2–1). This strict laboratory diagnosis has led to the identification of affected individuals who may be heterogeneous in terms of their clinical features. A particularly troublesome aspect of diagnosis is the categorization of certain patients with the physical and hematologic criteria of FA but who have negative chromosome breakage studies. Whether these cases, or patients with idiopathic "acquired" aplastic anemia, will eventually be found to have mutations in FA or FA-like genes is unknown.

FA usually presents with aplastic anemia, clini-

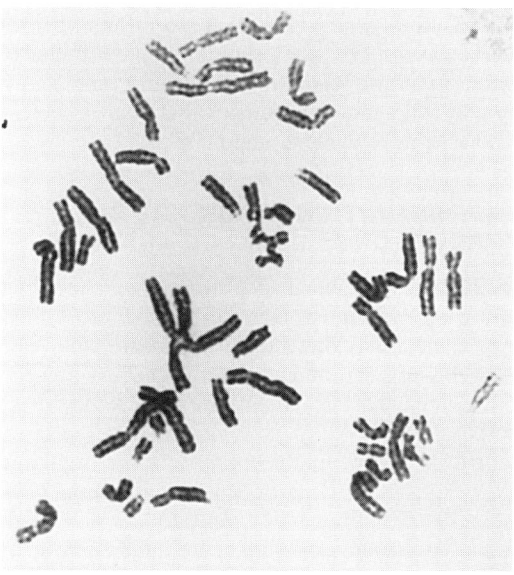

Figure 2–1 Mitomycin C–induced chromosome breaks in a patient with Fanconi's anemia.(Courtesy of Privatdozent Dr. Martin Digweed, Institut für Humangenetik, Humboldt-Universität zu Berlin.)

cally indistinguishable from the acquired form of the disease. Recent data from the International Fanconi Anemia Registry (IFAR) indicate that almost all FA patients will eventually develop hematologic abnormalities (thrombocytopenia or pancytopenia).[6] Nosologically, FA is thus linked with acquired aplastic anemia (although the hematologic manifestations are only a part of the FA syndrome). Similarities between the genetic disorder, FA, and acquired aplastic anemia may reflect common mechanistic pathways; initial findings regarding the function of FA genes suggest that this may indeed be true.

FA patients are susceptible to both hematologic and solid organ malignancy.[7] FA is usually grouped with the inherited cancer-prone syndromes such as ataxia telangiectasia, Bloom's syndrome, and xeroderma pigmentosum (XP). For some of these disorders, the genetic defect has been identified and correlated with a defect in DNA repair. For others, such as FA, the relationship to DNA repair is inferential. Although three FA genes have now been identified, the biochemical function of the encoded proteins remains elusive. Despite increasing experimental sophistication, controversy exists over the potential interaction between the different FA gene products and even their subcellular localization. At the heart of this debate is the novelty of the genes cloned thus far. It may be significant that FA genes seem not to have lower eukaryotic homologues. Possibly, FA genes have evolved relatively recently, and their function may be redundant with that of other genes. Despite these difficulties, research on the FA genes should eventually clarify their role in the regulation of chromosome stability and cell death mechanisms that bear on hematopoiesis, development, and neoplasia.

CASE DEFINITION: DIAGNOSIS BY CHROMOSOME BREAKAGE ANALYSIS

FA chromosome breakage, either spontaneous or following exposure to DNA alkylating (cross-linking) agents, was first recognized nearly 40 years after the original clinical description.[8] At present, cytogenetic analysis remains the basis for the diagnosis of FA. Testing is typically performed by scoring chromosome preparations for breakage after exposure to DEB or MMC[4, 5] (see Fig. 2–1). At a biochemical level, monoadducts and diadducts (interstrand cross-links) are induced in DNA by bifunctional cross-linking agents such as DEB, MMC, nitrogen mustard, cyclophosphamide, cisplatin, or activated psoralens. Interstrand cross-links are thought to block DNA replication and RNA transcription, with potent effects on cell survival and function. For FA, specific cellular defects following exposure to bifunctional cross-linking agents such as MMC include the induction of chromosomal aberrations (breaks and rearrangements)[9], delayed transit and arrest in the G_2 phase of the cell cycle,[10] with a consequent decrease in the numbers of cells synthesizing DNA[11], and cell death.[12] While chromosome breakage is most commonly performed to diagnose FA, flow cytometric assessment of G_2 phase arrest has also been used.[13]

A confounding factor in the diagnosis of FA by chromosome breakage analysis is "reverse mosaicism."[14–16] In the course of testing patients' lymphocytes for sensitivity to MMC, it was noted that approximately 25% of FA patients had evidence of spontaneously occurring mosaicism as manifested by the presence of two subpopulations of lymphocytes, one hypersensitive to MMC (as expected for FA) and a second behaving normally in response to this agent. In the initial report of eight FA patients with evidence of mosaicism, three were compound heterozygotes for a pathogenic FA gene, and the molecular mechanism of the mosaicism was attributed to recombination or gene conversion events.[15] Even FA patients initially diagnosed as a result of MMC breakage analysis could develop near-complete reversion in blood cells, raising the possibility that chromosome breakage tests would be interpreted as negative. In such circumstances, breakage analysis performed in nonhematopoietic tissues (presumably not subject to selective pressure for reversion) such as skin fibroblasts should allow for the correct diagnosis to be made.[16]

CLINICAL FEATURES

Diagnosis: Heterogeneity of Presentation

The classic features of FA are well-known to pediatric hematologists.[17] The diagnosis is suggested when a child presents with hyper- or hypopigmented skin lesions; short stature (poor growth); anomalies of the upper limb or thumb; male hypogonadism; microcephaly; characteristic facial features, including a broadened nasal base, epicanthal folds, and micrognathia; and structural renal abnormalities. When this constellation of physical anomalies is accompanied by bone marrow failure (which often triggers the initial medical evaluation), confirmation of the diagnosis can then be made by standard DEB or MMC chromosome breakage analysis. The mean age at diagnosis is usually 8 or 9 years.

With the advent of the chromosome breakage

test, however, has come increasing recognition of the heterogeneity of the clinical presentation of FA. Based solely on definition by the DEB test, nearly 40% of the first 200 patients analyzed in the IFAR were reported to be free of major physical anomalies.[4] Such normal-appearing patients had previously been identified by noting their familial presentation with hypoplastic or aplastic anemia: two such families were first described by Estren and Dameshek in 1947.[18] The diagnosis of FA was later confirmed by chromosome breakage analysis in a cousin of one of the original probands.[19] These cases of FA homozygotes with normal appearances may go unrecognized unless there is a high index of suspicion for familial disease.[20]

Another challenge is the diagnosis of FA in older patients. Although the mean age of diagnosis is in the first decade of life, FA has been described recently in a 56-year-old woman.[21] Whether older patients survive because of genetic heterogeneity—FA genes that predispose to a less severe phenotype—is unknown. Also unclear is the contribution of reverse mosaicism in these individuals, as the initial report described relatively mild disease in six of eight such patients.[15] Confirmation of these data with longer follow-up may have both diagnostic and therapeutic implications.

Symptoms, Signs, and Hematologic Indices: Severity Index

The symptoms and signs of FA typically relate to the hematologic presentation of cytopenias from marrow failure. Often thrombocytopenia or leukopenia is noted before full pancytopenia; furthermore, the pancytopenia typically worsens with time. Almost all FA patients will develop hematologic abnormalities in their lifetime.[6] Erythropoiesis is usually macrocytic, as was recognized by Fanconi when he initially described the anemia as *perniziösartige* or "pernicious-like."[1] Classically, the bone marrow is hypocellular and fatty, indistinguishable from that seen in acquired aplastic anemia. Microscopic examination of the marrow may show dyserythropoiesis and dysplasia. Some patients may develop or even present with a morphologically defined myelodysplastic syndrome (MDS) or frank acute myeloid leukemia (AML).[22]

There have been attempts to grade the severity of FA.[23] One system is based upon variables that discriminate for FA[4]: the score is calculated by adding 1 point each for growth retardation, birthmarks, kidney and urinary tract abnormalities, micro-ophthalmia, low platelet count, or thumb and radial abnormalities, and by subtracting 1 point each for learning disabilities and other skeletal abnormalities (these do not discriminate for FA).

The score thus ranges from -2 to $+6$; a score below 3 is defined as a mild phenotype. Such scoring systems would not be expected to be useful predictors of bone marrow failure or cancer susceptibility.

Cancer

The risk of developing MDS and AML[24] may be higher than previously thought: progression to AML occurs in at least 10% to 15% of cases, with increasing risk with age. Less commonly recognized is the probability of developing MDS, approximately 5%, which appears also to correlate with a poor prognosis for FA patients. Clonal karyotypic abnormalities, identical to those seen in non-FA MDS and secondary AML, are frequently found in FA patients, whether or not they meet marrow morphologic criteria for a defined MDS. The prognostic significance of these clonal chromosomal abnormalities in FA patients is not entirely clear, however, since cytogenetic changes can fluctuate over time in both number and variety.[25] Clonal hematopoiesis in this setting may simply reflect a reduced stem cell pool.

With better supportive care and the longer survival of FA patients, solid organ malignancies have been noted, with at least 5% of patients in a large retrospective series developing liver tumors.[7] In addition to these (presumed) de novo tumors, a subset of long-term survivors of stem cell transplantation will develop secondary malignancies, particularly involving the head and neck (see below). These clinical data may reflect an intrinsic propensity of mutant FA cells to undergo biologic transformation.[26]

GENETIC ANALYSIS OF FANCONI'S ANEMIA

Formal Genetics and Ethnic Variation

In the 1970s, FA was proved by formal genetic studies to be an autosomal recessive disorder.[27] FA is rare, occurring in approximately five per million births. All races and ethnic groups can suffer from FA. As the FA genes have been identified, predominant mutations have been associated with particular ethnic groups as a result of a founder effect. Because of these strong associations, the carrier frequency for certain mutations can be remarkably high in selected populations (see below), and for the general population has been estimated at approximately 1 in 300 in the United States, Europe, and Japan.

As of this writing, the three most common FA genes in the Western Hemisphere have been identified. Genotype-phenotype studies have only recently been possible, however, and except for *FANCC* (see below), it is not yet clear whether specific FA gene mutants are associated with a particular clinical outcome. Environmental influences and the genetic background of the FA patient are two other considerations that have not yet been systematically studied for their ability to influence the FA phenotype. As an example, the pathophysiology of bone marrow failure may involve sensitivity to apoptosis triggered by exogenous or endogenous stimuli, and the degree of sensitivity of each patient may be partially determined by that individual's genetic background.

Complementation Studies and *FANCC*

The variability of the clinical appearance in FA has long suggested genetic heterogeneity, since mutations in different genes could lead to alternative phenotypes. Complementation (correction of the increased sensitivity of FA cells to the cytotoxic action of DNA cross-linking agents) has been used to define this genetic heterogeneity. Many studies have been based on hybrid lymphoblast cell lines from patients. Selectable markers were introduced into FA cells and used to isolate hybrids after fusion. Complementation of the FA phenotype was assessed by analysis of spontaneous and MMC-induced chromosomal breakage and of growth inhibition by MMC. The initial studies led to the identification of two complementation groups, A and non-A.[28] Subsequent analysis of the non-A cell lines led to the description of four other complementation groups: B, C, D,[29] and E.[30] Currently, there is evidence for at least eight FA genes (FA-A through FA-H),[31] with more complementation groups likely to be found as the number of cell lines examined increases.

Several groups have attempted to clone the FA genes by exploiting the increased sensitivity of FA cells to DNA cross-linking agents. As first successfully applied to FA-C, complementary DNA (cDNA) libraries in episomal vectors were used to isolate a series of cDNAs that complement the cellular defects of FA-C cells.[32] The identity of these as true FA-C cDNAs was confirmed by showing first, that the defects in FA-A, FA-B, or FA-D cells were not complemented, and second, by detecting a mutation in this gene in the cell line used for the cloning. The cDNAs encode a novel protein, termed FANCC, of approximately 63 kD (Fig. 2–2).

Characteristics of *FANCC* Gene

FANCC has been mapped to 9q22.3 by in situ hybridization[29] (see Fig. 2–2). Portions of the gene have been cloned and preliminary studies suggest that *FANCC* is greater than 100 kb in length. The gene encodes alternatively processed transcripts, with differing 5′ and 3′ untranslated regions (UTRs), resulting in a 14-exon coding sequence[33] and a 558–amino acid polypeptide. FANCC shows no strong homologies to proteins of known func-

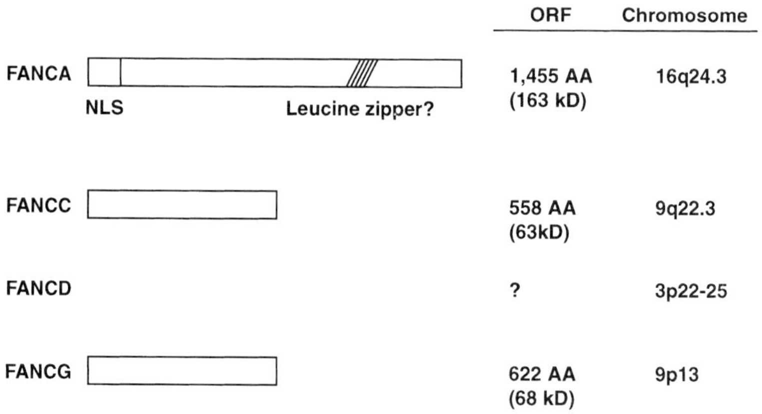

	ORF	Chromosome
FANCA (NLS, Leucine zipper?)	1,455 AA (163 kD)	16q24.3
FANCC	558 AA (63 kD)	9q22.3
FANCD	?	3p22-25
FANCG	622 AA (68 kD)	9p13

Figure 2–2 The FA genes and gene products. The newly identified *FANCA* gene encodes a 1455–amino acid polypeptide and is localized to chromosome 16q24.3. The FANCA protein has a putative nuclear localization signal (NLS) and a leucine zipper motif. *FANCC* encodes a 558–amino acid polypeptide with a molecular mass of 63 kD. Sequence analysis has revealed no consensus motifs that would be informative of the protein's function. *FANCC* maps to chromosome 9q22.3 and encodes a set of RNAs that share the same coding region but differ at both 5′ and 3′ untranslated regions. The *FANCD* gene has been mapped to 3p22–25. *FANCG* encodes a 622–amino acid polypeptide that is identical to XRCC-9.

tion but has consensus binding sites for serine and threonine phosphorylation and for binding to a molecular chaperone protein. The GRP94 chaperone interacts with FANCC in vitro and in vivo and appears to regulate the intracellular stability of FANCC.[34] Adult human and mouse tissues ubiquitously express FANCC at a low level, without any known induction patterns. In the developing mouse, however, murine Fancc messenger (mRNA) can be detected at high levels in undifferentiated mesenchyme and developing bones, as well as in lung, kidney, and gut mesenchyme, consistent with the location of congenital defects in FA patients.[35]

FANCC Mutations

The initial report on the cloning of the *FANCC* cDNAs showed that the one transcript present in the patient had a C-T transition that led to a leucine at position 554 being mutated to proline (L554P),[32] deleterious because of the changes in secondary structure of the protein. A cDNA in which the mutation was introduced by site-directed mutagenesis produced an inactive protein, suggesting that the C-terminus of the protein is important for its activity.[36] In addition, overexpression of the mutant L554P allele in a wild-type cellular background has been shown to induce the FA cellular phenotype, suggesting that the mutant protein might compete for proteins that bind to wild-type FANCC.[37] Other mutations have now been detected in FA-C patients. A splice mutation in intron 4 (IVS4+4 A→T) is the predominant genetic alteration in all FA patients of Ashkenazi Jewish origin.[38] The carrier frequency of this mutant allele in a selected Jewish population has been determined to be 1.1%.[39] Other *FANCC* mutations include 322delG, Q13X, and R185X.[40, 41]

Genotype-Phenotype Analysis for FANCC

FA-C patients can be divided into three subgroups based on results of genotype-phenotype analysis: patients with the intron 4 mutation; those with at least one exon 14 mutation (R548X or L554P); and those with at least one exon 1 mutation (322delG or Q13X) and no known exon 14 mutation.[42] Kaplan-Meier analysis suggested that patients with either an intron 4 or exon 14 mutation suffered from a significantly earlier onset of hematologic abnormalities and poorer survival as compared to exon 1 patients and to the non–FA-C IFAR population. The molecular basis for the milder phenotype of exon 1 patients may relate to the observation that cell lines with the 322delG mutation express a truncated isoform of FANCC, resulting in partial correction of MMC sensitivity,[23] whereas cell lines with the intron 4 mutation lack this isoform.

The Major FA Gene, FANCA

Approximately 65% of FA patients from Europe and North America appear to belong to complementation group A,[43–45] and this major FA mutant gene has recently been identified (see Fig. 2–2). By establishing a panel of families classified as FA-A by complementation analysis, a consortium of European investigators previously had localized *FANCA* to chromosome 16q24.3 by linkage analysis.[46] Employing the expression cloning strategy used to identify *FANCC*, an independent group of investigators isolated a cDNA representing the *FANCA* gene and found that it mapped to the same region of chromosome 16, thus strengthening the candidacy of this cDNA.[47] Mutation analysis of FA-A patients confirmed that the cDNA represented the *FANCA* gene. Concurrently, an international consortium used positional cloning methods and also identified *FANCA* as the disease gene that had been previously linked to chromosome 16q.[48]

FANCA Mutations

In contrast to *FANCC*, for which a few specific mutations account for nearly all cases, mutations in *FANCA* are widely dispersed through the gene and more likely to be unique to each patient. Single-strand conformational polymorphism analysis has been used to screen genomic DNA from a panel of 97 IFAR patients for mutations in the *FANCA* gene.[49] Forty variants were thought to represent pathogenic mutations. Seventeen of these were microdeletions or microinsertions associated with short direct repeats or homonucleotide tracts, a type of mutation that can be generated by a mechanism of slipped-strand mispairing during DNA replication. Two of these deletions (1115-1118del and 3788-3790del) are carried on about 2% and 5% of the FA alleles, respectively.

Microcell-Mediated Chromosome Transfer and FANCD

A third technique to localize FA genes is microcell-mediated chromosome transfer. A fibroblast line from an FA-D patient was used as a recipient for chromosome transfer and was complemented by genetic material from chromosome 3p, implying that *FANCD* maps to this region[50] (see Fig. 2–2).

FANCG

Using homozygosity mapping in a large consanguineous family, a fourth FA gene was mapped to chromosome 9p.[51] Shortly after this report, the *FANCG* gene was identified on the basis of complementation of an FA-G cell line and the presence of pathogenic mutations in four FA-G patients[52] (see Fig. 2–2). *FANCG* was found to be identical to human *XRCC9*, a gene which had initially been cloned based upon its ability to complement a Chinese hamster mutant cell line exhibiting hypersensitivity to MMC and other DNA-damaging agents.[53] *FANCG* was localized to chromosome band 9p13, corresponding to the previously described position.

PATHOPHYSIOLOGY

G_2 Phase Prolongation and Arrest

Cell cycle kinetics in FA have been studied using a specialized flow cytometric technique in that cells are labeled with bromodeoxyuridine, or BrdU (incorporated in place of thymidine) and stained with the DNA dyes Hoechst 33258 and ethidium bromide.[54, 55] These types of analyses determine the fraction of cells that enter but do not exit a particular cell compartment. FA cells accumulate not only in the G_2 phase of the first cell cycle but also within the G_2 compartments of the second and third consecutive cell cycles.[54] The phenomenon of G_2 phase prolongation and arrest seems to be a uniform characteristic of FA cells.[56] At least three other general features have been associated with the FA cellular phenotype: oxygen sensitivity, G_2 chromatid radiosensitivity, and overproduction of the multifunctional cytokine, tumor necrosis factor-α (TNF-α). The possible interrelationships among these phenomena are instructive in understanding the nature of the FA defect.

FA cells show abnormal sensitivity to oxygen; they grow very poorly at ambient (20%) but well at reduced (5%) oxygen tension.[55] Elegant BrdU-Hoechst flow cytometric studies have suggested that this oxygen sensitivity reflects a tendency of FA fibroblasts to accumulate in the G_2 phase of the cell cycle.[55] Interference with DNA topoisomerase function may underlie the mechanism of oxygen-exacerbated G_2 prolongation.[57] Oxygen and its reactive species also can modulate the proliferation of normal diploid fibroblasts, again characteristically inducing G_2 delay.[58]

Oxygen sensitivity in FA may involve either the complex system that controls excessive production of reactive oxygen species or the ability to tolerate oxygen-induced damage. There are data to support an intrinsic hypersensitivity to oxygen,[59] overproduction of reactive oxygen species,[60] as well as a deficient antioxidant defense[61, 62] (Fig. 2–3), but it seems doubtful that these events are causal for the FA defect. Since these topics have been the subject of several recent reviews,[63] they will not be detailed here except for two interesting findings. One of the first experiments linking FA with a defect in the enzymatic antioxidant defense system showed that CuZn superoxide dismutase (SOD), a key enzyme that detoxifies the superoxide anion (O_2^-), could suppress the cytotoxic effect of MMC on an FA primary fibroblast cell line.[64] These results prompted pilot clinical trials of CuZn-SOD that in turn suggested a beneficial effect on chromosomal breakage.[65, 66] However, a comparison of oxygen sensitivity between primary and transformed FA fibroblast lines has indicated that hypersensitivity to oxygen was lost following transformation with the SV40 large T antigen,[67] a result more compatible with a secondary, rather than primary, effect of mutations in FA genes.

Pathways for the bioactivation of MMC suggest another potential interrelationship with oxygen metabolism. Cellular enzymes activate the quinone group of MMC, resulting in the production of inter- and intrastrand DNA-DNA and DNA-protein cross-links.[68, 69] In addition, DNA strand breaks can be induced by redox cycling of MMC through its semiquinone intermediate. Under aerobic conditions, the semiquinone can react with molecular oxygen to form O_2^-, hydrogen peroxide (H_2O_2), and the hydroxyl radical (OH^-). FA lymphocytes pulsed with a low dose of MMC in the G_0 phase of the cell cycle are more sensitive to the subsequent clastogenic effect of O_2 than without MMC pretreatment.[70]

The effect of ionizing irradiation has been studied in two cell types. In contrast to cells from patients with the genetic disorder ataxia telangiectasia, FA fibroblasts and lymphocytes do not appear to be hypersensitive to ionizing irradiation, as measured by chromosome aberration or cell colony survival.[71] On the other hand, FA cells exhibit increased chromatid-type aberrations following irradiation in the G_2 phase of the cell cycle.[72] In this feature, FA shares similarities with other genetic cancer-predisposing disorders such as ataxia telangiectasia, Gardner's syndrome, Bloom's syndrome, and XP. G_2 chromatid radiosensitivity may result from a defect in G_2 repair of DNA damaged by reactive oxygen species.[73]

Several recent reports have documented overproduction of TNF-α from FA lymphoblasts[74] and high levels of TNF-α in patient serum samples.[75] Like oxygen sensitivity, TNF-α overproduction seems to be a general feature of the FA phenotype. Up to an eightfold increase in the cytokine was found in the growth media of FA lymphoblasts.[74] Addition of anti-TNF-α antibodies partially cor-

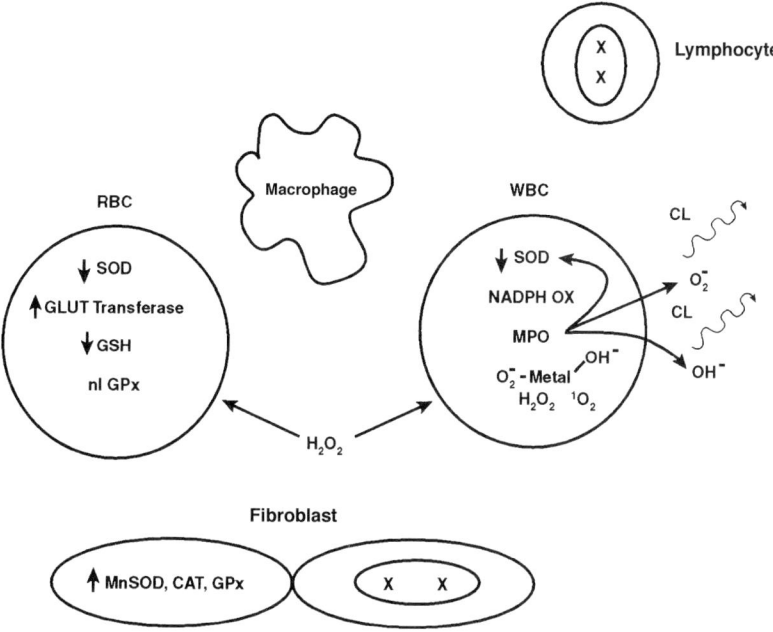

Figure 2–3 Schema of the cellular sources of reactive oxygen species and of the antioxidant defense system responsible for detoxifying these oxygen species. In Fanconi's anemia (FA) erythrocyte (RBC), levels of superoxide dismutase (SOD) and reduced glutathione (GSH) are decreased, whereas glutathione (GLUT) transferase levels are increased. In the FA leukocyte (WBC), levels of SOD are also decreased, and reactive oxygen species, including superoxide (O_2^-), the hydroxyl radical (OH^-), and singlet oxygen ($^1O_2$), may be generated and detected by chemiluminescent assays (CL). In the FA fibroblast, levels of manganese-SOD (MnSOD), catalase (CAT), and glutathione peroxidase (GPx) are paradoxically increased.

rected the FA cellular and chromosomal hypersensitivity to MMC, reminiscent of the experiments with SOD. TNF-α is a multifunctional cytokine and an important mediator of oxidative stress.[76] TNF-α overproduction might be a response to the stress of DNA damage. Eukaryotic cells are known to respond to genotoxic stress by the induction of genes involved in the control of cell proliferation and in the repair of DNA.[77] TNF-α is an example of a pleiotropic gene that is induced in response to DNA damage and, in turn, is able to control both cell growth and apoptosis. Sensitivity to oxygen (enhanced or exacerbated by TNF-α production) might possibly be a reflection of the type of damage that the FA gene product recognizes.

We began this analysis of some of the general features of FA by linking the oxygen hypersensitivity of FA cells to cell cycle disturbances. However, while G_2 phase prolongation and arrest seems to be a general characteristic of the FA phenotype, it need not be specific for oxygen stress. As noted, MMC is also able to cause a G_2 block in FA fibroblasts.[10] Arrest of mammalian cells in the G_2 phase of the cell cycle occurs after x-irradiation.[78] TNF-α acts preferentially during the G_2 phase and can lead to G_2 prolongation.[79] It seems plausible that G_2 delay and arrest may be triggered by DNA lesions, such as double-strand breaks, generated by the action of oxygen,[80] TNF-α, or clastogenic agents.[81] The G_2–M transition is genetically regulated in response to DNA damage and serves as a checkpoint to delay cell cycle progression and allow for the repair of damaged DNA.[82, 83] In FA, G_2 phase prolongation and arrest seems to be a consequence of DNA damage resulting from defective oxygen metabolism or clastogen-induced breakage, rather than a primary cell cycle disturbance. A defective response—recognition or processing—to DNA lesions seems to be a key feature of FA.[84]

Possible Function of Fanconi's Anemia Genes: Response or Repair of DNA Damage

Counteracting the effects of both exogenous and endogenous agents of DNA damage is the function of a complex cellular machinery[85] that includes both enzymes and transcription factors, as well as regulatory checkpoints that govern entry of the cell into cycle.[86] Unraveling these mechanisms has provided important insights into the etiology of genetic instability and malignancy. A key conclusion from these studies is that a defect in DNA repair can be responsible for genetic instability. DNA damage[87] can include lesions such as pyrimidine dimers, single- and double-strand breaks, adducts, deletions, base changes, and cross-links that must be recognized and repaired by specific sets of enzymes involved in either direct reversal of damage or excision of the damaged nucleotide or base. In addition to repair processes, the cell has evolved tolerance mechanisms that bypass DNA repair, sometimes allowing the introduction of errors in daughter DNA. Finally, recombination events can also be involved in repair and tolerance responses.

The hypersensitivity of FA cells to oxygen discussed above may reflect a defect in the repair of oxygen radical–damaged DNA. Reactive oxygen species can damage DNA at the base or sugar as well as form complex products such as cross-links and double-strand breaks. Excision repair of a base damaged by oxygen free radicals is mediated by specific DNA glycosylases[88] (Fig. 2–4, right panel). Specific apurinic/apyrimidinic endonucleases then break the phosphodiester backbone, resulting in a gap; this gap is subsequently filled and sealed by DNA polymerase and ligase. Assays have been developed that can detect the formation of radical-damaged DNA. For example, 8-hydrodeoxyguanosine (8OH-dG) is derived from deoxyguanosine (dG) by the action of radicals.[89] In two FA-A lymphoblast cell lines, two to three times more 8OH-dG was formed than in control cells following incubation with H_2O_2,[90] direct evidence of increased susceptibility to oxidative damage of these FA-A cells. Whether FA can be caused by a defect in an enzyme involved in the repair of oxidatively damaged DNA[88, 91, 92] is unknown.

The sensitivity of FA cells to bifunctional cross-linking agents suggested that the ability to repair DNA cross-links is impaired.[93–95] Handling of DNA cross-links is thought to be accomplished by the ubiquitous and versatile nucleotide excision repair (NER) pathway (Fig. 2–4, left panel). The steps in this pathway include recognition of damage, incision of the damaged DNA strand, excision of the defective site, repair replication, and ligation to replace the excised region with normal nucleotides.[85] Repair of vertebrate genomes is linked to transcriptional activity; transcribed regions are repaired quickly while untranscribed regions remain unrepaired.[96, 97] Some repair gene products actually constitute part of the transcription initiation complex. When RNA polymerase II encounters a DNA lesion, a helicase-like protein known as transcription initiation factor TFIIH may displace the stalled polymerase and unwind the region for entry of DNA repair enzymes and nucleases. XP is a well-studied paradigm disorder involving nucleotide excision repair.[98] XP can be due to mutations in any of at least seven different genes. The proteins encoded by two of the XP genes, XPB and XPD, are transient or integral components of TFIIH and apparently shuttle between transcribed and untranscribed regions of the genome.

The fidelity of excision repair has been studied in FA. At first, FA was thought to be comparable to XP in terms of inability to repair and remove DNA cross-links,[94] but in contrast to the situation in XP, FA cells apparently are not completely deficient,[99–101] exhibiting only a partial defect in the incision of interstrand cross-links.[102, 103] Two reports highlight some of the controversies over the nature of the FA defect in DNA repair. In one study, gene-specific repair was measured for DNA adducts induced by cisplatin in an FA-A cell line.[104] FA-A cells were found to repair these interstrand cross-links with only 50% to 60% of the efficiency of normal control cells. In contrast, another group of investigators using similar techniques was unable to differentiate FA cells from normal cells on the basis of comparing MMC-

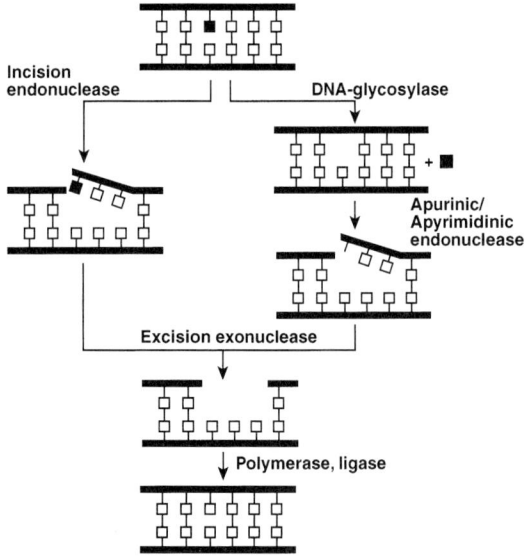

Figure 2–4 Nucleotide (left) and base (right) excision repair. See text for details.

induced cross-link repair efficiency at the level of the ribosomal RNA gene.[105]

The nature of the FA DNA excision repair defect has been further defined by measuring the activities of chromatin-associated DNA endonuclease extract.[106] In one FA-A cell line, an endonuclease activity showed markedly reduced ability to incise DNA containing interstrand cross-links produced by psoralens plus ultraviolet (UV) light; in addition, chromatin protein extracts were defective for a DNA-binding protein with specificity for interstrand cross-links.[107] Thus, the FA repair defect may be due in part to lack of this damage-recognition protein, as well as to a defect in the function of an endonuclease complex involved in the DNA incision process. FA cells from at least two defined complementation groups have been postulated to be deficient in repair of DNA damage, a defect that can be complemented by introduction of a normal endonuclease complex.[108]

Postreplication recombination repair and translesion replication represent two alternative pathways to excision repair. Recombinational repair is one of the major mechanisms for resolving double-strand breaks as well as DNA cross-links. In this pathway, the DNA polymerase enzyme stops upon encountering a DNA lesion and then resumes replication of DNA downstream; the postreplication gap may be filled by recombination. In bacteria, exposure to agents that interfere with DNA replication (UV damage, MMC, and others) leads to induction of the SOS response. Translesion synthesis is one of the components of the SOS response and refers to non–template-directed or error-prone replication across the DNA lesion, leading to a site of mismatch.[109] While the biochemistry of these types of repair and bypass has not been well characterized in eukaryotes, these pathways may be useful in conceptualizing the FA phenotype.

One of the ideas central to theories of cancer development is that genomic instability precedes tumorigenesis: an early step in carcinogenesis must be the development of a mutator phenotype, allowing cells to exhibit the required increased mutation rate.[110] Hypermutability has recently been linked to a deficiency in mismatch repair in a genetic cancer-predisposing disorder, hereditary nonpolyposis colorectal cancer.[111, 112] An association between hypermutability and other cancer-predisposing disorders would be direct evidence that the fidelity of DNA repair is impaired. Cells from XP patients show higher frequencies of mutations when compared with normal cells, suggesting that unexcised lesions are processed by an intact error-prone mechanism, since XP cells lack the error-free excision repair system[113] (in this case, an error-prone pathway includes a mechanism analogous to bacterial translesion synthesis, which leads to mismatch formation).

In FA, the situation is more complex. Although the rate of base pair substitutions was found to be low at the hypoxanthine phosphoribosyltransferase locus in FA-A and FA-D lymphoblasts and T lymphocytes,[114–116] the proportion of deletions was three to six times higher in mutants as compared to normal or XP cells.[115, 116] Furthermore, mutation frequency at the glycophorin A (GPA) locus was found to be markedly elevated in FA erythrocytes.[116] Hypermutability at the GPA locus again could be attributed to a predisposition to deletion or chromosome loss as opposed to point mutation, suggesting chromosomal but not nucleotide instability.[117] Allelic loss can lead to the dysregulation of cell proliferation by deletion or inactivation of tumor suppressor genes.[118] In this sense, the chromosome instability of FA may be causally related to predisposition to leukemia and other solid tumors. For *FANCA*, the large number and variety of mutations has led to the suggestion that *FANCA* is hypermutable and susceptible to slipped-strand mispairing (a mechanism involved in the generation of mutations in *p53*, retinoblastoma, and *BRCA 1*, among others)[49]; this implies that a gene that regulates chromosome stability may itself be susceptible to mutation.

Fanconi's Anemia Proteins: Search for a Function

FANCC and FANCA Interactions

Of the eight FA groups determined by somatic cell hybridization and complementation analysis, *FANCC*[32] and *FANCA*[47, 48] were the first to have been identified. Since the two genes are not homologous with each other and yet mutations in either gene lead to FA, FANCC and FANCA (and perhaps other FA proteins) have been postulated either to function in a common pathway (e.g., as members of an enzymatic cascade), to physically associate, or to interact in some indirect manner.

If the primary defect in FA is in DNA repair, at least part of the time FA proteins should be located in the nucleus (Fig. 2–5). Surprisingly, FANCC was initially bound primarily to the cytoplasm.[119, 120] Recently, however, Kupfer et al.[121] reported that the FANCC and FANCA proteins interact to form a nuclear complex. A patient-derived mutant FANCC (L554P) failed to bind FANCA, suggesting that the formation of this complex was functionally important. Mutation or deletion of the N-terminal nuclear localization signal (NLS) of FANCA resulted in loss of functional activity, absence of FANCC binding, and cyto-

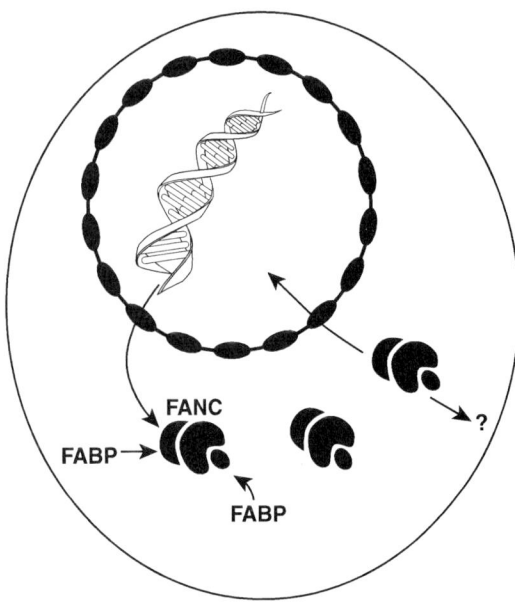

Figure 2–5 The precise biochemical function of the FANC polypeptides is currently unknown. The susceptibility of Fanconi's anemia (FA) cells to DNA cross-linking agents such as mitomycin C suggests that the FA phenotype involves defective recognition or repair of damaged DNA. However, direct evidence of a defect in cross-link repair has been difficult to establish. Localization of the FANCC polypeptide primarily to the cytoplasm has suggested that mechanisms other than direct repair of DNA may be operative. In addition, the cellular pathophysiology of FA suggests other disturbances, such as sensitivity to oxygen and oxygen metabolites. The FANCC protein has been shown to bind to at least three cytoplasmic proteins (denoted FABP for *FA binding protein*). The FANCC protein may also form a complex with the FANCA protein that is translocated to the nucleus.

plasmic retention of FANCA.[122] Finally, these investigators determined that FANCA is phosphorylated.[123] All these data suggested that the FA proteins are directly involved in a nuclear pathway (such as DNA repair).

In contrast, a second group has been unable to confirm any interaction between FANCA and FANCC, either in vivo or in vitro.[124] With the technique of enforced cytoplasmic localization, FANCA lost its ability to complement FA-A cells on export to the cytoplasm. Conversely, earlier work had established that enforced nuclear expression of FANCC abolished its ability to complement FA-C cells, consistent with a cytoplasmic function for FANCC.[125] These results argue that if FANCA and FANCC are functionally linked, they are more likely to be in a linear pathway because they function in separate subcellular compartments.

FANCC Protein Function

Knowledge about the primary function of FANCC is still rudimentary, but concrete laboratory findings point to a cytoplasmic action that may not directly involve DNA repair. MMC is an antibiotic that both generates reactive oxygen species and is itself capable of cross-linking DNA. Experiments varying oxygen tension to favor either oxygen radical generation or DNA cross-linking have suggested that radicals account for the induction of apoptotic cell death in FA-C cells exposed to MMC.[126] Recently, in experiments testing MMC-induced cross-link formation in FA-C cells, the predominant abnormality was in initial processing of interstrand cross-links.[125] This "prerepair" molecular defect was corrected by the cytoplasmic action of FANCC, suggesting that FANCC might act as a cytoplasmic sensor of DNA cross-linker damage. Alternatively, FANCC might participate in a metabolic pathway to detoxify or defend against such damage. One way this could occur has recently been discovered: FANCC was shown to bind to NADPH cytochrome P-450 reductase, a microsomal membrane protein involved in electron transfer.[127] Expression of FANCC suppressed the ability of the P-450 enzyme to reduce cytochrome c in the presence of NADPH. Consequently, FANCC appears to play a key role in vivo by attenuating the activity of the P-450 reductase enzyme, thereby regulating a major detoxification pathway in mammalian cells.[127]

DNA Repair and FANCG

The recent identification of the FANCG protein as being identical to the human XRCC9 (*x-ray cross-complementing*) protein has led to renewed speculation about a direct DNA repair function for the FA proteins.[52] Unfortunately, the *XRCC9* gene product itself has not been well characterized biochemically. *XRCC9* was originally cloned as a cDNA that was able to partially correct the hypersensitivity of a Chinese hamster ovary mutant cell line to a variety of chemical agents and UV and gamma radiation.[53] However, as with the other FA proteins, the translated XRCC9 sequence is not similar to that of any other GENBANK database protein of known biochemical function. XRCC9 may play a role in postreplication repair or function in regulating a cell cycle checkpoint.[53]

Cell Death Mechanisms: Data from FANCC

There is mounting evidence that at least one important function of the wild-type FANCC protein is in the modulation of apoptosis, or programmed cell death. FANCC was first shown to suppress a DNA cross-linker–inducible apoptosis pathway in FANCC-mutant lymphoblastoid cell lines.[128] Overexpression of the wild-type FANCC protein was reported to protect hematopoietic cells from apoptosis.[129] However, lymphoblastoid cell lines and peripheral blood lymphocytes from FANCC-mutant patients have appeared to resist apoptosis induced by various stimuli.[130] One possible explanation for these contradictory findings is that FANCC (and possibly other FA proteins) may act at a decision fork between apoptotic and non-apoptotic (necrotic) cell death.[131] A prediction from this hypothesis is that overexpression of the FANCC protein might promote cell survival through suppression of apoptosis pathways.

Loss of Function: Knock-out Mouse Model of FA-C

Fancc knock-out mice have been created by two groups of investigators. When mice were generated with targeted inactivation of the Fancc gene, the nullizygous genotype did not exhibit developmental abnormalities up to 9 months of age.[132] As predicted, spleen cells from the knock-out mice developed increased numbers of chromosomal aberrations in response to MMC, and hematopoietic progenitors were also hypersensitive to MMC.[133] Homozygous male and female mice also exhibited compromised gametogenesis and markedly impaired fertility, mimicking some of the features of the human disease.[134] Surprisingly, however, the animals did not exhibit gross hematologic defects.[132, 135]

Although the mice had normal peripheral blood counts, the colony-forming capacity of progenitor cells from the knock-out mice was markedly diminished by the addition of interferon-γ (IFN-γ).[135, 136] IFN-γ was previously implicated as an inhibitory cytokine present in the bone marrow of patients with acquired aplastic anemia (reviewed in Chapter 1). In tissue culture, IFN-γ and TNF-α (see above) suppress the proliferation of early and late hematopoietic progenitor and stem cells.[137, 138] The mechanism by which these cytokines suppress hematopoiesis involves upregulation of the Fas death receptor (Fas) on hematopoietic cells.[139] A member of the TNF superfamily of death receptors, Fas is a key molecule involved in the induction of apoptosis of Fas-bearing cells.[140] Fas ligand (Fas-L) binds to Fas and initiates the sequential activation of the caspases.[141, 142] The exaggerated sensitivity of progenitor cells from Fancc mutant mice to IFN-γ may be an important clue regarding the pathophysiologic mechanism of bone marrow failure in FA. Currently, there is no information regarding the levels of Fas-L or IFN-γ in FA patients. However, as mentioned above, abnormally high levels of TNF-α have been reported to be associated with the FA genetic background, with detectable levels in serum from both homozygotes and obligate heterozygotes.[74, 75] Addition of antibodies to TNF-α was found to partially correct the cytotoxic hypersensitivity to MMC.[74]

Gain of Function: Complementation and Overexpression of FANCC

To better understand the function of FANCC in hematopoiesis, we created transgenic mice to overexpress human FANCC protein.[143] We tested the effect of inducing apoptosis in FANCC-transgenic mouse cells by incubating bone marrow cells in methylcellulose culture with IFN-γ, TNF-α, or a Fas-triggering antibody. Hematopoietic progenitors from FANCC-transgenic mice were up to 10-fold less sensitive to the cytolytic effect of Fas ligation. These studies complement the Fancc knock-out model, in that overexpression of human FANCC protected against Fas-mediated cell death, whereas disruption of murine Fancc led to sensitivity to the inhibitory effects of IFN-γ,[135, 136] TNF-α,[144] and Fas ligand.[145]

In sum, these experiments suggest that FANCC acts in a downstream pathway regulating apoptosis; when FANCC is absent or defective, mutant cells may be unusually susceptible to various forms of apoptotic stimuli (death receptor, growth factor deprivation, DNA damage). Bone marrow failure would be secondary to continuing and cumulative apoptosis of hematopoietic stem cells (HSCs). Some of the physical anomalies may be due to inappropriate cell apoptosis in developing tissues. FA may therefore be a disorder of dysregulated apoptosis, with unknown triggering mechanisms.

An important and unresolved paradox, given our model for FA pathophysiology, relates to the tendency of FA patients to develop leukemias.[24] We previously reported that wild-type FANCC gene transfection decreased the susceptibility of mutant fibroblasts to transformation by the oncogenic SV40 virus, consistent with a role for wild-type FANCC in tumor suppression.[146] If, as suggested, wild-type FANCC functions to suppress apoptosis, then defective FANCC function manifested by a greater sensitivity to cell death would not account for the proclivity to malignant transformation. Possibly, incomplete cell death of hematopoietic cells leads to the outgrowth of damaged preleukemic clones. Alternatively, second genetic mutations may be necessary for transformation events.

Hematopoietic Defects in Fanconi's Anemia

Some hypotheses about the bone marrow failure in FA patients include qualitative or quantitative defects in HSCs or defects in the auxiliary cells of the hematopoietic microenvironment, resulting in reduced or even absent colony formation (as measured by myeloid[147] and erythroid[148] progenitor assays). Of course, these clonogeneic assays do not provide direct information regarding the stem cell compartment.

With respect to stromal cells, the FA mutation does not seem to consistently abrogate the formation of an adherent layer in long-term bone marrow culture,[149] although the layer may develop slowly. The capacity of FA fibroblasts to produce stem cell factor (SCF) and macrophage colony-stimulating factor (M-CSF) is normal, but the interleukin-1 (IL-1-)–induced expression of granulocyte colony-stimulating factor (G-CSF), granulocyte-macrophage colony-stimulating factor (GM-CSF), and interleukin-6 (IL-6) varies among individuals, ranging from blunted responses to hypersensitivity,[150] a variability that may reflect the heterogeneity of the disorder but does not seem to be a direct effect of the FA mutation. By inference, the FA defect is not a primary stromal dysfunction but a disorder affecting the HSC.

Assessment of human HSC reserve is technically difficult. HSCs are classically defined by their ability to reconstitute multilineage hematopoiesis after transplantation into marrow-ablated animals. Enrichment of these rare cells is now based upon identifying unique surface antigens such as the CD34 molecule. No direct assay to identify and quantitate true HSCs exists, although the long-term culture–initiating cell (LTC-IC) test has been proposed as a surrogate. The LTC-IC is defined as a primitive hematopoietic cell capable of producing clonogeneic progenitor cells after 5 weeks of long-term bone marrow culture.[151, 152] Several investigators have examined FA hematopoiesis in long-term culture.[149, 153] Secondary colonies were reported to develop from the nonadherent population of cells,[153] but no studies have systematically assessed LTC-IC (from the adherent population) numbers in FA patients.

Progress in defining the hematopoietic defect in FA has recently been made by studying the in vivo effects of MMC in *Fancc* nullizygous mice.[154] As previously mentioned, these knock-out mice do not spontaneously develop marrow failure. However, acute exposure to MMC induced marked bone marrow hypoplasia and degeneration of proliferative tissues, causing death within a few days. Sequential, nonlethal doses of MMC caused a progressive decrease in all peripheral blood values, specifically targeting the bone marrow compartment without effects on other proliferative tissues. Reduction in the number of early and committed hematopoietic progenitors was noted. This model of hematopoietic failure in FA should also prove useful in testing novel therapies.

STANDARD AND EXPERIMENTAL THERAPIES

Stem Cell Transplantation and Supportive Care

Allogeneic bone marrow transplantation (BMT) from an HLA-matched sibling donor is the only curative therapy for the hematologic manifestations of FA (aplasia or myelodysplasia). Typically, decreased doses of cyclophosphamide and irradiation must be used to avoid severe toxicity due to the chemo- and radiosensitivity of FA patients. In early reports, FA patients undergoing BMT suffered a uniformly poor outcome as a result of toxicity of the preparative regimen, severe-graft-versus host disease (GvHD), and infection.[155] Based on biologic and clinical observations, investigators from Paris championed the use of a conditioning regimen of low-dose (20 mg/kg) cyclophosphamide and 5-Gy thoracoabdominal irradiation (TAI).[156, 157] Single transplantation centers, which generally adopted this modified conditioning regimen with or without TAI, have reported good early results for FA patients who did not present with leukemia or preleukemic transformation (Table 2–1). Collected data from multiple institutions (with over 150 FA patients) yielded an

TABLE 2–1 Single-Institution Bone Marrow Transplantation Experience in Fanconi's Anemia (10 or More Patients)

Reporting Group	Survival (N)
Hows et al. (1989)[186]	6/10 MSD, 2/9 alternative
Kohli-Kumar et al. (1994)[187]	17/18 MSD
Zanis-Neto et al. (1995)[188]	8/10 MSD
Flowers et al. (1996)[162]	8/9 MSD

MSD, matched sibling donor; alternative, alternative donor.

overall 2-year survival rate of 66% (range 58% to 73%), with lower-dose cyclophosphamide and limited field irradiation correlated with improved survival.[158] Older age at transplantation and low platelet count prior to BMT were also associated with a lower rate of survival, mostly as a result of increased graft failure and chronic GvHD.

Despite success in treating the aplasia of FA by stem cell replacement, some survivors will later develop secondary malignancies, particularly of the head and neck.[159-161] On long-term follow-up, 7 of a cohort of 50 patients receiving transplants according to the French conditioning regimen developed late cancer (8-year projected incidence, 24%). Presumably, these cancers reflect the continued genetic susceptibility of host nonhematopoietic tissues to carcinogenesis. The role of irradiation as a cofactor could not be excluded, as transplant patients at Seattle who did not receive irradiation also developed late cancers (two cases among the long-term survivors).[162]

Umbilical cord blood transplantation from related donors has also been successfully applied to a small number of FA patients.[163, 164] There is a suggestion from the initial cases reported that the incidence of GvHD may be lower than in allogeneic BMT, but no comprehensive analysis in FA patients has been reported yet in the literature. A few FA patients have also undergone successful stem cell transplantation with cord blood from unrelated donors.[165]

Clearly, young patients with an HLA-compatible sibling should be treated by stem cell transplantation (either from bone marrow or umbilical cord blood) at the earliest stages of marrow failure in preference to other therapies. However, most patients do not have an HLA-identical donor and are dependent upon the identification of a suitably matched nonsibling relative or unrelated donor. A small number of FA patients have undergone BMT from such alternative sources (matched unrelated and haploidentical family donors) to treat either aplasia or myelodysplasia, with or without clonal chromosomal abnormalities. The initial analysis of 48 patients undergoing BMT from alternative donors showed a 29% 2-year survival rate.[158] To date, the largest single-institution experience with mismatched related or unrelated donor stem cell transplantation for FA has been at the University of Minnesota (John Wagner, personal communication, 1998), and a subset of this cohort has been reported in the literature.[166] A total of 29 patients were treated with cyclophosphamide 40 mg/kg and total body irradiation (4.0 to 6.0 Gy) followed by stem cell transplantation using marrow or umbilical cord blood from related (nonsibling) or unrelated donors. The overall probability of marrow and white blood cell (WBC) recovery was 63% (37% failed engraftment with donor cells). The Kaplan-Meier estimate of overall survival was 35% at 1 year. At this time, graft failure remains the single most important complication limiting the successful use of alternative donor transplantation, and this therapy must still be considered as a late or last resort.

Patients lacking a suitable HLA-compatible donor (either sibling or matched unrelated) may benefit from chronic administration of androgens or hematopoietic growth factors (HGFs), which serve as temporizing measures until improvements in unrelated BMT offer a better probability of long-term survival.

Androgens

First used to treat FA in 1959,[167] androgens have been shown to induce hematologic responses in approximately 50% of FA patients, although their effectiveness in raising blood counts may be neither durable nor complete in all lineages. In one large series that included mostly patients with acquired aplastic anemia, 75% showed some initial response.[168] Typically, androgen therapy is initiated when the platelet count is consistently below 30,000/μL or the hemoglobin less than 7 g/dL. Orally administered oxymetholone 2 to 5 mg/kg/day is usually combined with prednisone 5 to 10 mg every other day to counterbalance the anabolic properties of oxymetholone with the catabolic actions of corticosteroids.[169] Androgen therapy is associated with liver toxicities, including transaminase enzyme elevation, cholestasis, peliosis hepatitis, and hepatic tumors. The last complication has only rarely appeared in patients not previously treated with androgens, thus suggesting that androgen therapy itself predisposes FA patients to liver disease. Injectable androgens are associated with a decreased risk of hepatotoxicity, but pediatricians have sometimes objected to their use over concerns of pain and local bleeding: one standard formulation is nandrolone decanoate, administered by intramuscular injection at a dose of 1 to 2 mg/kg/week. Despite years of experience with androgens, the scientific rationale for their use in FA is still unclear; possibly, new insights regarding the role of FA genes in regulating apoptosis or the immune system may explain their effectiveness.

Hematopoietic Growth Factors

Levels of most growth factors, including the stem or progenitor cell–active Flt3 ligand,[170] are markedly increased in FA as they are in acquired aplastic anemia, likely as a compensatory physiologic response to pancytopenia. One worrisome aspect of chronic growth factor administration is the theoretical risk of stimulating a leukemic clone, particularly in patients prone to developing MDS or AML, or speeding the process of stem cell exhaustion.

Phase I and II clinical trials of HGFs have been conducted to determine if the marrow failure of FA would respond to pharmacologic doses.[171] In one study, seven patients (median WBC count of 2.24×10^9/L and absolute neutrophil count [ANC] of 0.24×10^9/L) were entered on a trial of subcutaneous GM-CSF treatment. Most of the patients were initially dependent on red blood cell (RBC) and platelet transfusions. Therapy consisted of 21-day cycles of GM-CSF 2.5 to 10 µg/kg/day with a dose escalation if the response was judged inadequate. The median WBC count of responding patients at the end of the study was increased more than threefold, to 7.3×10^9/L, and the ANC by more than 12-fold, to 3.05×10^9/L. One patient became RBC transfusion–free, but no improvement in platelet count was noted in any cases. At the end of the study, no patient had developed excess blasts, and cytogenetics remained nonclonal in all. Two of six patients treated with subcutaneous IL-3 also had an improvement in both median WBC count and ANC, and one patient had decreased RBC and platelet requirements.

Chronic therapy with G-CSF has also been reported in 12 FA patients with neutropenia (ANC less than 1×10^9/L).[172] G-CSF was started at 5 µg/kg/day. All showed an increase in ANC at week 8, with a median ANC during therapy of 5×10^9/L. Four patients had an increase in their platelet count by week 8 without transfusion; however, platelet counts fell toward baseline levels as the G-CSF dose was reduced. Four patients who did not require RBC transfusions had an increase in their hemoglobin level of at least 2.0 g/dL. Thus, chronic administration of G-CSF had transient beneficial effects on multiple hematopoietic lineages in some patients.

Gene Therapy

In view of the limited therapeutic options available for patients lacking a suitable BMT donor, experimental trials of hematopoietic cell transduction (with *FANCC* and other FA genes when identified) seem reasonable. However, such trials have unknown long-term consequences and should be considered only in carefully selected patients.

Gene Transduction and Hematopoiesis

Recombinant vectors to transfer foreign genes have been engineered from both DNA and RNA viruses. Currently, murine retroviruses are still the best-characterized vectors adapted to stable integration of foreign genetic material, a process referred to as transduction. Retroviruses are single-stranded RNA viruses that bind to a specific surface receptor; inside the cell, viral RNA is converted into double-stranded DNA and integrated into the host cell genome as provirus. The main advantage of retroviral vectors is their ability to integrate into the host cell genome and to confer long-term expression of the transgene; their major limitation is that the target cell must be actively replicating in order for the vector to integrate into the host chromosome.

Adeno-associated viruses (AAVs) are single-stranded DNA parvoviruses. In the absence of a helper virus such as adenovirus, AAV causes a latent infection characterized by the integration of viral DNA into the cellular genome. Recombinant AAV vector production involves cotransfection of a permissive cell line (such as the 293-cell line) with a recombinant plasmid containing the gene to be transferred (with a promoter and polyadenylation signal) flanked by the AAV inverted terminal repeats (ITRs) and a helper plasmid carrying the other required viral genes but lacking the AAV ITRs. The 293 cells are coinfected with adenovirus to generate AAV virion particles.

We have used both recombinant retroviral and AAV vectors to transfer copies of the normal *FANCC* cDNA to cells from patients with *FANCC* mutations[173–175] (Fig. 2–6). Phenotypic correction followed viral transduction, as shown by resistance to MMC-induced cell death and insusceptibility to induced chromosomal aberrations. CD34-enriched hematopoietic progenitors isolated from FA patients, which exhibit the same hypersensitivity to MMC as do cultured FA cells, also showed improved colony formation in clonogeneic assays in the absence as well as in the presence of low concentrations of MMC, after gene transduction with a viral vector containing the wild-type *FANCC* cDNA.[173, 174] Similarly, transduction with a *FANCA* vector also improved the viability of hematopoietic progenitor colonies from patients with *FANCA* mutations.[176] These experiments implied that both FANCC and FANCA proteins are involved in the maintenance of hematopoietic progenitor cell viability, perhaps by countering programmed cell death.

Hematopoietic Stem Cell Targets and Rationale for Gene Therapy

Theoretically, HSCs represent an ideal target for gene therapy since they can be harvested from bone marrow, peripheral blood, or umbilical cord blood and transduced outside the body. Replica-

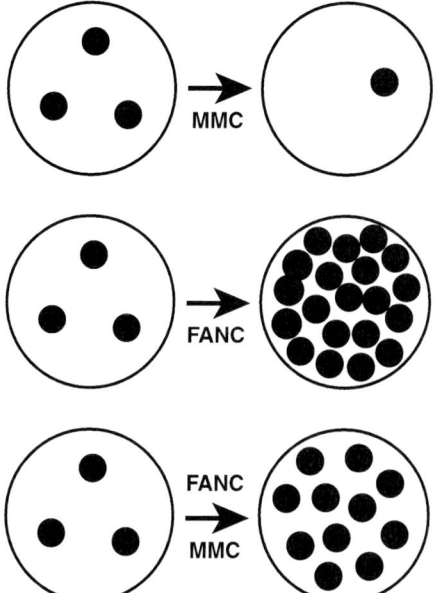

Figure 2–6 Fanconi's anemia hematopoietic progenitor growth and the influence of *FANC* gene transduction. Typically, poor colony growth is observed in the absence or presence of mitomycin C (MMC). However, following transduction by a viral vector containing the normal *FANCC* or *FANCA* complementary DNA (cDNA), colony growth was markedly enhanced in the absence and presence of low concentrations of MMC.

tion (self-renewal) of stem cells and repopulation with progeny blood cells should result in the continuous maintenance of the transgene in blood cells of the patient. In practice, many technical obstacles limit gene transfer to HSCs. First, as discussed above, no direct assay to identify and quantitate true human stem cells exists. For example, no direct correlation exists between transduction of LTC-IC and HSCs. Second, HSCs may be predominantly quiescent and insusceptible to proviral integration and transduction. Third, since chromosomal integration is necessary for delivery of the transgene to progeny cells, vector systems that do not lead to integration will result in only transient expression. Gene-marking studies, conducted as part of autologous bone marrow or peripheral blood stem cell transplantation protocols for the treatment of malignancies,[177, 178] have confirmed that transfer of genes to human HSCs is very inefficient.[179]

It has been possible to model HSC gene therapy with computer simulation studies in which the contribution of labeled (genetically marked) progenitor cells to hematopoiesis is assessed under various circumstances.[180] For this purpose, HSCs are assumed to undergo either self-renewal, differentiation, or apoptosis, and these parameters are assigned probabilities. Gene transfer experiments that confer on the transduced HSCs either a proliferative (replication rate) or survival (anti-apoptosis) advantage can significantly increase the number of marked cells in these simulations. However, transplantation of small numbers of HSCs led to dramatic variation in terms of the contribution of marked clones to hematopoiesis, whereas variability was minimized when large numbers of HSCs were transplanted.[180] These predictions highlight the difficulties in devising effective HSC gene therapy, since the large numbers of HSCs needed for successful transplantation may be inefficiently transduced. This problem is magnified in FA, in one sense, as the numbers of HSCs are so low. On the other hand, if FA gene transfer conferred a survival advantage to the corrected HSCs, these clones might become dominant contributors to hematopoiesis. As mentioned above, FA patients may develop spontaneous reversion of the cellular phenotype.[15] In one of the patients described, the degree of reversion was sufficient to allow replacement of the majority of the mutant cells, implying that a single revertant stem cell gradually gained clonal dominance over the mutant cell.

Experimental Trial of *FANCC* Gene Therapy

Based upon our preclinical data,[175] as well as safety studies conducted in animals,[181] we undertook an experimental trial of gene therapy for FA-C patients. This ongoing study is meant to test two questions: (1) Could the known inefficiency of retroviral vectors in transducing human HSCs be improved by multiple cycles of gene therapy in a nonmyeloablated host? (2) Can *FANCC* gene–complemented stem and progenitor cells outcompete defective mutant cells in vivo and selectively repopulate patient bone marrow?

Our trial used mobilized peripheral blood progenitor cells, which can contribute to long-term engraftment after autologous transplantation.[179] The progenitor cells were collected by apheresis following mobilization with G-CSF. G-CSF–mobilized cell populations may not be quiescent[182] and may therefore be more susceptible to retroviral gene transduction, a process that requires cell division. Because of the inefficiency of retroviral transduction of HSCs, we designed our study to include four cycles of mobilization, collection, transduction, and infusion, in an attempt to increase the number of gene-corrected cells. The addition of exogenous HGFs (SCF, IL-3, IL-6) was necessary for efficient progenitor transduction.[175] Because of the hypoplastic state of the FA host bone marrow, ablative chemotherapy was not included prior to cell infusion.

Three FA patients, each bearing a different *FANCC* mutation (exon 1, exon 14, intron 4), participated in the initial trial. The *FANCC* transgene was demonstrated in transduced CD34-enriched progenitor cells. Following infusion, *FANCC* was also present transiently in peripheral blood cells. Function of the normal *FANCC* transgene was suggested by a marked increase in hematopoietic colonies following successive transduction cycles in all patients. Transient improvement in bone marrow cellularity coincided with this expansion of hematopoietic progenitors. Apparently, transduction of the normal *FANCC* gene into hematopoietic cells from patients with *FANCC* mutations was able to improve the pathologic process affecting FA hematopoiesis. However, despite the in vitro selective advantage resulting from *FANCC* gene transfer, we did not observe long-term hematopoietic reconstitution with gene-corrected clones.

Future Directions

Genetic manipulation of true human HSCs continues to be an elusive goal. Although our small trial was able to confirm that relatively long-lived hematopoietic progenitors can be genetically altered, the number of peripheral blood mononuclear cells transduced by the *FANCC* transgene was only 1 in 1000, remaining relatively constant following an initial 10-fold increase. Despite the apparent growth advantage of corrected cells in vitro, we were unable to confirm selective amplification of the transfected clone in vivo. One of the fundamental problems with current gene therapy protocols is the low efficiency of transduction to multipotential HSCs. Since HSCs do not replicate often, they may be insusceptible to retroviral transduction. Future efforts to address these problems may include the use of new combinations of stem cell–active cytokines,[183] vectors that can transduce quiescent HSCs,[184] and ex vivo HSC expansion.[185]

For FA, a number of conclusions can be drawn from our pilot study. First, our work suggests that gene transduction has at least transient positive effects on FA hematopoiesis as measured by progenitor growth and marrow cellularity, suggesting that collection of hematopoietic stem cells in FA patients prior to the outgrowth of dysplastic clones may be desirable. Those stem cells might then be transduced and reinfused at a later point should leukemia develop. Second, amplification of the transduced clone may require additional selective pressure, perhaps from the use of DNA cross-linking agents to select for resistant (transduced) clones or to purge dysplastic cells. An important unanswered question is whether autologous bone marrow cells transduced with the FA transgene can be used to reconstitute FA patients who have developed graft failure following allogeneic stem cell transplantation from an unrelated donor. In theory, additional selective pressure for FA gene–modified cells may exist because the recipient will have received immunosuppression and chemotherapy.

CONCLUSIONS

With the identification of two more FA genes, *FANCA* and *FANCG*, transduction strategies should become applicable to a larger number of patients within the context of carefully designed research trials. As the field of hematopoietic cell gene transfer continues to evolve, with both minor alterations in transduction conditions (to include newer and more potent cytokines), as well as radical improvements in vector development and HSC growth, persistent expression of the FA genes in HSCs may become feasible. As for more conventional therapies, improvements in transplantation of HSCs from mismatched and unrelated donors appear likely in the next few years. With greater knowledge about the function of FA genes and resultant insights into cellular processes, there is every expectation that effective gene, protein, or cell therapies will soon be developed.

REFERENCES

1. Fanconi G: Familiäre infantile perniziösartige Anämie (perniziöses Blutbild und Konstitution). Jahrb Kinderheilkd 1927; 117:257–280.
2. Alter BP: Fanconi's anaemia and its variability. Br J Haematol 1993; 85:9–14.
3. Fanconi G: Familial constitutional panmyelopathy, Fanconi's anemia (F.A.). I. Clinical aspects. Semin Hematol 1967; 4:233–240.
4. Auerbach AD, Rogatko A, Schroeder-Kurth TM: International Fanconi Anemia Registry: Relation of clinical symptoms to diepoxybutane sensitivity. Blood 1989; 73:391–396.
5. Auerbach AD: Fanconi anemia diagnosis and the diepoxybutane (DEB) test (editorial). Exp Hematol 1993; 21:731–733.
6. Butturini A, Gale RP, Verlander PC, et al: Hematologic abnormalities in Fanconi anemia: An International Fanconi Anemia Registry study. Blood 1994; 84:1650–1655.
7. Alter BP: Fanconi's anemia and malignancies. Am J Hematol 1996; 53:99–110.
8. Schroeder TM, Anschutz F, Knopp A: Spontane

Chromosomenaberrationen bei familiärer Panmyelopathie. Humangenetik 1964; 1:194–196.
9. Latt SA, Stetten G, Juergens LA, et al: Induction by alkylating agents of sister chromatid exchanges and chromatid breaks in Fanconi's anemia. Proc Natl Acad Sci USA 1975; 72:4066–4070.
10. Kaiser TN, Lojewski A, Dougherty C, et al: Flow cytometric characterization of the response of Fanconi's anemia cells to mitomycin C treatment. Cytometry 1982; 2:291–297.
11. Claassen F, Kortbeek H, Arwert F: Effects of mitomycin C on the rate of DNA synthesis in normal and Fanconi anaemia cells. Mutat Res 1986; 165:15–19.
12. Ishida R, Buchwald M: Susceptibility of Fanconi's anemia lymphoblasts to DNA-cross-linking and alkylating agents. Cancer Res 1982; 42:4000–4006.
13. Seyschab H, Friedl R, Sun Y, et al: Comparative evaluation of diepoxybutane sensitivity and cell cycle blockage in the diagnosis of Fanconi anemia. Blood 1995; 85:2233–2237.
14. Dokal I, Chase A, Morgan NV, et al: Positive diepoxybutane test in only one of two brothers found to be compound heterozygotes for Fanconi's anaemia complementation group C mutations. Br J Haematol 1996; 93:813–816.
15. Lo TFJ, Kwee ML, Rooimans MA, et al: Somatic mosaicism in Fanconi anemia: Molecular basis and clinical significance. Eur J Hum Genet 1997; 5:137–148.
16. Joenje H, Arwert F, Kwee ML, et al: Confounding factors in the diagnosis of Fanconi anaemia (letter). Am J Med Genet 1998; 79:403–404.
17. Alter BP, Potter NU, Li FP: Classification and aetiology of the aplastic anaemias. Clin Haematol 1978; 7:431–465.
18. Estren S, Dameshek W: Familial hypoplastic anemia of childhood. Report of eight cases in two families with beneficial effect of splenectomy in one case. Am J Dis Child 1947; 73:671–687.
19. Li FP, Potter NU: Classical Fanconi anemia in a family with hypoplastic anemia. J Pediatr 1978; 92:943–944.
20. Liu JM, Auerbach AD, Young NS: Fanconi anemia presenting unexpectedly in an adult kindred with no dysmorphic features (letter). Am J Med 1991; 91:555–557.
21. Kwee ML, van der Kleij JM, van Essen AJ, et al: An atypical case of Fanconi anemia in elderly sibs. Am J Med Genet 1997; 68:362–366.
22. Auerbach AD, Weiner MA, Warburton D, et al: Acute myeloid leukemia as the first hematologic manifestation of Fanconi anemia. Am J Hematol 1982; 12:289–300.
23. Yamashita T, Wu N, Kupfer G, Corless C, et al: Clinical variability of Fanconi anemia (type C) results from expression of an amino terminal truncated Fanconi anemia complementation group C polypeptide with partial activity. Blood 1996; 87:4424–4432.
24. Auerbach AD, Allen RG: Leukemia and preleukemia in Fanconi anemia patients. A review of the literature and report of the International Fanconi Anemia Registry. Cancer Genet Cytogenet 1991; 51:1–12.
25. Alter BP, Scalise A, McCombs J, et al: Clonal chromosomal abnormalities in Fanconi's anaemia: What do they really mean? Br J Haematol 1993; 85:627–630.
26. Todaro GJ, Green H, Swift MR: Susceptibility of human diploid fibroblast strains to transformation by SV40 virus. Science 1966; 153:1252–1254.
27. Schroeder TM, Tilgen D, Kruger J, et al: Formal genetics of Fanconi's anemia. Hum Genet 1976; 32:257–288.
28. Duckworth-Rysiecki G, Cornish K, Clarke CA, et al: Identification of two complementation groups in Fanconi anemia. Somat Cell Mol Genet 1985; 11:35–41.
29. Strathdee CA, Duncan AM, Buchwald M: Evidence for at least four Fanconi anaemia genes including FACC on chromosome 9. Nat Genet 1992; 1:196–198.
30. Joenje H, Lo TFJ, Oostra AB, et al: Classification of Fanconi anemia patients by complementation analysis: Evidence for a fifth genetic subtype. Blood 1995; 86:2156–2160.
31. Joenje H, Oostra AB, Wijker M, et al: Evidence for at least eight Fanconi anemia genes. Am J Hum Genet 1997; 61:940–944.
32. Strathdee CA, Gavish H, Shannon WR, et al: Cloning of cDNAs for Fanconi's anaemia by functional complementation. Nature 1992; 356:763–767.
33. Gibson RA, Buchwald M, Roberts RG, et al: Characterisation of the exon structure of the Fanconi anaemia group C gene by vectorette PCR. Hum Mol Genet 1993; 2:35–38.
34. Hoshino T, Wang J, Devetten MP, Iwata N, et al: Molecular chaperone GRP94 binds to the Fanconi anemia group C protein and regulates its intracellular expression. Blood 1998; 91:4379–4386.
35. Krasnoshtein F, Buchwald M: Developmental expression of the Fac gene correlates with congenital defects in Fanconi anemia patients. Hum Mol Genet 1996; 5:85–93.
36. Gavish H, dos SC, Buchwald M: A Leu554-to-Pro substitution completely abolishes the functional complementing activity of the Fanconi anemia (FACC) protein. Hum Mol Genet 1993; 2:123–126.
37. Youssoufian H, Li Y, Martin ME, Buchwald M: Induction of Fanconi anemia cellular phenotype in human 293 cells by overexpression of a mutant FAC allele. J Clin Invest 1996; 97:957–962.
38. Whitney MA, Saito H, Jakobs PM, et al: A common mutation in the FACC gene causes Fanconi anaemia in Ashkenazi Jews. Nat Genet 1993; 4:202–205.
39. Verlander PC, Kaporis A, Liu Q, et al: Carrier frequency of the IVS4 + 4 A→T mutation of the Fanconi anemia gene FAC in the Ashkenazi Jewish population. Blood 1995; 86:4034–4038.
40. Verlander PC, Lin JD, Udono MU, et al: Mutation

analysis of the Fanconi anemia gene FACC. Am J Hum Genet 1994; 54:595–601.
41. Gibson RA, Hajianpour A, Murer-Orlando M, et al: A nonsense mutation and exon skipping in the Fanconi anaemia group C gene. Hum Mol Genet 1993; 2:797–799.
42. Gillio AP, Verlander PC, Batish SD, et al: Phenotypic consequences of mutations in the Fanconi anemia FAC gene: An International Fanconi Anemia Registry study. Blood 1997; 90:105–110.
43. Buchwald M: Complementation groups: One or more per gene? Nat Genet 1995; 11:228–230.
44. Joenje H: Fanconi anaemia complementation groups in Germany and the Netherlands. European Fanconi Anaemia Research group. Hum Genet 1996; 97:280–282.
45. Savoia A, Zatterale A, Del Principe D, et al: Fanconi anaemia in Italy: High prevalence of complementation group A in two geographic clusters. Hum Genet 1996; 97:599–603.
46. Pronk JC, Gibson RA, Savoia A, et al: Localisation of the Fanconi anaemia complementation group A gene to chromosome 16q24.3. Nat Genet 1995; 11:338–340.
47. Foe JR, Rooimans MA, Bosnoyan-Collins L, et al: Expression cloning of a cDNA for the major Fanconi anaemia gene, FAA. Nat Genet 1996; 14:488.
48. The Fanconi Anaemia/Breast Cancer Consortium. Positional cloning of the Fanconi anaemia group A gene. Nat Genet 1996; 14:324–328.
49. Levran O, Erlich T, Magdalena N, et al: Sequence variation in the Fanconi anemia gene FAA. Proc Natl Acad Sci USA 1997; 94:13051–13056.
50. Whitney M, Thayer M, Reifsteck C, et al: Microcell mediated chromosome transfer maps the Fanconi anaemia group D gene to chromosome 3p. Nat Genet 1995; 11:341–343.
51. Saar K, Schindler D, Wegner RD, et al: Localisation of a Fanconi anaemia gene to chromosome 9p. Eur J Hum Genet 1998; 6:501–508.
52. de Winter JP, Waisfisz Q, Rooimans MA, et al: The Fanconi anaemia group G gene *FANCG* is identical with *XRCC9*. Nat Genet 1998; 20:281–283.
53. Liu N, Lamerdin JE, Tucker JD, et al: The human *XRCC9* gene corrects chromosomal instability and mutagen sensitivities in CHO UV40 cells. Proc Natl Acad Sci USA 1997; 94:9232–9237.
54. Kubbies M, Schindler D, Hoehn H, et al: Endogenous blockage and delay of the chromosome cycle despite normal recruitment and growth phase explain poor proliferation and frequent endomitosis in Fanconi anemia cells. Am J Hum Genet 1985; 37:1022–1030.
55. Schindler D, Hoehn H: Fanconi anemia mutation causes cellular susceptibility to ambient oxygen. Am J Hum Genet 1988; 43:429–435.
56. Dutrillaux B, Aurias A, Dutrillaux AM, et al: The cell cycle of lymphocytes in Fanconi anemia. Hum Genet 1982; 62:327–332.
57. Poot M, Hoehn H: DNA topoisomerases and the DNA lesion in human genetic instability syndromes. Toxicol Lett 1993; 67:297–308.
58. Balin AK, Goodman DB, Rasmussen H, et al: Oxygen-sensitive stages of the cell cycle of human diploid cells. J Cell Biol 1978; 78:390–400.
59. Joenje R, Arwert F, Eriksson AW, et al: Oxygen-dependence of chromosomal aberrations in Fanconi's anaemia. Nature 1981; 290:142–143.
60. Korkina LG, Samochatova EV, Maschan AA, et al: Release of active oxygen radicals by leukocytes of Fanconi anemia patients. J Leuk Biol 1992; 52:357–362.
61. Gille JJ, Wortelboer HM, Joenje H: Antioxidant status of Fanconi anemia fibroblasts. Hum Genet 1987; 77:28–31.
62. Joenje H, Frants RR, Arwert F, et al: Erythrocyte superoxide dismutase deficiency in Fanconi's anaemia established by two independent methods of assay. Scand J Clin Lab Invest 1979; 39:759–764.
63. Clarke AA, Marsh JC, Gordon-Smith EC, et al: Molecular genetics and Fanconi anaemia: New insights into old problems. Br J Haematol 1998; 103:287–296.
64. Nagasawa R, Little JB: Suppression of cytotoxic effect of mitomycin-C by superoxide dismutase in Fanconi's anemia and dyskeratosis congenita fibroblasts. Carcinogenesis 1983; 4:795–799.
65. Izakovic V, Strbakova E, Kaiserova E, et al: Bovine superoxide dismutase in Fanconi anaemia. Therapeutic trial in two patients. Hum Genet 1985; 70:181–182.
66. Liu JM, Auerbach AD, Anderson SM, et al: A trial of recombinant human superoxide dismutase in patients with Fanconi anaemia. Br J Haematol 1993; 85:406–408.
67. Saito H, Hammond AT, Moses RE: Hypersensitivity to oxygen is a uniform and secondary defect in Fanconi anemia cells. Mutat Res 1993; 294:255–262.
68. Pritsos CA, Sartorelli AC: Generation of reactive oxygen radicals through bioactivation of mitomycin antibiotics. Cancer Res 1986; 46:3528–3532.
69. Krishna MC, DeGraff W, Tamura S, et al: Mechanisms of hypoxic and aerobic cytotoxicity of mitomycin C in Chinese hamster V79 cells. Cancer Res 1991; 51:6622–6628.
70. Joenje H, Oostra AB: Effect of oxygen tension on chromosomal aberrations in Fanconi anaemia. Hum Genet 1983; 65:99–101.
71. Duckworth-Rysiecki G, Taylor AM: Effects of ionizing radiation on cells from Fanconi's anemia patients. Cancer Res 1985; 45:416–420.
72. Bigelow SB, Rary JM, Bender MA: G2 chromosomal radiosensitivity in Fanconi's anemia. Mutat Res 1979; 63:189–199.
73. Parshad R, Sanford KK, Jones GM: Chromatid damage after G2 phase x-irradiation of cells from cancer-prone individuals implicates deficiency in DNA repair. Proc Natl Acad Sci USA 1983; 80:5612–5616.
74. Rosselli F, Sanceau J, Gluckman E, et al: Abnormal lymphokine production: a novel feature of the

genetic disease Fanconi anemia. II. In vitro and in vivo spontaneous overproduction of tumor necrosis factor alpha. Blood 1994; 83:1216–1225.
75. Schultz JC, Shahidi NT: Tumor necrosis factor-alpha overproduction in Fanconi's anemia. Am J Hematol 1993; 42:196–201.
76. Bazzoni F, Beutler B: The tumor necrosis factor ligand and receptor families. N Engl J Med 1996; 334:1717–1725.
77. Holbrook NJ, Fornace AJ Jr: Response to adversity: Molecular control of gene activation following genotoxic stress. New Biol 1991; 3:825–833.
78. Sinclair WK: Cyclic x-ray responses in mammalian cells in vitro. Radiat Res 1968; 33:620–643.
79. Darzynkiewicz Z, Williamson B, Carswell EA, et al: Cell cycle–specific effects of tumor necrosis factor. Cancer Res 1984; 44:83–90.
80. Seyschab H, Sun Y, Friedl R, et al: G2 phase cell cycle disturbance as a manifestation of genetic cell damage. Hum Genet 1993; 92:61–68.
81. Tobey RA: Different drugs arrest cells at a number of distinct stages in G2. Nature 1975; 254:245–247.
82. Weinert TA, Hartwell LH: The RAD9 gene controls the cell cycle response to DNA damage in *Saccharomyces cerevisiae*. Science 1988; 241:317–322.
83. Weinert TA, Kiser GL, Hartwell LH: Mitotic checkpoint genes in budding yeast and the dependence of mitosis on DNA replication and repair. Genes Dev 1994; 8:652–665.
84. Buchwald M, Moustacchi E: Is Fanconi anemia caused by a defect in the processing of DNA damage? Mutat Res 1998; 408:75–90.
85. Barnes DE, Lindahl T, Sedgwick B: DNA repair. Curr Opin Cell Biol 1993; 5:424–433.
86. Hartwell L: Defects in a cell cycle checkpoint may be responsible for the genomic instability of cancer cells. Cell 1992; 71:543–546.
87. Bohr VA, Evans MK, Fornace AJJ: DNA repair and its pathogenetic implications. Lab Invest 1989; 61:143–161.
88. Laval J, Jurado J, Saparbaev M, et al: Antimutagenic role of base-excision repair enzymes upon free radical–induced DNA damage. Mutat Res 1998; 402:93–102.
89. Kasai H: Analysis of a form of oxidative DNA damage, 8-hydroxy-2′-deoxyguanosine, as a marker of cellular oxidative stress during carcinogenesis. Mutat Res 1997; 387:147–163.
90. Takeuchi T, Morimoto K: Increased formation of 8-hydroxydeoxyguanosine, an oxidative DNA damage, in lymphoblasts from Fanconi's anemia patients due to possible catalase deficiency. Carcinogenesis 1993; 14:1115–1120.
91. Wang D, Kreutzer DA, Essigmann JM: Mutagenicity and repair of oxidative DNA damage: Insights from studies using defined lesions. Mutat Res 1998; 400:99–115.
92. Moller P, Wallin H: Adduct formation, mutagenesis and nucleotide excision repair of DNA damage produced by reactive oxygen species and lipid peroxidation product. Mutat Res 1998; 410:271–290.
93. Sasaki MS, Tonomura A: A high susceptibility of Fanconi's anemia to chromosome breakage by DNA cross-linking agents. Cancer Res 1973; 33:1829–1836.
94. Sasaki MS: Is Fanconi's anaemia defective in a process essential to the repair of DNA cross links? Nature 1975; 257:501–503.
95. Fujiwara Y, Tatsumi M: Cross-link repair in human cells and its possible defect in Fanconi's anemia cells. J Mol Biol 1977; 113:635–649.
96. Buratowski S: DNA repair and transcription: The helicase connection [see comments]. Science 1993; 260:37–38.
97. Drapkin R, Sancar A, Reinberg D: Where transcription meets repair. Cell 1994; 77:9–12.
98. Cleaver JE: It was a very good year for DNA repair. Cell 1994; 76:1–4.
99. Fornace AJJ, Little JB, Weichselbaum RR: DNA repair in a Fanconi's anemia fibroblast cell strain. Biochim Biophys Acta 1979; 561:99–109.
100. Sognier MA, Hittelman WN: Loss of repairability of DNA interstrand crosslinks in Fanconi's anemia cells with culture age. Mutat Res 1983; 108:383–393.
101. Poll EH, Arwert F, Kortbeek HT, et al: Fanconi anaemia cells are not uniformly deficient in unhooking of DNA interstrand crosslinks, induced by mitomycin C or 8-methoxypsoralen plus UVA. Hum Genet 1984; 68:228–234.
102. Papadopoulo D, Averbeck D, Moustacchi E: The fate of 8-methoxypsoralen-photoinduced DNA interstrand crosslinks in Fanconi's anemia cells of defined genetic complementation groups. Mutat Res 1987; 184:271–280.
103. Matsumoto A, Vos JM, Hanawalt PC: Repair analysis of mitomycin C–induced DNA crosslinking in ribosomal RNA genes in lymphoblastoid cells from Fanconi's anemia patients. Mutat Res 1989; 217:185–192.
104. Zhen W, Evans MK, Haggerty CM, et al: Deficient gene specific repair of cisplatin-induced lesions in xeroderma pigmentosum and Fanconi's anemia cell lines. Carcinogenesis 1993; 14:919–924.
105. Rey JP, Scott R, Muller H: Induction and removal of interstrand crosslinks in the ribosomal RNA genes of lymphoblastoid cell lines from patients with Fanconi anemia. Mutat Res 1993; 289:171–180.
106. Lambert MW, Tsongalis GJ, Lambert WC, et al: Defective DNA endonuclease activities in Fanconi's anemia cells, complementation groups A and B. Mutat Res 1992; 273:57–71.
107. Hang B, Yeung AT, Lambert MW: A damage-recognition protein which binds to DNA containing interstrand cross-links is absent or defective in Fanconi anemia, complementation group A, cells. Nucleic Acids Res 1993; 21:4187–4192.
108. Lambert MW, Tsongalis GJ, Lambert WC, et al: Correction of the DNA repair defect in Fanconi anemia complementation groups A and D cells.

Biochem Biophys Res Commun 1997; 230:587–591.
109. Defais M, Lesca C, Monsarrat B, et al: Translesion synthesis is the main component of SOS repair in bacteriophage lambda DNA. J Bacteriol 1989; 171:4938–4944.
110. Loeb LA: Mutator phenotype may be required for multistage carcinogenesis. Cancer Res 1991; 51:3075–3079.
111. Parsons R, Li GM, Longley MJ, et al: Hypermutability and mismatch repair deficiency in RER+ tumor cells. Cell 1993; 75:1227–1236.
112. Leach FS, Nicolaides NC, Papadopoulos N, et al: Mutations of a mutS homolog in hereditary nonpolyposis colorectal cancer. Cell 1993; 75:1215–1225.
113. Maher VM, Ouellette LM, Curren RD, et al: Frequency of ultraviolet light–induced mutations is higher in xeroderma pigmentosum variant cells than in normal human cells. Nature 1976; 261:593–595.
114. Papadopoulo D, Porfirio B, Moustacchi E: Mutagenic response of Fanconi's anemia cells from a defined complementation group after treatment with photoactivated bifunctional psoralens. Cancer Res 1990; 50:3289–3294.
115. Papadopoulo D, Guillouf C, Mohrenweiser H, et al: Hypomutability in Fanconi anemia cells is associated with increased deletion frequency at the HPRT locus. Proc Natl Acad Sci USA 1990; 87:8383–8387.
116. Sala-Trepat M, Boyse J, Richard P, et al: Frequencies of HPRT-lymphocytes and glycophorin A variants erythrocytes in Fanconi anemia patients, their parents and control donors. Mutat Res 1993; 289:115–126.
117. Lengauer C, Kinzler KW, Vogelstein B: Genetic instabilities in human cancers. Nature 1998; 396:643–649.
118. Sager R: Tumor suppressor genes: The puzzle and the promise. Science 1989; 246:1406–1412.
119. Yamashita T, Barber DL, Zhu Y, et al: The Fanconi anemia polypeptide FACC is localized to the cytoplasm. Proc Natl Acad Sci USA 1994; 91:6712–6716.
120. Youssoufian H: Localization of Fanconi anemia C protein to the cytoplasm of mammalian cells. Proc Natl Acad Sci USA 1994; 91:7975–7979.
121. Kupfer GM, Naf D, Suliman A, et al: The Fanconi anaemia proteins, FAA and FAC, interact to form a nuclear complex. Nat Genet 1997; 17:487–490.
122. Naf D, Kupfer GM, Suliman A, et al: Functional activity of the Fanconi anemia protein FAA requires FAC binding and nuclear localization. Mol Cell Biol 1998; 18:5952–5960.
123. Yamashita T, Kupfer GM, Naf D, et al: The Fanconi anemia pathway requires FAA phosphorylation and FAA/FAC nuclear accumulation. Proc Natl Acad Sci USA 1998; 95:13085–13090.
124. Kruyt FA, Youssoufian H: The Fanconi anemia proteins FAA and FAC function in different cellular compartments to protect against cross-linking agent cytotoxicity. Blood 1998; 92:2229–2236.
125. Youssoufian H: Cytoplasmic localization of FAC is essential for the correction of a prerepair defect in Fanconi anemia group C cells. J Clin Invest 1996; 97:2003–2010.
126. Clarke AA, Philpott NJ, Gordon-Smith EC, et al: The sensitivity of Fanconi anaemia group C cells to apoptosis induced by mitomycin C is due to oxygen radical generation, not DNA crosslinking. Br J Haematol 1997; 96:240–247.
127. Kruyt FA, Hoshino T, Liu JM, et al: Abnormal microsomal detoxification implicated in Fanconi anemia group C by interaction of the FAC protein with NADPH cytochrome P450 reductase. Blood 1998; 92:3050–3056.
128. Kruyt FA, Dijkmans LM, van den Berg TK, et al: Fanconi anemia genes act to suppress a crosslinker-inducible p53-independent apoptosis pathway in lymphoblastoid cell lines. Blood 1996; 87:938–948.
129. Cumming RC, Liu JM, Youssoufian H, et al: Suppression of apoptosis in hematopoietic factor–dependent progenitor cell lines by expression of the FAC gene. Blood 1996; 88:4558–4567.
130. Ridet A, Guillouf C, Duchaud E, et al: Deregulated apoptosis is a hallmark of the Fanconi anemia syndrome. Cancer Res 1997; 57:1722–1730.
131. Guillouf C, Wang TS, Liu J, et al: Fanconi anemia C protein acts as a switch between apoptosis and necrosis in mitomycin C–induced cell death. Exp Cell Res 1999; 246:384–394.
132. Chen M, Tomkins DJ, Auerbach W, et al: Inactivation of Fac in mice produces inducible chromosomal instability and reduced fertility reminiscent of Fanconi anaemia. Nat Genet 1996; 12:448–451.
133. Otsuki T, Wang J, Demuth I, et al: Assessment of mitomycin C sensitivity in Fanconi anemia complementation group C gene (Fac) knock-out mouse cells. Int J Hematol 1998; 67:243–248.
134. Alter BP, Frissora CL, Halperin DS, et al: Fanconi's anaemia and pregnancy. Br J Haematol 1991; 77: 410–418.
135. Whitney MA, Royle G, Low MJ, et al: Germ cell defects and hematopoietic hypersensitivity to gamma-interferon in mice with a targeted disruption of the Fanconi anemia C gene. Blood 1996; 88:49–58.
136. Rathbun RK, Faulkner GR, Ostroski MH, et al: Inactivation of the Fanconi anemia group C gene augments interferon-gamma–induced apoptotic responses in hematopoietic cells. Blood 1997; 90:974–985.
137. Selleri C, Maciejewski JP, Sato T, et al: Interferon-gamma constitutively expressed in the stromal microenvironment of human marrow cultures mediates potent hematopoietic inhibition. Blood 1996; 87:4149–4157.
138. Selleri C, Sato T, Anderson S, Young NS, et al: Interferon-gamma and tumor necrosis factor-alpha suppress both early and late stages of hematopoiesis and induce programmed cell death. J Cell Physiol 1995; 165:538–546.
139. Maciejewski J, Selleri C, Anderson S, et al: Fas antigen expression on CD34+ human marrow

139. cells is induced by interferon gamma and tumor necrosis factor alpha and potentiates cytokine-mediated hematopoietic suppression in vitro. Blood 1995; 85:3183–3190.
140. Nagata S: Apoptosis by death factor. Cell 1997; 88:355–365.
141. Enari M, Hug H, Nagata S: Involvement of an ICE-like protease in Fas-mediated apoptosis. Nature 1995; 375:78–81.
142. Vaux DL, Strasser A: The molecular biology of apoptosis. Proc Natl Acad Sci USA 1996; 93:2239–2244.
143. Wang J, Otsuki T, Youssoufian H, et al: Overexpression of the Fanconi anemia group C gene (FAC) protects hematopoietic progenitors from death induced by Fas-mediated apoptosis. Cancer Res 1998; 58:3538–3541.
144. Haneline LS, Broxmeyer HE, Cooper S, et al: Multiple inhibitory cytokines induce deregulated progenitor growth and apoptosis in hematopoietic cells from Fac-/-mice. Blood 1998; 91:4092–4098.
145. Otsuki T, Nagakura S, Wang J, et al: Tumor necrosis factor-alpha and CD95 ligation suppress erythropoiesis in Fanconi anemia C gene knock-out mice. J Cell Physiol 1999; 179:79–86.
146. Liu JM, Poiley J, Devetten M, et al: The Fanconi anemia complementation group C gene (FAC) suppresses transformation of mutant fibroblasts by the SV40 virus. Biochem Biophys Res Commun 1996; 223:685–690.
147. Daneshbod-Skibba G, Martin J, Shahidi NT: Myeloid and erythroid colony growth in non-anaemic patients with Fanconi's anaemia. Br J Haematol 1980; 44:33–38.
148. Alter BP, Knobloch ME, Weinberg RS: Erythropoiesis in Fanconi's anemia. Blood 1991; 78:602–608.
149. Stark R, Thierry D, Richard P, et al: Long-term bone marrow culture in Fanconi's anaemia. Br J Haematol 1993; 83:554–559.
150. Bagby GCJ, Segal GM, Auerbach AD, et al: Constitutive and induced expression of hematopoietic growth factor genes by fibroblasts from children with Fanconi anemia. Exp Hematol 1993; 21:1419–1426.
151. Eaves CJ, Sutherland HJ, Cashman JD, et al: Regulation of primitive human hematopoietic cells in long-term marrow culture. Semin Hematol 1991; 28:126–131.
152. Sutherland HJ, Eaves CJ, Eaves AC, et al: Characterization and partial purification of human marrow cells capable of initiating long-term hematopoiesis in vitro. Blood 1989; 74:1563–1570.
153. Butturini A, Gale RP: Long-term bone marrow culture in persons with Fanconi anemia and bone marrow failure. Blood 1994; 83:336–339.
154. Carreau M, Gan OI, Liu L, et al: Bone marrow failure in the Fanconi anemia group C mouse model after DNA damage. Blood 1998; 91:2737–2744.
155. Gluckman E, Devergie A, Schaison G, et al: Bone marrow transplantation in Fanconi anaemia. Br J Haematol 1980; 45:557–564.
156. Gluckman E, Devergie A, Dutreix J: Radiosensitivity in Fanconi anaemia: Application to the conditioning regimen for bone marrow transplantation. Br J Haematol 1983; 54:431–440.
157. Gluckman E: Radiosensitivity in Fanconi anemia: Application to the conditioning for bone marrow transplantation. Radiother Oncol 1990; 18(suppl 1):88–93.
158. Gluckman E, Auerbach AD, Horowitz MM, et al: Bone marrow transplantation for Fanconi anemia. Blood 1995; 86:2856–2862.
159. Socié G, Henry-Amar M, Cosset JM, et al: Increased incidence of solid malignant tumors after bone marrow transplantation for severe aplastic anemia. Blood 1991; 78:277–279.
160. Deeg HJ, Socié G, Schoch G, et al: Malignancies after marrow transplantation for aplastic anemia and Fanconi anemia: A joint Seattle and Paris analysis of results in 700 patients. Blood 1996; 87:386–392.
161. Socié G, Devergie A, Girinski T, et al: Transplantation for Fanconi's anaemia: Long-term follow-up of fifty patients transplanted from a sibling donor after low-dose cyclophosphamide and thoraco-abdominal irradiation for conditioning. Br J Haematol 1998; 103:249–255.
162. Flowers ME, Zanis J, Pasquini R, et al: Marrow transplantation for Fanconi anaemia: Conditioning with reduced doses of cyclophosphamide without radiation. Br J Haematol 1996; 92:699–706.
163. Gluckman E, Broxmeyer HA, Auerbach AD, et al: Hematopoietic reconstitution in a patient with Fanconi's anemia by means of umbilical-cord blood from an HLA-identical sibling. N Engl J Med 1989; 321:1174–1178.
164. Kohli-Kumar M, Shahidi NT, Broxmeyer HE, et al: Haemopoietic stem/progenitor cell transplant in Fanconi anaemia using HLA-matched sibling umbilical cord blood cells. Br J Haematol 1993; 85:419–422.
165. Kurtzberg J, Laughlin M, Graham ML, et al: Placental blood as a source of hematopoietic stem cells for transplantation into unrelated recipients. N Engl J Med 1996; 335:157–166.
166. Davies SM, Khan S, Wagner JE, et al: Unrelated donor bone marrow transplantation for Fanconi anemia. Bone Marrow Transplant 1996; 17:43–47.
167. Shahidi NT, Diamond LK: Testosterone-induced remission in aplastic anemia. Am J Dis Child 1959; 98:293–302.
168. Sanchez-Medal L: The hemopoietic action of androstanes. Prog Hematol 1971; 7:111–136.
169. Shahidi NT, Crigler JFJ: Evaluation of growth and of endocrine systems in testosterone-corticosteroid–treated patients with aplastic anemia. J Pediatr 1967; 70:233–242.
170. Lyman SD, Seaberg M, Hanna R, et al: Plasma/serum levels of flt3 ligand are low in normal individuals and highly elevated in patients with Fanconi anemia and acquired aplastic anemia. Blood 1995; 86:4091–4096.
171. Guinan EC, Lopez KD, Huhn RD, et al: Evaluation of granulocyte-macrophage colony–stimu-

lating factor for treatment of pancytopenia in children with Fanconi anemia. J Pediatr 1994; 124:144–150.
172. Rackoff WR, Orazi A, Robinson CA, et al: Prolonged administration of granulocyte colony–stimulating factor (filgrastim) to patients with Fanconi anemia: A pilot study. Blood 1996; 88:1588–1593.
173. Walsh CE, Grompe M, Vanin E, et al: A functionally active retrovirus vector for gene therapy in Fanconi anemia group C. Blood 1994; 84:453–459.
174. Walsh CE, Nienhuis AW, Samulski RJ, et al: Phenotypic correction of Fanconi anemia in human hematopoietic cells with a recombinant adeno-associated virus vector. J Clin Invest 1994; 94:1440–1448.
175. Walsh CE, Mann MM, Emmons RV, et al: Transduction of CD34-enriched human peripheral and umbilical cord blood progenitors using a retroviral vector with the Fanconi anemia group C gene. J Invest Med 1995; 43:379–385.
176. Fu KL, Foe JR, Joenje H, et al: Functional correction of Fanconi anemia group A hematopoietic cells by retroviral gene transfer. Blood 1997; 90:3296–3303.
177. Brenner MK, Rill DR, Moen RC, et al: Gene-marking to trace origin of relapse after autologous bone-marrow transplantation. Lancet 1993; 341:85–86.
178. Brenner MK, Rill DR, Holladay MS, et al: Gene marking to determine whether autologous marrow infusion restores long-term haemopoiesis in cancer patients. Lancet 1993; 342:1134–1137.
179. Dunbar CE, Cortler-Fox M, O'Shaughnessy JA, et al: Retrovirally marked CD34-enriched peripheral blood and bone marrow cells contribute to long-term engraftment after autologous transplantation. Blood 1995; 85:3048–3057.
180. Abkowitz JL, Catlin SN, Guttorp P: Strategies for hematopoietic stem cell gene therapy: Insights from computer simulation studies. Blood 1997; 89:3192–3198.
181. Liu JM, Kim S, Walsh CE: Retroviral-mediated transduction of the Fanconi anemia C complementing (FACC) gene in two murine transplantation models. Blood Cells Mol Dis 1995; 21:56–63.
182. Lemoli RM, Tafuri A, Fortuna A, et al: Cycling status of CD34+ cells mobilized into peripheral blood of healthy donors by recombinant human granulocyte colony-stimulating factor. Blood 1997; 89:1189–1196.
183. Kiem HP, Andrews RG, Morris J, et al: Improved gene transfer into baboon marrow repopulating cells using recombinant human fibronectin fragment CH-296 in combination with interleukin-6, stem cell factor, FLT-3 ligand, and megakaryocyte growth and development factor. Blood 1998; 92:1878–1886.
184. Miyoshi H, Smith KA, Mosier DE, et al: Transduction of human CD34+ cells that mediate long-term engraftment of NOD/SCID mice by HIV vectors. Science 1999; 283:682–686.
185. Emerson SG: Ex vivo expansion of hematopoietic precursors, progenitors, and stem cells: The next generation of cellular therapeutics. Blood 1996; 87:3082–3088.
186. Hows JM, Chapple M, Marsh JC, et al: Bone marrow transplantation for Fanconi's anaemia: The Hammersmith experience 1977–89. Bone Marrow Transplant 1989; 4:629–634.
187. Kohli-Kumar M, Morris C, DeLaat C, et al: Bone marrow transplantation in Fanconi anemia using matched sibling donors. Blood 1994; 84:2050–2054.
188. Zanis-Neto J, Ribeiro RC, Medeiros C, et al: Bone marrow transplantation for patients with Fanconi anemia: A study of 24 cases from a single institution. Bone Marrow Transplant 1995; 15:293–298.

3

Myelodysplastic Syndromes

Cynthia E. Dunbar, M.D.
Yogen Saunthararajah, M.B.B.Ch.

The myelodysplastic syndromes (MDSs) are a group of disorders in which the clonal proliferation of a pluripotent hematopoietic cell results in a clinical syndrome characterized by cytopenias; qualitative (including morphologic) abnormalities of erythroid, myeloid, and megakaryocytic lineages; and a tendency to evolve into acute leukemia. This broad definition encompasses biologic, clinical, and pathologic criteria, although in the absence of specific cytogenetic abnormalities, confirmation of cellular clonality is not a practical option in most cases of MDS. Patients with MDS come to clinical attention due to incidentally discovered blood count depression or because of symptomatic cytopenias. The initial evaluation generally involves a careful examination of peripheral blood and bone marrow morphology, supplemented by more specialized testing such as cytogenetics of bone marrow cells, and exclusion of other potential causes such as folate or vitamin B_{12} deficienciy. It is most important to realize that the MDSs are a very heterogeneous group of diseases. The current deficits in our understanding of the underlying pathophysiology of these syndromes result in imperfect classification and prognostication systems. Laboratory and clinical research goals must be to identify common basic molecular defects determining the behavior of hematologic syndromes in groups of patients.

Clinical and possibly pathophysiologic overlap with aplastic anemia, myeloproliferative disorders, and acute leukemia (Fig. 3–1) can make the diagnosis of MDS difficult. Once a patient with MDS is identified, medical care may be complex, and many difficult treatment decisions must be made, often with little directly applicable clinical trial data to guide the physician and the patient. Evolving schemas for classification and prognosis, such as the French-American-British (FAB) system, and more recently the International Prognostic Scoring System (IPSS), do provide predictions regarding clinical course, but more rational approaches to treatment will require better understanding of the pathophysiology of these disorders.[1,2]

The only curative therapy for patients with true MDS is allogeneic stem cell transplantation, but for many patients this aggressive approach is either unavailable or inappropriate, and selecting among other options, including supportive care only, requires careful assessment of the individual patient over time. Newer therapies continue to be explored, including immunosuppression, antiapoptotis and differentiation agents, and high-dose chemotherapy, but these should in general be employed only in formal clinical trials, given the paucity of data showing clear efficacy. Over the next decade, it seems likely that advances in the understanding of the biology of MDS will make an impact on treatment, as has been the case in the approach to acute myelogenous leukemia (AML).

HISTORICAL PERSPECTIVE AND DEFINING CRITERIA

Two separate lines of clinical investigation converged at the current conceptual framework for understanding MDS. In the 1920s and 1930s, as the nutritional requirements for erythropoiesis came to be understood, patients with chronic anemia unresponsive to folate, vitamin B_{12}, and iron were described. Rhoads and Barker[3] reported 60 such patients with what they called refractory anemia (RA), one third of whom would have met the current diagnostic criteria for MDS. Further studies in the late 1950s drew attention to a form of

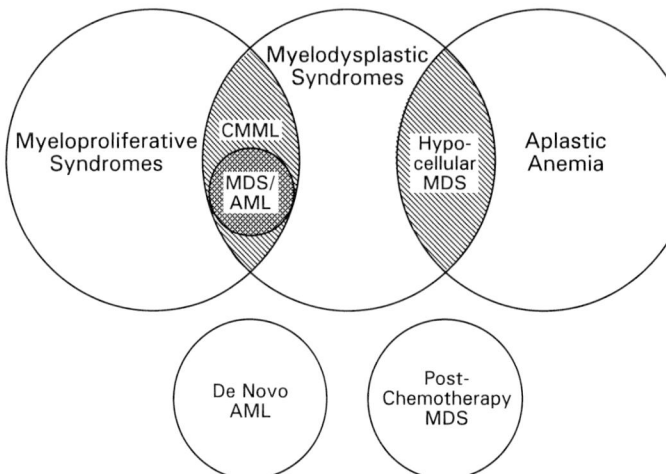

Figure 3–1 Schematic representation of current understanding of the relationships between bone marrow failure syndromes. There is both clinical and biologic overlap between the characteristics of some patients with myelodysplastic syndromes (MDS) and other bone marrow failure states, especially aplastic anemia and myeloproliferative syndromes. This may confuse diagnosis, but provides increasing insight into pathophysiology. CMML, chronic myelomonocytic leukemia; AML, acute myelogenous leukemia.

chronic RA in elderly patients, in which the bone marrow showed erythroid hyperplasia, some megaloblastic changes, and numerous coarse siderotic granules in many of the erythroblasts.[4] Around the same time, clinicians caring for patients with acute leukemias noted that some patients had a chronic phase of cytopenias preceding development of overt AML. In 1949, Hamilton-Patterson[5] described three patients with acute leukemia preceded by an anemic phase. Crosby et al.[6] reported in 1959 that of 26 patients with "sidero-achrestic anaemia," five subsequently developed a frankly leukemic or erythroleukemic state. Intrigued by these reports, and wanting to explore the possibility that what they called "refractory sideroblastic anemia" might be a phase in the development of erythroleukemia, Hayhoe and Quaglino[7] compared the cytochemical staining properties in these two conditions and found sufficient similarities to suggest a relationship between them. That the "primary refractory anemias," "refractory anemia with hyperplastic marrow," "chronic refractory anaemia with sideroblastic bone marrow," and other chronic cytopenias described by many authors might actually be identical to the preleukemic syndromes, variously designated as Di Guglielmo syndrome and erythremic myelosis, was first suggested by Dameshek in 1965[8] with Dreyfus et al.[9] and Saarni and Linman[10,11] later making this connection explicit.

French-American-British Classification

In 1975, the FAB cooperative group used the term "dysmyelopoietic" or "myelodysplastic" syndrome to distinguish this group of disorders, in which immediate cytotoxic therapy may not be indicated, from the acute leukemias.[12] In the initial proposal, two subtypes were defined: RA with excess of blasts (RAEB) and chronic myelomonocytic leukemia (CMML). In 1982, this same group published peripheral blood and bone marrow morphologic criteria for the diagnosis and classification of the MDSs into the five subtypes generally used today[1] (Table 3–1). The use of the FAB system has since become universal, and the understanding of what is meant by giving a patient the diagnosis of "MDS" much clearer. However, minimal diagnostic criteria for MDS remain a subject of some controversy.[13–15]

Rather than representing separate biologic entities, some FAB subtypes may more usefully be seen as stages in the evolution of MDS. For example, an initial diagnosis of CMML may need to be modified to RAEB based on a subsequent increase in the marrow blast percentage, or a patient originally meeting the criteria for RA may progress through RAEB, RAEB-T (RAEB in transformation), and finally into frank AML over the course of months to years. However, not all patients with RA, refractory anemia with ringed sideroblasts (RARS), or CMML necessarily evolve to RAEB, RAEB-T, or AML. Many cases of RARS do not progress. Clinicomorphologic criteria will undoubtedly remain important in the initial diagnosis of MDS, though biologic subtyping will eventually supersede a purely morphologic approach. Indeed, the advent of the IPSS in 1997, incorporating biologic criteria such as cytogenetics, is an important first step in this direction.[2]

EPIDEMIOLOGY

Based on the cases of MDS diagnosed in the catchment area of a district general hospital in

Bournemouth, England, the incidence of the MDS was estimated at 5.3 per 100,000 for the 50- to 59-year-old age group, rising to 15 per 100,000 for ages 60 to 69, 49 per 100,000 for ages 70 to 79, and 89 per 100,000 for ages 80 and above.[16] As many cases of MDS are diagnosed as a result of abnormalities noted only incidentally on blood counts, the true incidence of MDS may be higher: patients with asymptomatic and stable disease may never come to medical attention. The annual incidence in the United States is probably on the order of 10,000 to 20,000 newly diagnosed cases. The aging of the population will likely result in an overall increase in MDS in Europe, Japan, and North America. There is no clear evidence that the incidence of primary MDS is increasing, other than that due to changing demographics and populations skewed toward the elderly.[17] The rates in men and women are approximately even, though the 5q- syndrome has a female preponderance and CMML has a male bias. No ethnic associations have been identified.

MDS is not confined to the elderly, and children and young adults occasionally present with clinically similar syndromes.[18] In a large proportion of pediatric cases, a family history of hematologic disorders may be elicited. Series of familial MDS have been reported, although Fanconi's anemia has not always been rigorously excluded.[19, 20] Secondary or therapy-related MDS (t-MDS), following chemotherapy or radiation therapy for another disorder, tends to occur in younger patients, since they are the long-term survivors of disorders such as Hodgkin's disease or testicular cancer. As treatment of these malignancies improves, the incidence of t-MDS is expected to increase.

Data regarding epidemiologic associations of MDS have been limited to case descriptions, uncontrolled surveys, or small case-control studies. The strongest evidence involves benzene. Many reports have indicated an association between occupational exposure to benzene and AML.[21–23] A preceding MDS phase was common, with an average latency time from the start of exposure until diagnosis of 10 to 11 years. Contact with concentrations as low as 1 ppm for prolonged periods were believed to be possibly significant. There are indications that use of other organic solvents may also increase the risk of MDS and AML: ammonia and diesel fuel and other petrochemicals have been implicated.[24, 25] In a case-control study of 116 Japanese MDS patients, a significant correlation with alcohol consumption was found.[26] Associations with cigarette smoking, use of hair dye products, and exposure to organic solvents also were noted but did not achieve statistical significance.

Therapy-Related Myelodysplastic Syndromes

The only unequivocal risk factor for MDS is prior exposure to chemotherapy or radiation. As many as 15% of MDS patients in large series have a

TABLE 3–1 The French-American-British (FAB) Classification of the Myelodysplastic Syndromes

Abbreviation	Category	Peripheral Blood		Bone Marrow
RA	Refractory anemia*	Blasts ≤ 1% Monocytes ≤ 1 × 10⁹/L	and	Blasts < 5% Ringed sideroblasts ≤ 15% of erythroblasts
RARS	Refractory anemia* with ringed sideroblasts	Blasts ≤ 1% Monocytes ≤ 1 × 10⁹/L	and	Blasts < 5% Ringed sideroblasts > 15% of erythroblasts
RAEB	Refractory anemia* with excess blasts	Monocytes ≤ 1 × 10⁹/L, blasts > 1% Blasts < 5%	or and	Blasts ≥ 5% Blasts ≤ 20%
RAEB-T	Refractory anemia* with excess blasts in transformation	Blasts ≥ 5% or Auer rods in blasts		Blasts > 20% but < 30%, or Auer rods in any blasts
CMML	Chronic myelomonocytic leukemia	Blasts < 5% Monocytes > 1 × 10⁹/L Granulocytes often increased		Blasts ≤ 20% Promonocytes increased

*Despite "anemia" in the title, any cytopenia with dysplastic marrow changes would qualify.

history of cytotoxic drug or radiation treatments.[27] The association between MDS and alkylating agents is a strong one, increasing nonlinearly with the duration and intensity of treatment. Up to 13% of patients treated with alkylating agents for Hodgkin's disease developed t-MDS or therapy-related AML (t-AML) within 10 years of therapy; the mean time to symptomatic presentation was 48 to 68 months.[28] The risk of developing t-MDS or t-AML does not appear to extend more than 10 years beyond completion of therapy for Hodgkin's disease. MDS following epipodophyllotoxins, anthracyclines, and radiation therapy has also been described, although the potential for radiation therapy alone to result in an increased risk of t-MDS or t-AML is controversial.[29, 30] Recent reports have also implicated purine analogues and hydroxyurea.[31, 32] No other type of chemotherapy appears, however, to result in risks as high as these seen with either repeated cycles or chronic administration of alkylating agents. Treatment of essential thrombocythemia with hydroxyurea alone was associated with a leukemic or t-MDS culmulative risk of approximately 4%. Patients undergoing autologous transplantation for lymphoma, multiple myeloma, or other malignancy also have been reported to be at risk for t-MDS or t-AML, at rates as high as 10% to 15% in some studies.[33] Standard chemotherapy given prior to cell harvesting and transplantation appears to determine risk, instead of the conditioning drugs or the transplant itself. Thus, patients being considered as candidates for autologous transplantation should have their exposure to alkylating agents minimized.

t-MDS tends to be a much more aggressive disease than primary or idiopathic MDS, justifying a separate classification category.[29] Proper classification is particularly critical in the design and analysis of clinical trials. The progression from t-MDS to t-AML is generally so rapid that these patients are often grouped together in the literature, a lumping that is justified, especially

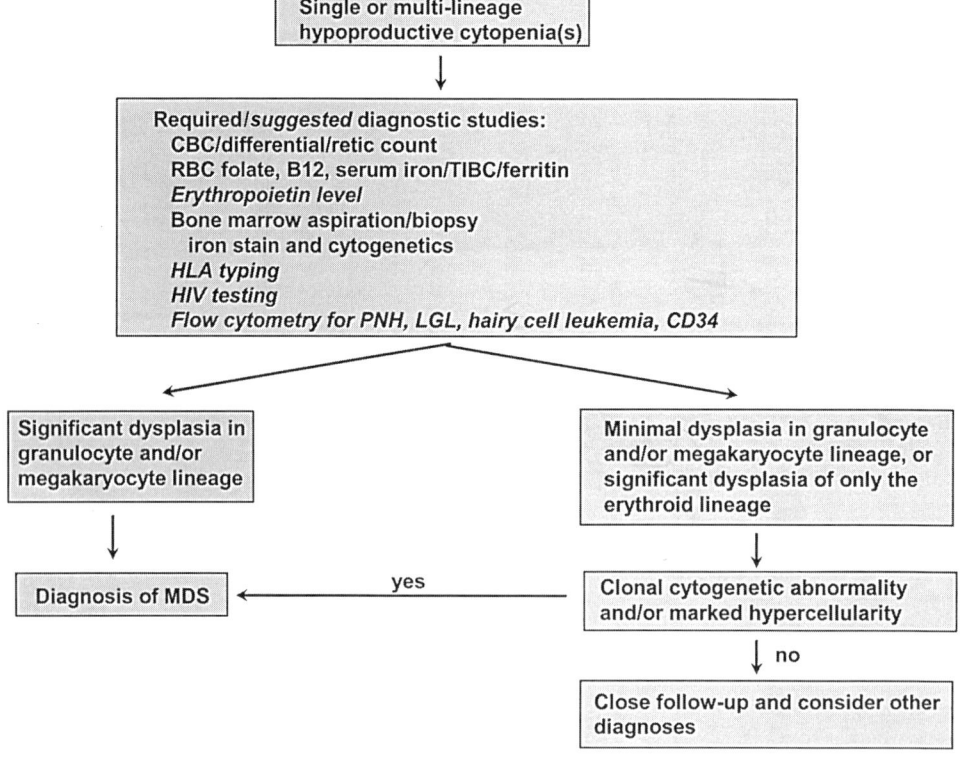

Figure 3–2 Initial diagnostic approach to a patient with possible myelodysplastic syndrome. Tests given in italics may not be appropriate for every patient; those given in regular type should always be performed when MDS is suspected. CBC, complete blood count; retic, reticulocyte; RBC, red blood cell, TIBC, total iron-binding capacity; HIV, human immunodeficiency virus; PNH, paroxysmal nocturnal hemoglobinuria; LGL, large granular lymphocytic disease.

since cytogenetic abnormalities such as −5 and −7 are detected both in patients first diagnosed with t-MDS and initially with t-AML.[34]

CLINICAL PRESENTATION AND SUGGESTED DIAGNOSTIC STUDIES

Symptoms and Signs

The symptoms and signs in MDS result primarily from cytopenias and abnormal hematologic cell function, although currently many patients with MDS are diagnosed during an asymptomatic phase, after performance of a complete blood count during health screening. The most common symptoms relate to anemia, such as fatigue and dyspnea, but bleeding complaints are also frequent.[27, 35] Infections are unusual at presentation. Occasionally patients complain of diffuse arthralgia or intermittent fever without documented infection. Weight loss or other B-type symptoms are rare and generally indicate disease progression or leukemic transformation.

There are few specific findings on physical examination: splenomegaly is found in about 20%, most often in patients with CMML, and is sometimes accompanied by hepatomegaly and lymphadenopathy. The skin may show petechiae, or rarely unusual infiltrative rashes, such as neutrophilic dermatosis (Sweet's syndrome) or granulocytic sarcoma (leukemia cutis).[36]

Initial Evaluation and Differential Diagnosis

A suggested algorithm for the initial evaluation of a cytopenic patient with possible MDS is given in Figure 3–2, and results of specific analyses are discussed below. Few if any pathognomonic features of MDS exist. The process of diagnosis requires two approaches. First, other primary hematologic conditions must be excluded (Table 3–2), especially aplastic anemia, myeloproliferative disorders, nutritional deficiencies, de novo leukemia, and systemic diseases such as systemic lupus erythematosis or human immunodeficiency virus type 1 (HIV-1) infection, with hematologic manifestations that may be similar to MDS. Second, specific morphologic features of dysplasia in the peripheral blood and bone marrow are required to support the diagnosis of MDS. Recognizing significant dysplasia involves qualitative and often subjective judgments. The presence of clonal marrow cytogenetic abnormalities is the single most useful test in establishing the diagnosis of MDS, but these are only present in 50% to 70% of patients. For a young patient outside the typical age range for MDS, a vigorous search for other, rare hematologic disorders, including congenital marrow failure syndromes or sideroblastic anemias, is appropriate. Review of prior blood counts can be very useful in this regard: anemia (even if mild) present since childhood is very unlikely to be due to acquired MDS. When the marrow is hypoplastic, differentiation from aplastic anemia can be extremely difficult (see below). Longitudinal observation can prove helpful in cases that do not at first meet strict criteria for diagnosis, and it

TABLE 3–2 Disorders to Be Considered as Causes of Hypoproductive Cytopenias Before Diagnosing Myelodysplastic Syndromes

Hematologic conditions
  Congenital
    Hereditary sideroblastic anemia
    Congenital dyserythropoietic anemia
    Fanconi's anemia
    Diamond-Blackfan syndrome
    Shwachman syndrome
    Kostmann's syndrome
  Nutritional
    Vitamin B_{12} deficiency
    Folate deficiency
    Iron deficiency
  Aplastic anemia
  Paroxysmal nocturnal hemoglobinuria
  Systemic mastocytosis
  Hairy cell leukemia
  Large granular lymphocyte disease
  Myeloproliferative syndromes
    Idiopathic myelofibrosis
    Polycythemia vera (spent phase)
    Chronic myelogenous leukemia
    Essential thrombocytosis (advanced)

Nonhematologic conditions
  Toxins
    Alcohol
    Postchemotherapy or radiation
    Medications
  Chronic diseases
    Renal failure
    Collagen-vascular diseases
    Chronic infections
  Viral infections
    Parvovirus B19
    Cytomegalovirus
    Human immunodeficiency virus
  Malignancies
    Marrow infiltration
    Paraneoplastic syndrome

is important not to label a patient with a diagnosis as intimidating as "preleukemia" or MDS without firm data. Many of the tests useful in diagnosis, most notably cytogenetics, are also important for determining the prognosis. MDS is extremely heterogeneous, and accurate assessment is critical for making treatment decisions (see below).

Blood Chemistry Tests

Standard chemical analyses of metabolic, renal, and hepatic function may show nonspecific abnormalities, but none are clinically relevant or diagnostic. Assessment of iron is of more importance. Patients with MDS, especially RARS, may have increased total body iron stores at presentation, even without or with only minimal prior transfusions.[37] This phenomenon may partly be due to earlier inappropriate empirical treatment of anemia with iron. In addition, patients with a large but ineffective erythroid compartment in the marrow can inappropriately increase intestinal iron absorption.[38] The contribution of homozygous or especially heterozygous mutated hemochromatosis genes is unknown but under active investigation given the very high prevalence of these mutations in some populations. Accurate assessment of iron status at the time of diagnosis and throughout the course of the disease is important in MDS, since so many patients ultimately require transfusion therapy. Early institution of chelation therapy may be necessary in low-risk MDS to prevent morbidity and mortality from iron overload. Determination of folate and vitamin B_{12} levels is performed to exclude vitamin deficiencies as causative of cytopenias.

Hematologic Abnormalities

Anemia is present in most patients, in 45% to 93% of cases in large studies, but anemia as an isolated cytopenia has been reported in only 30% to 35% of MDS. More than half of MDS patients have an absolute neutrophil counts (ANC) of less than 2500/μL, and 20% to 35% have more severe neutropenia with counts less than 1000 to 1500/μL.[27, 35, 39] Only about 10% of patients present with evidence of active infection.[40] Those at highest risk have an ANC of less than 1000/μL, although neutrophil or more global immunodeficiencies result in infections even in those with seemingly adequate neutrophil counts. Bacterial infections are most common; infections usually associated with T cell deficiencies, such as viral or protozoal infections, are rare. Except in patients with CMML, the total leukocyte count is rarely increased. Twenty-five percent to 50% of patients have thrombocytopenia, but only in about 5% are platelets the only lineage affected.[39, 41] In rare cases, primarily in the 5q- syndrome, the platelet count may be increased. Platelets are often dysfunctional, whatever their numbers, as evidenced by abnormal platelet aggregation studies, prolonged bleeding time, and a clinical bleeding tendency despite seemingly adequate levels.[42]

Peripheral Blood Morphology

Abnormalities of peripheral blood morphology are a hallmark of MDS[1, 39] (Table 3–3). Macrocytosis is very common, as is anisopoikilocytosis. Reticulocytosis is rare: MDS patients generally have ineffective erythropoiesis and inappropriately low reticulocyte counts, but occasional patients develop a hemolytic component to their anemia and may show polychromasia on the peripheral smear.[43, 44] Patients with MDS and increased marrow reticulin can have circulating teardrop cells, erythrocyte fragments, and nucleated red blood cells (RBCs), but an overwhelming preponderance of these cells suggests an underlying diagnosis of myelofibrosis (see Chapter 5). Giant platelets, sometimes approaching the size of a lymphocyte, are frequent in MDS, and they may also be hypogranulated.[45] The most striking abnormalities on the peripheral smear are generally in the myeloid lineage: hypogranulated neutrophils with very abnormal nuclei, such as Pelger-Huët anomalies and hypo- or hypersegmentation. Even in the absence of circulating myeloblasts, immature myeloid cells may be seen, but these are frequent mainly in CMML. A marked left shift in the myeloid series may point to another diagnosis.

Ham's test traditionally was indicated to rule out paroxysmal nocturnal hemoglobinuria (PNH) as an alternative or coexisting diagnosis (see Chapter 4). Recently, flow cytometric evaluation of glycosylphosphatidylinositol (GPI)-linked cell surface proteins has been found to be more sensitive, specific, and reproducible than Ham's test. A high percentage of MDS patients have been reported to have PNH-like cells in their ciruclation.[46]

Bone Marrow Examination

Typical defining dysplastic features seen in MDS marrow are listed in Table 3–3 and examples are illustrated in Plate 4.[1, 47] Much can be learned from standard morphologic review of Wright's-stained aspirate smears. The FAB did not specify the proportion of examined cells that need to be dysplastic in order to establish a diagnosis of dysplasia; most authors settle for 10%. The FAB did

TABLE 3–3 Dysplastic Features of Peripheral Blood and Marrow Cells

Erythroid lineage
Bone marrow
   Megaloblastoid changes
   Nuclear abnormalities, including multinucleated forms
   Ringed sideroblasts
Peripheral blood
   Polychromasia

Platelet lineage
Bone marrow
   Micromegakaryocytes
   Abnormal megakaryocyte nuclei: single nuclei or few small, round separated nuclei
Peripheral blood
   Giant platelets
   Agranular platelets

Granulocyte lineage
Bone marrow
   Megaloblastoid changes
   Left shift, ± increased myeloblasts (5%–30%)
   Abnormal localization of immature precursors
   Hypogranulated promyelocytes (sparse azurophilic granules)
   Hypogranulated myelocytes, metamyelocytes, and bands (secondary granules)
Peripheral blood
   Circulating myeloblasts
   Pelger-Huët-type nuclear abnormalities
   Hypogranulation of neutrophils and eosinophils
   Ring nuclei of eosinophils

Monocyte lineage
Bone marrow
   Increased monoblasts
   Abnormal nuclei of monoblasts and monocytes: elongated shapes
   Giant forms
   Hemophagocytosis
   Abnormal granulation, with persistence of azurophilic granules
Peripheral blood
   Increased monocytes and monoblasts

recommend examining 10 megakaryocytes and counting at least 500 cells to establish the differential count used for MDS classification. Peroxidase or Sudan black B stains can be used to confirm the myeloid origin of blasts, but peroxidase levels can be anomalously decreased in cells from MDS patients.[48] Dyserythropoiesis can be seen in a number of other disorders, including aplastic anemia and congenital sideroblastic anemia. The presence of Auer rods indicates de novo AML. Other bone marrow studies include immunohistochemistry to identify micromegakaryocytes and a reticulin stain, especially of a hypoplastic marrow, in which positive studies favor a diagnosis of hypoplastic MDS over aplastic anemia.[48] Marrow fibrosis may be prominent in t-MDS.

Cytogenetic Analysis

The presence of clonal cytogenetic abnormalities in marrow cells from MDS patients has yielded important clues to pathophysiology, and chromosomal analysis may be the single most useful test to aid in diagnosis. The presence or absence of specific abnormalities has also been found to have powerful prognostic significance (see below).[2] A cytopenic patient whose low blood counts do not have an immediately apparent cause, such as vitamin deficiency, should have cytogenetic analysis performed on the initial diagnostic marrow aspiration, unless the contribution of a chronic disease such as rheumatoid arthritis is obvious or strongly suspected. Of patients with primary MDS, 30% to 79% have been reported to have detectable, clonal cytogenetic abnormalities, with the variability due to whether only patients studied at diagnosis are included and the use of high-resolution banding techniques.[49, 50] In general, informative analyses must involve at least 10 metaphases, and to be labeled "clonal" the same abnormality must be present in at least two metaphases. The performance of cytogenetics requires aspiration of adequate numbers of immature and thus dividing cells from the marrow; insufficient cells may make chromosome studies unsuccessful in patients with fibrosis or marked marrow hypocellularity. Patients with t-MDS have a higher incidence of abnormalities, 80% to 100% in some studies, and they often show multiple abnormalities within a single clone.[51] Even patients with initially normal cytogenetics may acquire new abnormalities with disease progression.[52]

Almost every chromosome has been reported to be affected in MDS, although most common are loss (less frequently gain) of segments of chromosomes 5, 7–9, 11, 12, and 18–21.[34] Translocations such as t(15;17), t(8;21), inv(16), t(16;16), t(9;11), t(11;17), t(6;9), t(1;22), and t(8;16) are typical of de novo AML rather than MDS, and they carry different prognostic and therapeutic implications in these two diseases.

Flow Cytometry

Flow cytometry is an alternative method of determining myeloblast percentage, using CD45 side scatter plot or by measuring the number of CD34+ cells.[53] However, it is important to realize that all current classifications and prognostic scoring systems are based on blast percentage as estimated morphologically, and the relationship between morphologic and flow cytometric blast determinations has not been formally defined. The presence of aberrant maturation also can make flow enumeration of cells at various stages of development very difficult. Conversely, the presence of dysplasia can be supported by the observation of cells in various lineages with aberrant antigen expression. Flow cytometry can also be used to diagnose PNH by revealing GPI-linked protein deficiencies on neutrophil and RBC lineages (see Chapter 4). In general, flow cytometry, while currently a research technique, eventually will supplant conventional morphologic methods for the diagnosis and evaluation of MDS.

SPECIFIC SYNDROMES, MDS VARIANTS, AND DIAGNOSTIC DIFFICULTIES

Hypoplastic Myelodysplastic Syndromes

The original FAB criteria required at least a normocellular marrow for the diagnosis of MDS. Many subsequent observations indicated the artificiality of such distinctions.[35, 54–56] First, stereotypic clonal cytogenetic abnormalities, such as 5q-syndrome, have been detected in patients with peripheral cytopenias and hematopoietic cell dysplasia but frankly hypocellular marrows. Second, even in patients who have hypocellular bone marrows, the presence of marked dysplasia of more than one lineage, especially of micromegakaryocytes, was associated with a high risk of progression to AML, as compared to patients with hypocellular marrows but no dysplasia. Third, laboratory and clinical studies have increasingly linked aplastic anemia and MDS as pathophysiologically related (see below). Patients with aplastic anemia treated with immunosuppression have a risk of 10% to 30% of developing late clonal hematopoiesis, including PNH, MDS, and AML.[57–60] Conversely, patients with both hypo- and hypercellular MDS have been reported to respond to antithymocyte globulin (ATG) or cyclosporine (CSA), the same immunosuppressive agents used to treat aplastic anemia.[61–63] There may be a crucial role for the immune system in the suppression of marrow function in both syndromes.[64] Nonetheless, an effort to distinguish MDS from aplastic anemia is important for prognosis and treatment decisions[14] (Table 3–4).

MDS With Fibrosis

The finding of marrow fibrosis in a cytopenic patient does not necessarily establish the diagnosis of idiopathic myelofibrosis.[65, 66] Some studies show that up to 25% of MDS patients have increased marrow reticulin. If trilineage dysplasia or typical cytogenetic abnormalities are also present there is less difficulty in diagnosis. The distinction from classic myelofibrosis has prognostic implications. It may also be difficult to distinguish fibrotic MDS from acute megakaryocytic leukemia, especially if the marrow is inaspirable and morphologic analysis is difficult; megakaryocytic blasts can be identified by staining marrow biopsies for lineage-specific antigens such as the integrin gpIIb/IIIa.[48]

Childhood MDS

Pediatric acquired MDS is rare, and the clinical course is usually more aggressive in children than for corresponding FAB categories in adults.[18] Congenital syndromes such as Fanconi's anemia, neurofibromatosis, Down syndrome, or familial monosomy 7 must be considered and excluded.

TABLE 3–4 Clues to Help Distinguish Hypocellular Myelodysplastic Syndrome (MDS) From Aplastic Anemia

Hypocellular MDS	Aplastic Anemia	Both
Easily identified megakaryocytes	Absent or rare megakaryocytes	Megaloblastic erythroid precursors
Dysplastic megakaryocytes	Normal megakaryocyte morphology	PNH-type cells in marrow or blood
Left shift in myeloid lineage	Reduced myeloid precursors	
Clonal cytogenetic abnormalities	Increased lymphocytes in marrow	
Older adults	Increased mast cells in marrow	
Gradual onset	Children and young adults	
	Sudden onset	

PNH, paroxysmal nocturnal hemoglobinuria.

Because progression of childhood MDS to acute leukemia is frequent and rapid, aggressive therapies such as bone marrow transplantation (BMT) should be considered early after diagnosis. One exception may be MDS-AML in patients with Down syndrome; these leukemias are very responsive to conventional antileukemic chemotherapy, with 4-year survival rates of over 80%.[67]

Dysplasia in Patients with HIV Marrow Disease

Many patients who are infected with HIV-1 develop blood count abnormalities and examination of the marrow can show sometimes quite striking dysplastic morphology of hematopoietic cells.[68, 69] However, such patients should not be labeled as having MDS, or included in clinical trials or natural history studies of MDS. There is no evidence to date that these patients have clonal hematopoiesis, nor are they at risk of developing AML. The cytopenias and dysplasia are most likely results of a combination of factors, including infections, drug effects, and immune dysregulation. Patients with HIV lymphoma who are treated with cytotoxic chemotherapy are, of course, at risk for t-MDS.

Chronic Myelomonocytic Leukemia

The appropriateness of the inclusion of CMML in the larger category of MDS, rather than its consideration as a unique syndrome with more myeloproliferative characteristics, has been debated.[70] Indeed, the recent IPSS excluded CMML patients with high WBC.[2] There are few pathophysiologic or biologic clues to help in more precise classification. However, the morphologic features of marked trilineage dysplasia and cytopenias of all lineages, despite absolute monocytosis, have argued for inclusion of CMML in MDS.[71] The clinical course is predicted by the marrow blast percentage, also typical of MDS in general.[72] Further distinction depends on better understanding of the underlying pathophysiology. Difficulties are most often encountered in distinguishing between CMML, chronic myelogenous leukemia (CML), and atypical CML (a myeloproliferative syndrome lacking the bcr/abl translocation and without a propensity to blast crisis), but careful attention to morphology and cytogenetic analysis usually resolve the diagnosis.[73]

5q- Syndrome

Patients with 5q- syndrome and no prior chemotherapy have a stereotypic clinical syndrome.[74, 75] Most patients are female; they present with anemia, accompanied by normal leukocyte counts and normal or even elevated platelet numbers. The marrow generally does not show increased myeloblasts but rather markedly dysplastic megakaryocytes, including micromegakaryocytes or cells with very separated nuclei. Patients with 5q- syndrome have a good prognosis, with slow progression and only rare transformation to acute leukemia.

Therapy-Related Myelodysplastic Syndrome

As noted in the epidemiology section above, patients with MDS who are diagnosed subsequent to treatment with cytotoxic chemotherapy, chemo- and radiation therapy, or even radiation alone have a distinct syndrome that should not be grouped with idiopathic primary MDS in either clinical studies or laboratory investigations.[76] FAB classification and prognostic systems derived from primary MDS data do not apply to t-MDS. The prognosis, even for patients seeming to meet criteria for the more favorable subgroups RARS or RA, is uniformly grim, with almost invariable rapid progression to severe cytopenias or leukemic transformation.[29] Patients with complex cytogenetic abnormalities or monosomy 7 do particularly poorly. Allogeneic transplantation should be considered immediately if a donor is available, but even with this intervention survival is low owing to high transplant-related mortality, compounded by prior chemotherapy-related organ damage and frequent relapse.[77, 78]

PATHOPHYSIOLOGY

The underlying pathophysiology and ultimately the molecular basis of MDS remain elusive. Among the obstacles to identifying causal factors are the heterogeneous nature of the disease and the difficulty of distinguishing between inciting events that produce the MDS phenotype and secondary manifestations of disordered hematopoietic cell maturation. Any model must account for the preponderance of clonal hematopoiesis in multiple lineages, in most cases without evidence for simply accelerated proliferation or "overgrowth" of an abnormal clone, as exists in the myeloproliferative syndromes. Suppression of normal hematopoiesis also must be explained. Most traditional models have postulated a multistep mechanism in which genetic alterations confer on the abnormal clone and its progeny survival advantages, which progressively accumulate and may eventually lead to full-blown leukemic transformation.[79–81] An alternative and possibly complementary model has recently been proposed, based on the association of MDS with aplastic anemia and the differences between MDS and de novo AML (see below).[63, 64, 82]

Clonality

A fundamental property of malignancy is clonal and dysregulated proliferation that presumably results from acquired genetic events which confer a proliferative or survival advantage to the progeny of the initially affected cell. As noted above, clonal cytogenetic abnormalities are common on analysis of marrow metaphases from MDS patients, but they may represent relatively late events in pathogenesis. Chromosome analysis is relatively crude, and gross cytogenetic alterations may occur due to general chromosomal instability, long after clonal hematopoiesis has been established. Thus other research laboratory techniques have been utilized to study clonality.[83]

X-inactivation analysis in somatic cells of females has proved informative. Early in embryogenesis, one of the two X chromosomes in each cell of a female embryo is randomly inactivated through a process termed lyonization. After lyonization, every progeny cell maintains the same X-inactivation pattern, presumably to prevent overexpression of X chromosome genes in females. After birth, each tissue or cell lineage should on average have approximately equal numbers of cells containing either an active maternally derived or paternally derived X chromosome. The paternal vs. maternal derivation of a locus can be defined using known common genetic allelic markers, and the inactive compared with the active X chromosome by study of the expression of one of these loci or analysis of the methylation patterns of genes, which differ between the active and inactive chromosome.[84, 85]

The first evidence for clonal hematopoiesis using X chromosome inactivation in MDS was obtained by isozyme analysis of glucose-6-phosphate dehydrogenase (G6PD)–heterozygous females.[83] Early reports showed that granulocytes, erythrocytes, platelets, and B and even T lymphocytes expressed a single dominant G6PD isoenzyme and were thus monoclonal in origin.[86, 87] More recently, molecular analyses of other loci such as the androgen receptor gene have allowed investigation of clonality in much larger numbers of women with MDS.[88] By using one or more of these markers, over 90% of women can be informative: in the majority of such patients, clonal origin of granulocytes and erythroid precursors has been confirmed.[89, 90] Clonality of B lymphocytes has been more variable, and T lymphocytes have generally not been found to be part of the clone; whether lymphocytes are indeed affected remains controversial.[91–95] Unlike CML, progression to acute lymphocytic leukemia (ALL) does not occur in MDS, supporting the hypothesis that MDS is an abnormality of myeloid but not lymphoid progenitor cells. Several studies have detected significant numbers of residual polyclonal immature cells in MDS marrow, suggesting that normal hematopoiesis is not destroyed but suppressed, a finding with important pathophysiologic and therapeutic implications in this disease.[93, 96, 97] Clonality appears to be an early event in MDS, and patients destined to develop t-MDS may manifest clonal hematopoiesis or cytogenetic abnormalities long before any morphologic or hematologic changes.[98–100]

However, there are a number of important caveats to consider when assessing X-inactivation studies of patients with MDS.[84] First, with increasing age a significant number of normal persons display monoclonal or oligoclonal hematopoiesis, in the absence of cytopenias or other signs of MDS.[101, 102] These patients might have very-early-stage MDS, perhaps analogous to monoclonal gammopathy of uncertain significance as related to multiple myeloma. Alternatively, the same finding might result from a gene on one X chromosome that gives a slight advantage to progeny cells, as has been reported for a cat model.[103] Second, some normal females have very skewed clonality patterns in all their tissues from birth, presumably resulting from very early lyonization or some inherited genetic cause.[84] Skewed lyonization of normal tissues can be excluded by concurrent analysis of skin fibroblasts or other nonhematopoietic tissue, but many studies omit this important control. Third, the finding of residual polyclonal hematopoiesis at quite significant levels in some patients with unequivocal morphologic and clinical MDS, and even clonal cytogenetic abnormalities in some metaphases, requires explanation in any pathophysiologic model.[93, 96]

Cytogenetic Clues

As discussed above, about half of patients with primary MDS and almost all patients with t-MDS have cytogenetic abnormalities. These chromosomal aberrations can be acquired or evolve as disease progresses over time, and they may be more relevant to the evolution toward leukemia than to the initial MDS phenotype.[52] The nature of the cytogenetic abnormalities in MDS suggests a number of hypotheses regarding pathogenesis.[104] Clonal somatic acquired abnormalities developing over time is inconsistent with genetic changes resulting in altered growth and survival of hematopoietic cells.[105] In many types of de novo AML, specific balanced chromosomal translocations have been identified, and the abnormal fusion gene product has been implicated in leukoneogenesis. In contrast, the most common abnormalities in MDS are either full or partial chromosomal deletions: loss of a tumor suppressor gene on the deleted chromosome combined with a microdeletion or an inactivating mutation on the other allele could result in a malignant phenotype.[106] However, this hypothesis has not yet been supported by firm data in MDS, due partly to the difficulty of identifying individual putative tumor suppressor genes within the huge deleted areas.

Deletions of chromosomes 5 and 7 have been the focus of investigation because of their high incidence in MDS. As described above, the clinically stereotypic 5q- syndrome is characterized by diminished erythroid activity, thrombocytosis, and abnormal megakaryocytic maturation.[75, 107] Many genes with presumed roles in hematopoiesis are localized on 5q, including those for some cytokine receptors, cytokines themselves, and potential tumor suppressors. However, some of these genes lie outside the now well-defined critical region that is deleted uniformly in all patients with 5q- syndrome (5q31–5q33).[108, 109] Redundancy in cytokine function indicates the absence of one or both cytokine gene or receptor alleles unlikely to result in an MDS phenotype, and loss of heterozygosity has not been unequivocally demonstrated for any potential tumor suppressor gene.[110] Interferon regulatory factor 1 (IRF-1) lies within the deleted region in some patients and was implicated in early studies in patients with 5q- and either primary or secondary MDS or AML.[111] Since the gene product is a transcription factor acting on interferon-α (IFN-α), tumor necrosis factor-α (TNF-α), the major histocompatibility complex, and other growth-regulatory genes, it was an exciting candidate if loss of heterozygosity could be confirmed.[112] However, gene dosage experiments have shown no or only hemizygous loss of IRF-1 in 12 5q- patients.[113] Even less is known about critical deleted regions on chromosome 7, although the areas around 7q22 or 7q32–34 deserve examination as critical areas because of their common loss in most patients with chromosome 7 abnormalities.[114]

There has been more progress in identifying involved genes in the rarer MDS translocations. In de novo AML, the gene *MLL* is involved in translocations involving 11q23, and this region has been implicated in patients with MDS or AML following exposure to topoisomerase inhibitors. In t(11;16)(q23;p13) *MLL* is joined to the transcriptional coactivator CREB binding protein (CBP): widespread gene dysregulation might be expected.[115, 116] The t(3;21)(q26;q22) translocation has been found in patients with t-MDS or t-AML and normal or elevated platelet counts, marked hyperplasia and dysplasia of megakaryocytes, and very short survival.[117] The *AML1* gene on chromosome 21 is joined to one or several genes on chromosome 3.[118] The abnormality (5;12)(q31;p12) is associated with the rare syndrome of CMML with eosinophilia, and this translocation results in part of the gene encoding the platelet-derived growth factor (PDGF) receptor β fusing to the *TEL* transcription factor gene.[119, 120] This fusion gene can cause leukemia in mice. Specific inhibitors of the PDGF receptor kinase are being studied as potential therapies based on identification of this molecular defect.

Mutations in Oncogenes and Tumor Suppressor Genes

Activating point mutations in oncogenes such as *ras* or dominant negative mutations in tumor suppressor genes such as the adenomatous polyposis coli (*APC*), retinoblastoma (*RB*), or *p53* in germ line cells or somatic tissues have been implicated in familial cancer syndromes, sporadic human solid tumors, and in many animal models of carcinogenesis. Similar analyses have provided only limited insights into MDS.[121] Thirty percent to 40% of MDS patients were reported in early studies to have activating mutations of the oncogene *ras*, but more recent investigations have reported a much lower rate.[122–125] The frequency of these abnormalities increases with advanced disease and N-*ras* mutations absent at diagnosis have appeared later.[126, 127] While *ras* mutations alone are likely neither sufficient nor necessary for the MDS phenotype, they nonetheless may contribute as early or late pathogenic events.

Mutations of other oncogenes or of dominant negative tumor suppressor genes have also been investigated. Abnormalities of the *p53* gene have been observed infrequently.[128] Loss of the normal *NF1* (neurofibromatosis) allele is associated with an MDS, AML, or myeloproliferative disease in patients with inherited abnormalities of this gene, but *NF1* mutations were not detected in adults with acquired MDS.[129] The significance of mutation screening is clouded by the polymerase chain reaction (PCR) technology used, as this method of mutation analysis is prone to false-positive results and is difficult to perform quantitatively: even the presence of a *ras* mutation in a very small fraction of marrow cells would score the patient as "positive," even if there is no evidence that the mutation resulted in a selective advantage for the cells carrying it. Point mutations in almost every growth-regulatory gene examined may reflect overall genetic instability of the MDS clone, not causality.

Apoptosis

As in almost all diseases involving either abnormal survival or increased proliferation of cells, abnormalities in apoptosis have been pursued in patients with MDS. The data are conflicting to date. Moderate to marked increases in the overall number of apoptotic cells in MDS marrow compared to controls has been reported; however, often the entire marrow cell population has been tested, and it is unclear which cells, mature or immature, normal or part of the affected clone, are undergoing programmed cell death.[130–133] Conversely, purified primitive CD34 cells from patients with MDS have been shown to be more resistant to Fas-mediated apoptosis than are normal CD34 cells.[134] This discrepancy could be explained by a model in which primitive cells of the MDS clone are relatively resistant to apoptotic signals, conferring a survival advantage on their progeny. Residual normal primitive cells would suffer either indirectly by competition with the MDS apoptosis-resistant clone or directly by death signals secreted or presented by the MDS clone. Possibly a hyperactive immune response against hematopoietic cells could result in preferential survival of the abnormal cells (see below). An overall increased level of apoptosis also could be explained by disordered maturation of lineage-committed cells, rendering them more susceptible to apoptosis as they differentiate.[135]

The Immune Milieu

There is both clinical and experimental evidence for an abnormal immune milieu in MDS, despite the probable lack of clonal involvement of the T cell and even B cell lineage in most patients.[136] Clinical responses to immunomodulating therapies such as antithymocyte (ATG) and cyclosporine (see below) implicate immune mechanisms, at least in part, in the origin of MDS cytopenias. Lymphocytes can release cytokines such as TNF-α with dual effects on hematopoietic cells, stimulating immature CD34 cells to proliferate while inducing apoptosis of more mature cells.[137] Increased expression of TNF-α, transforming growth factor-β (TGF-β), and interleukin-1β (IL-1β) have been reported in MDS marrow, and there may be an association between TNF-α levels and apoptosis.[138, 139] Patients with MDS have a high cyotoxic–T helper lymphocyte ratio, as has been reported in aplastic anemia, where the presence of cytotoxic CD8 cells producing IFN-γ has been linked to the suppression of hematopoiesis by active destruction of progenitor and stem cells (see Chapter 1).[140–142] Consistent with a heightened immune response, which can induce Fas expression by target cells, both Fas and Fas-ligand expression appear to be increased in MDS marrow.[130, 143] The hypothetical role of autoreactive T cells, which preferentially destroy normal stem cells as a component of MDS pathogenesis, is depicted in the model shown in Figure 3–3.

Functional Consequences of Disordered Maturation

Whatever the basic genetic or marrow microenvironmental defect(s) in MDS, the clinical conse-

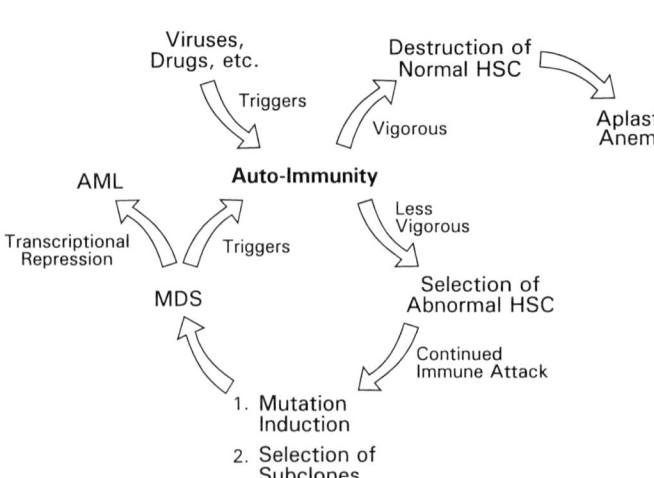

Figure 3–3 A new model for myelodysplastic syndrome pathogenesis. A role for autoimmunity in selecting, expanding, and even inducing an abnormal dysplastic clone is proposed. HSC, hematopoietic stem cells; AML, acute myelogenous leukemia.

quences to the patient result in part from dysfunction of circulating mature cells of all lineages. Many biochemical, phenotypic, and functional abnormalities of cells from patients with MDS have been described; some may be important in designing clinical and therapeutic approaches to this disease.

Erythroid Cells. Erythropoiesis in the marrow of MDS patients may be hypo- or hyperactive but is almost always ineffective.[144] Even if anucleate mature RBCs are released from the marrow, they may have abnormalities that result in a short circulation time, including frank hemolysis.[44] A number of biochemical abnormalities have been described that could result in hemolysis or oxygen-carrying limitations, including increased adenosine deaminase, G6PD, 6-phosphogluconate dehydrogenase, hexokinase, aldolase, and enolase activity, and decreased pyruvate kinase, phosphofructokinase, adenylate kinase, and diphosphoglycerate mutase activity.[145, 146] A significant percentage of MDS patients have PNH-type cells in all lineages when tested using sensitive flow techniques, but they rarely manifest clinically significant hemolysis.[46]

Iron metabolism in MDS patients has been much investigated, especially in RARS. The pathognomonic feature of RARS is the ring sideroblast, in which iron is aberrantly trapped within the mitochondria. These cells can be detected at lower frequency in many other MDS patients who do not fulfill criteria for RARS.[147] Iron accumulation could be due to normal or increased iron uptake by the erythroid progenitor, accompanied by decreased iron incorporation into hemoglobin. In RARS, heme synthetic dysfunction is not responsible for ring sideroblast formation, as abnormal mitochondrial iron deposition is present in early erythroid progenitors even prior to heme synthesis.[148] Nor is there evidence that increased and inappropriate uptake of iron by erythroblasts leads to ring sideroblast formation.[149] On the other hand, generalized mitochondrial dysfunction has been demonstrated in both erythroblasts and granulocytes of patients with RARS; the presence of the defects in both cell types suggests that mitochondrial dysfunction may be causative rather than a result of abnormal iron deposition.[150] These processes are probably secondary consequences of disordered maturation in MDS and not responsible for leukemic transformation. Acquired or inherited pure sideroblastic anemia, which is pyridoxine-responsive, differs from the true myelodysplastic entity of RARS.[151] Patients with acquired RARS of MDS may not have the same pathophysiology of ringed sideroblast formation that exists in patients with congenital sideroblastic anemia or lead poisoning. Patients with X-linked inherited sideroblastic anemia have mutations in the erythroid-specific synthase 5-amino levulinate (ALAS) gene, and they do not have trilineage dysplasia, marrow failure, or an increased risk of leukemia.[151]

Platelets. Many functional abnormalities of platelets in MDS have been described: decreased aggregation with agonists such as adenosine diphosphate, epinephrine, and collagen, low platelet ADP content, diminished adenosine triphosphate release consistent with a storage pool deficiency, and defective release of dense granule contents during platelet aggregation.[152, 153] Consistent with platelet dysfunction, the bleeding time is increased in as many as half of MDS patients, even in those with normal platelet counts.[152] There are no specific platelet abnormalities associated with an FAB subtype or clinical syndrome such as t-MDS or the 5q- syndrome. However, patients with more advanced and higher-risk disease usually appear to have the more compromised platelet function, although coexistent thrombocytopenia often confuses interpretation of the cause of clinical bleeding. Regardless, thrombocytopenic MDS patients are more likely to bleed than patients with aplastic anemia or idiopathic thrombocytopenic purpura, and they may need more aggressive transfusion therapy at a higher threshold platelet count.

Leukocytes. Clinically, dysfunction of WBCs has the most impact on MDS patients. Functional abnormalities of neutrophils include abnormal chemotaxis, phagocytosis, adhesion, chemiluminescence, and microbicidal capacity.[154] The granule content of myeloperoxidase may be decreased in MDS to the extent that myeloid cells do not stain for this enzyme.[155] Granulocyte dysfunction can place patients who have seemingly adequate neutrophil counts at increased risk of infection, and patients should be considered functionally neutropenic, especially if they have advanced or high-risk disease.[156] Patients with RARS or RA and normal neutrophil counts are less likely to suffer infectious complications.

CLINICAL COURSE AND PROGNOSIS

The overall median survival for all patients diagnosed with primary acquired MDS is only about 2 years.[2, 157] Spontaneous complete remission or even significant hematologic improvement without therapy rarely, if ever, occurs—such an event should call the original diagnosis into doubt. However, the clinical course in MDS is very heterogeneous, and many patients can lead normal lives

82 Bone Marrow Failure Syndromes

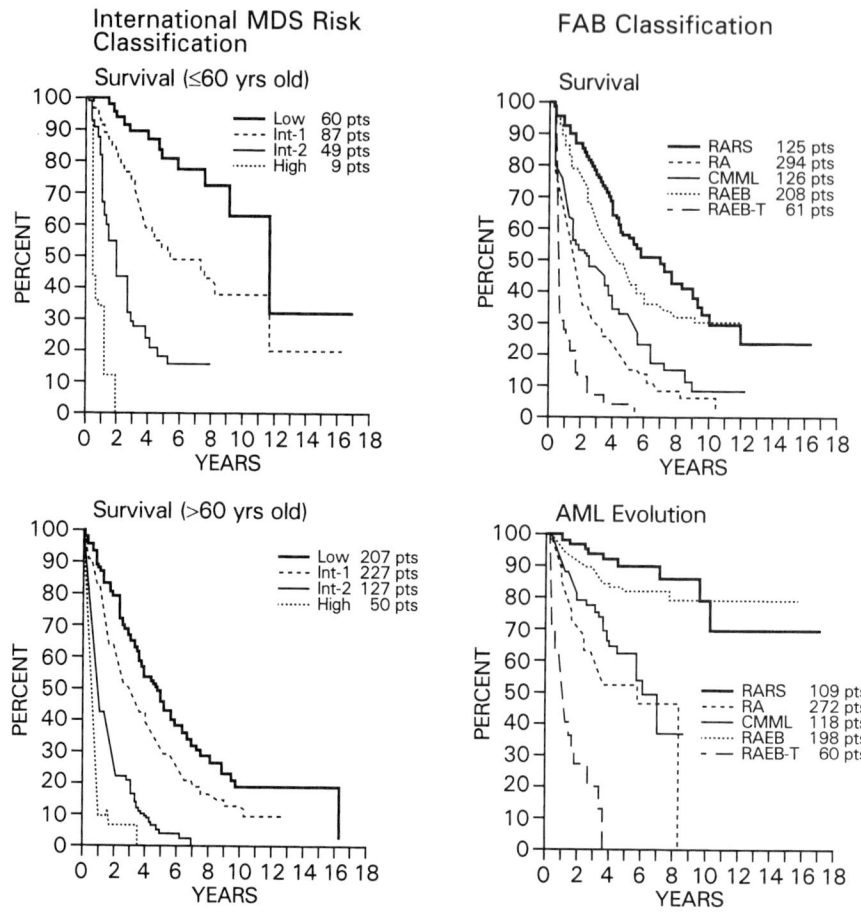

Figure 3–4 Kaplan-Meier survival and leukemia progression curves for patients with primary myelodysplastic syndromes (MDS) classified by French-American-British (FAB) subtype or International Prognostic Scoring System (IPSS) risk category; see Greenberg et al.[2] AML, acute myelogenous leukemia; RARS, refractory anemia with ring sideroblasts; RA, refractory anemia; CMML, chronic myelomonocytic leukemia; RAEB, refractory anemia with excess blasts; RAEB-T, RAEB in transformation; Int, intermediate.

despite the diagnosis and without the need for treatment. Despite the historic use of the term "preleukemia" for MDS, only about 30% of patients ultimately die of leukemic transformation. A slightly larger number instead succumb to complications of cytopenias or related abnormal hematopoietic cell dysfunction, leading to fatal bleeding or infection.[40] But fully one third of MDS patients do not die of their disease, and mortality from unrelated causes reflects the advanced age of most MDS patients and the often indolent clinical course.

The wide variability in time to leukemic transformation and in overall survival, in combination with the fact that the only curative therapy, allogeneic stem cell transplantation, carries significant risk, has magnified the importance of assessing an individual patient's prognosis. A number of increasingly useful algorithms have been developed. Patients in low-risk groups may have median survival times of greater than 5 years, as compared with high-risk groups with median survival of less than 3 to 6 months.[2] Accurate placement of patients in well-defined risk categories has obvious importance for treatment decisions in the individual and for the design of clinical trials.

The FAB classification was not originally developed as a prognostic aid, but because the FAB subtypes were essentially distinguished by the percentage of blasts in the marrow, their application did produce useful prognostic information[1] (Figure 3–4). Large studies have reported quite variable survival times for the FAB categories, except for

TABLE 3–5 International Prognostic Scoring System

Prognostic Variable	Score Value				
	0	0.5	1.0	1.5	2.0
Bone marrow blasts	< 5%	5%–10%		11%–20%	21%–30%
Karyotype*	Good	Intermediate	Poor		
Cytopenias†	0 or 1 lineage	2 or 3 lineages			

*Good = normal, −Y, del(5q), del (20q); Poor = complex (≥ 3 abnormalities) or chromosome 7 abnormalities; Intermediate = all other abnormalities.
†Cytopenias defined as hemoglobin < 10 g/dL, platelet count < 100,000/μL, absolute neutrophil count < 1500/μL.

Risk Group Scores

Risk group	Score
Low	0
Intermediate-1	0.5–1.0
Intermediate-2	1.5–2.0
High	≥ 2.5

From Greenberg P, Cox C, LeBeau MM, et al: International scoring system for evaluating prognosis in myelodysplastic syndromes. Blood 1997; 89:2079.

the uniformly bleak outlook in RAEB-T.[27, 158–160] Disparities may reflect differences in referral populations, inclusion or exclusion of patients with t-MDS, and subjectivity in applying diagnostic criteria. In an attempt to improve on morphology alone, a number of prognostic systems were devised in the 1980s that added clinical information such as hemoglobin level or degree of thrombocytopenia, but they provided only marginally better accuracy and have not been widely utilized.[159, 161]

As in acute leukemias, the most useful single additional factor contributing to prognosis has been the presence and type of clonal cytogenetic abnormalities, as detected on standard metaphase spreads of bone marrow cells[2, 162] Both structural anomalies such as translocations and loss or gain of entire chromosomes have been found in MDS. Although every chromosome has been reported to be affected, cytogenetic alterations are not random, with abnormalities of chromosomes 5, 7, 8, and 20 most common.[49, 163] The occurrence of single nonspecified karyotypic abnormalities in most studies did not predict a worse outcome than normal karyotypes; however, complex karyotypic changes, usually multiple chromosomal abnormalities within one clone or coexisting multiple clones and subclones, did predict shorter survival.[50] The utility of cytogenetic studies dramatically increased with the recognition that some specific and frequent common single cytogenetic abnormalities had very clear negative or positive impacts on survival, which had been masked when they were grouped for analysis.[164] For instance, in primary MDS an isolated 5q- abnormality has a more favorable prognosis than any other karyotype in MDS, including even a normal karyotype.[74, 165, 166] Loss of Y and 20q- also carry a good prognosis, while instead loss of part or all of chromosome 7 augurs a very poor outcome.[50, 167]

In 1997, an International MDS Risk Analysis Workshop used a large patient data set to investigate the prognostic power gained by adding various factors to models, and investigators then validated the resulting new scoring system in an independent cohort of patients. The factors found to be most relevant were various low- and high-risk cytogenetic abnormalities, degree of cytopenias, and further subdivision of bone marrow myeloblast percentages: the model resulted in the International Prognostic Scoring System (IPSS)[2] (Table 3–5). Patients who had previously received intensive chemotherapy and patients with the "myeloproliferative" type of CMML (WBC count greater than 12,000/μL) were excluded from the analysis, and the IPSS may not be applicable to them. The IPSS has been particularly useful for differentiating widely disparate patient types within what had previously been a very heterogeneous group, particularly RA (Fig. 3–5). At the present time, this scoring system is the best available guide to decision making in individual MDS cases and is extensively utilized in clinical trials.

A number of other biologic and clinical factors have been reported as significant in the prognosis

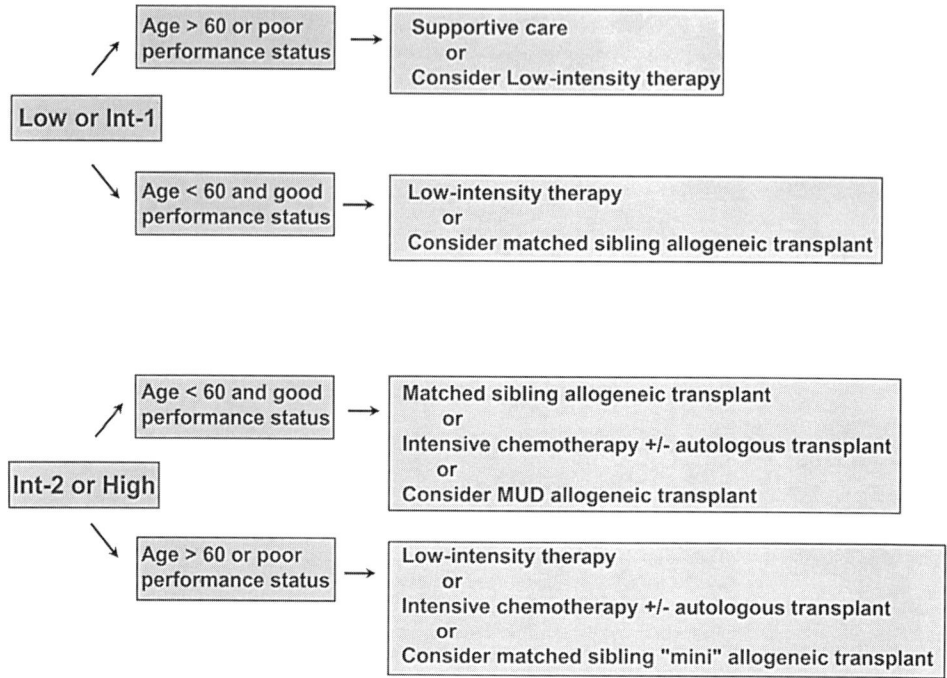

Figure 3–5 Suggested treatment approaches based on International Prognostic Scoring System (IPSS) risk category and age. See Table 3–5 for information on placing patients into IPSS risk categories; see also Greenberg et al.[2]

of MDS patients, but they have either not added to standard multivariate analyses or have proved impractical in general application. For instance, in vitro marrow myeloid clonogenic culture shows two patterns of growth in MDS: (1) a leukemic type with microcluster and macrocluster formation and defective maturation of blasts within aggregates resulting in persistence of single blasts or (2) normal-appearing colonies with very low plating efficiency.[168] There is an increase in the risk of leukemic transformation in patients with the leukemic-type colony pattern.[169] Flow cytometry may be more practical as a method for assessment of the state of differentiation and the degree of aberrancy of marrow and blood cells.[53] Increased numbers of CD34+ cells have identified a subset of RAEB patients who have decreased survival.[170] As the pathophysiology of MDS comes to be better understood, molecular measurements, such as detection of mutations in or deletions of oncogenes and tumor suppressor genes may play an important role in predicting clinical course.

Prognosis of Therapy-Related Myelodysplastic Syndrome

t-MDS has an extremely poor prognosis, with median survival of 3 to 8 months and death occurring from cytopenias or leukemic transformation.[171, 172] Patients developing MDS following chemotherapy or radiation therapy (or treatment of aplastic anemia) must be separated from primary MDS patients in analyses of prognostic factors or in clinical trials, and failure to make this distinction has confounded the results of many studies. Even t-MDS patients scored as having apparently "low-risk" disease by IPSS or FAB criteria nevertheless have very high rates of rapid progression to AML. It is more appropriate to group t-MDS patients with t-AML patients, since median survivals are similar in the two groups, whether or not the actual criteria for leukemia are met at the time of diagnosis.[29] Likewise, once AML has evolved from t-MDS, the FAB morphologic classification has little meaning: undifferentiated M0 or M1 morphology is typical. The only group with a somewhat better prognosis may be patients developing t-MDS or t-AML after epipodophyllotoxin therapy, which is associated with abnormalities of chromosome 11q23.[30]

TREATMENT

Therapy decisions in MDS should be carefully individualized, incorporating age and overall clinical condition; prognosis using the best available scoring system, now the IPSS; and the preferences of the patient. These factors are especially important in MDS, since curative options such as allogeneic transplantation are not available or appropriate for the majority, and many newer therapies have serious or uncertain side effects and should probably not be administered except in monitored clinical protocols. A major difficulty in the interpretation of published studies is the heterogeneity of the patient populations, especially the inclusion of patients with t-MDS (see above). A second methodologic problem is the definition of "response": many statistically or numerically significant responses have no clinical importance, as, for instance, an increase in neutrophil count from 1200 to 4000/µL. A more valid endpoint may be documentation of transfusion-independence in patients previously receiving regular RBC or platelet transfusion, but very few trials use or report on this result: even transfusion independence may be complicated by subjective and changing thresholds for transfusion. Thus many published clinical studies do not provide much practical information on appropriate treatment approaches. Based on our own review of the literature and substantial clinical experience, a suggested approach to the treatment of MDS patients is shown in Figure 3–5. As patients progress into higher-risk categories over time, treatment strategies must be adjusted accordingly.

Transfusion and Other Supportive Care

A careful approach to supportive care is critical to maintaining a good quality of life and allowing successful application of more aggressive therapies such as transplantation. Transfusion support is central to the management of cytopenic MDS patients and is required in the vast majority at some point during their disease. Patients with symptomatic anemia should be transfused on a regular schedule that allows normal daily activity even at the nadir hemoglobin value. Many patients tolerate hemoglobin concentrations as low as 6 to 7 g/DL, but others require higher levels to remain asymptomatic, especially the elderly with complicating conditions such as coronary artery disease or chronic pulmonary dysfunction. Most MDS patients do not require platelet transfusions to treat thrombocytopenia in the absence of active bleeding, even with counts below 20,000/µL. Occasionally a bleeding tendency may be manifested, even with baseline counts greater than 20,000 to 50,000/µL, due to platelet dysfunction; in such cases prophylactic or therapeutic platelet transfusions may be appropriate regardless of the count.[152, 153] Platelet transfusions should be ABO and Rh compatible, if possible. Leukocyte depletion of RBC and platelet transfusions minimizes allosensitization in the platelet transfusion–dependent patient. Irradiation of blood products is only indicated for those receiving intensive chemotherapy or undergoing transplantation; otherwise, MDS patients have not been reported to be at risk for transfusion-associated graft-versus-host disease, (GvHD).

Iron chelation with chronic desferrioxamine given as a subcutaneous or intravenous nightly infusion should be considered for patients with a transfusion burden exceeding 20 to 50 units of packed red blood cells or with ferritin levels consistently above 2500 ng/mL.[173] Aggressive chelation therapy has dramatically increased survival in the transfusion-dependent congenital anemias, such as thalassemia.[174] The decision to institute chelation therapy in MDS can be difficult: chelation therapy involves discomfort and some risks, and it is not indicated in patients with a very poor prognosis, who are unlikely to die of iron overload. However, when the prognosis is good or intermediate, early institution of chelation therapy in transfusion-dependent patients is almost always advisable. Patients with sideroblastic anemias have been reported to hyperabsorb iron and present with evidence of iron overload even with minimal or no RBC transfusions.[37, 38] They should be aggressively chelated, and there have been reports of improved marrow function with chelation alone, suggesting a deleterious effect of excessive iron on hematopoiesis.

Many MDS patients, even with adequate neutrophil counts, are susceptible to serious bacterial and fungal infections.[40] Patients and their primary care physicians should be counseled about the importance of seeking rapid medical evaluation and treatment for fevers or other symptoms of infection. Prophylactic chronic oral antibiotics may be useful in selected cases, although they should not be given routinely to neutropenic patients who lack a history of infectious complications.

Hematopoietic Growth Factors

Hematopoietic growth factors that have had varying degrees of success in alleviating the cytopenias of MDS include erythropoietin (Epo), granulocyte colony-stimulating factor (G-CSF), and granulocyte-macrophage colony-stimulating factor (GM-CSF), alone or in combination. Epo has been studied extensively; while the anemia in MDS is generally hyporegenerative, it can be accompanied by an inappropriately low serum Epo level.[175] The overall response rate to this hormone is about 20%, as measured by decreased anemia, using Epo at doses ranging from 200 units/kg three times per week to 1000 units/kg daily.[176] Unfortunately, a lower percentage of patients become transfusion independent. Ironically, it is the non–transfusion-dependent patients who seem to respond best. Other predictors of response include serum Epo levels of less than 200 to 500 units/L, the absence of ring sideroblasts, normal cytogenetics, and a marrow blast percentage of less than 10%. Hematopoietic responses are usually seen within the first 4 to 8 weeks of treatment. In patients with symptomatic or transfusion-dependent anemia, especially if the serum Epo is less than 500 units/L, a 2-month trial of high-dose Epo (300 units/kg/day or greater) may be considered, and with response the dose can be titrated. Iron repletion should be documented before instituting Epo therapy, especially in thrombocytopenic patients with a history of significant bleeding.

GM-CSF or G-CSF administration results in increased neutrophil counts in as many as 80% of MDS patients, although severely neutropenic patients are less likely to respond.[177-179] Response is usually dependent on continued drug administration, and it may be accompanied by worsening thrombocytopenia. With few exceptions, cytogenetic abnormalities persist, suggesting stimulation of the abnormal clone.[180] However, improvement in neutrophil counts with these two agents has not translated into improved survival or other clinically significant outcomes in phase III trials.[181, 182] The possibility that G-CSF or GM-CSF could hasten progression to acute leukemia has been a continuing concern, but there is no evidence for a role of cytokine treatment in transformation. In individual patients with neutropenia and recurrent or serious infections, it may be reasonable to consider G-CSF administration together with antibiotics.

The combinations of G-CSF and Epo or GM-CSF and Epo have been reported to synergistically increase the erythroid response rate over Epo alone to 34% to 38%.[183-185] A model for predicting response to the combination of Epo and G-CSF has been proposed.[186] One approach to growth factor therapy may be to add G-CSF if there is no response to Epo alone and to treat with the combination for another 2 to 3 months. The doses of G-CSF required are relatively low, on average 1 µg/kg/day. Most studies predict that the response rate in patients with Epo levels greater than 500 units/L is so low as to argue against a trial of Epo alone or in combination with G-CSF. Patients with the 5q- abnormality appear less likely to respond to this combination.

Allogeneic Bone Marrow or Peripheral Blood Stem Cell Transplantation

Allogeneic transplantation, the only curative option for patients with MDS, should be considered for any patient aged less than 55 to 60 years with a fully HLA-matched sibling, regardless of disease risk category. However, treatment-related morbidity and mortality are significant, making decisions regarding timing of transplantation, especially in patients with low-risk disease, very difficult.[187] Information on the availability of a matched sibling donor is helpful in planning an approach to treatment and expedites transplantation if disease progression occurs. We recommend that all patients under age 60 and their full siblings be HLA-typed. Immediate transplantation for patients with IPSS low-risk disease should only be considered in very young patients (under 20) or those with life-threatening cytopenias.

Most published series contain heterogeneous patient populations, including those with t-MDS, and differing transplantation regimens. In a retrospective analysis of a large cohort of 251 patients transplanted for MDS between 1981 and 1996 in Seattle, the overall disease-free survival rate was 40%.[77, 78] In a retrospective analysis of 131 patients, the European Group for Blood and Bone Marrow Transplantation (EBMT) reported 34% 5-year disease-free survival and 41% overall survival.[188] In the Seattle series, the IPSS score correlated with survival: the 5-year disease-free survival was 60% for intermediate-1 (and a very few low-risk) patients; 36% for intermediate-2 risk; and 28% for high-risk patients.[78] Older age (greater than 50 years), increasing disease duration, mismatched donors, male sex, and t-MDS each independently predicted greater transplant-related mortality. Disease duration, morphology (more advanced FAB subgroups), and high-risk cytogenetic abnormalities each correlated with relapse. The relapse rate in patients transplanted while in FAB RA appears to be extremely low, but the prolonged survival in this subtype or in IPSS low-risk patients without any aggressive therapy precludes the routine application of allogeneic transplantation.

The data for matched unrelated donor (MUD) transplantation are much more limited. The two largest series reported a 3-year survival of 30% (EBMT) or a 2-year survival of 38% (Seattle), not significantly different from that obtained with matched siblings. However, the median age of patients undergoing unrelated donor transplantation was lower (mainly less than 35 years of age).[78, 189] Nonrelapse mortality has been high with MUD, 48% in the Seattle and European series. With the advent of DNA-based HLA typing to supplement serologic typing, survival should improve, but at the cost of a diminished donor pool for each patient. Patients with IPSS high-risk or intermediate-2 disease under the age of 40 to 50 years should consider MUD transplantation if a suitable donor is available. A mismatched family donor can also be considered as a second choice. Patients with lower-risk disease or adverse factors for transplantation should pursue nontransplant options instead, especially if no DNA-matched unrelated donor is available.

In patients with increased marrow blasts (greater than 5% to 10%), the benefit of AML-type induction chemotherapy for cytoreduction prior to allogeneic transplantation conditioning is unclear. MDS patients with no response to antileukemic chemotherapy have a much lower likelihood of disease-free survival with transplantation. Patients with t-MDS have lower rates of disease-free survival compared with patients with de novo MDS, owing primarily to increased transplant-related mortality resulting from prior chemotherapy or irradiation, as well as to higher relapse rates.[190] There is no clear preference regarding conditioning therapy for MDS patients undergoing allogeneic transplantation: cyclophosphamide and total body irradiation or cyclophosphamide and busulfan have been most frequently utilized.[191] More intensified conditioning with busulfan, cyclophosphamide, and total body irradiation has failed to show benefit. Nonmyeloablative or "mini"-transplants are beginning to be studied as an option for patients older than 50 who have matched sibling donors.[192, 193] Transplant-related morbidity and mortality is reduced with these less intensive conditioning regimens, and success depends on immunologically mediated gradual replacement of host hematopoiesis by engrafted cells. Early reports of MDS patients responding to immunotherapy with donor lymphocyte infusions at the time of relapse post allogeneic transplantation imply that some graft-versus-leukemia effect may exist in this disease.

Intensive Chemotherapy

The justification for high-dose chemotherapy in MDS comes from the relative success of such therapy in younger patients with some types of de novo AML. Such data cannot be applied uncritically to treating older patients with high-risk MDS or MDS-AML. Unfortunately, as summarized above, MDS and de novo AML in the elderly are likely biologically different diseases compared with de novo AML of the young, where many patients fall into good prognosis categories (like M3 with t15;17 or M4-eo with inv16). AML in patients older than 55 years of age is associated with an increased frequency of unfavorable cytogenetic abnormalities, multidrug resistance (*MDR1*) gene expression, and CD34+ blast cells.[194,195] Remission rates with conventional or high-dose antileukemic chemotherapy tend to be lower than in younger patients. In addition, older patients with AML or MDS tolerate infections and other complications of chemotherapy poorly. Studies of intensive chemotherapy for high-risk MDS or MDS-AML have shown complete remission rates in a broad range from 18% to 79% (Table 3–6); variability may be due to differing chemotherapy regimens, differences in the aggressiveness of supportive care, statistical variance due to small study sizes, and the heterogeneity of MDS and MDS-AML types, especially the inclusion or exclusion of patients with t-MDS or t-AML. The use of G-CSF or other cytokines post chemotherapy and both before and after chemotherapy has not been shown to affect response or survival rates, or even the duration of hospitalization, despite fewer neutropenic days.[196, 197] Regardless of the response rate, the median remission duration is typically less than 6 to 12 months, with only rare instances of prolonged disease-free survival. Patients with chromosome 5 or 7 abnormalities have especially low rates of response and brief durations of remission, similar to patients in poor-risk categories of de novo AML with similar cytogenetic abnormalities.[198] Recent trials with newer combinations of agents, such as the addition of fludarabine, are preliminarily reporting higher remission rates, but relapse still occurs early.[199, 200]

High treatment-related morbidity and mortality and the brief duration of response are compelling reasons not to proceed to intensive chemotherapy in every patient with high-risk MDS or MDS-AML, but patients fitting criteria for MDS at the time of antileukemia treatment do no worse with induction than do poor-risk de novo AML patients.[198, 201] It is important to note that a survival benefit has not been shown for intensive chemotherapy, even with full hematologic and cytogenetic remissions. Nonetheless, given the poor prognosis, it is appropriate to apply aggressive strategies selectively, preferably in the setting of clinical research protocols. Any impact on survival is likely to come from improvement in postremission therapy to prolong responses, making consolidation strategies such as autologous transplantation attractive.

TABLE 3–6 Representative Trials of High-Dose Chemotherapy in Myelodysplastic Syndromes

Regimen	N	Complete remission	Reference
High-dose cytarabine C + topotecan	35	63%	Beran et al. (1996)[199]
Daunorubicin/idarubicin + cytarabine	47	47%	Fenaux et al. (1991)[236]
Daunorubicin + cytarabine ± G-CSF	211	50% (−) vs 41% (+)	Godwin et al. (1998)[197]
Fludarabine + cytarabine C + G-CSF + idarubicin	19	63%	Parker et al. (1997)[200]
Cytarabine C + idarubicin + etoposide 16 + G-CSF	19	47%	Ganser et al. (1993)[237]
High-dose cytarabine	11	18%	Preisler et al. (1986)[238]
Idarubicin + etoposide + cytarabine C ± G-CSF	105	33% (−) vs. 43% (+)	Bernasconi et al. (1998)[196]

G-CSF, granulocyte colony-stimulating factor.

Autologous Bone Marrow or Peripheral Blood Stem Cell Transplantation

Until recently, very few patients with MDS or MDS-AML were eligible for autologous transplantation, mainly due to the problem of very slow engraftment with infusion of insufficient numbers of residual normal hematopoietic stem cells.[202] However, because intensive chemotherapy can result in at least transient loss of clonal cytogenetic abnormalities and a polyclonal pattern on X chromosome inactivation studies, autologous transplantation has recently been employed as a consolidation therapy in young patients with intermediate- or high-risk MDS who lack appropriate allogeneic donors.[203, 204] A complete remission must first be achieved with intensive chemotherapy, before collection of the patient's own stem cells. Aggressive consolidation with transplantation is warranted by the short median duration of remission after standard induction chemotherapy alone. One hundred fourteen MDS or secondary MDS-AML patients undergoing autologous transplantation were reported to the EBMT: 2 year survival for the 79 patients receiving transplants in first complete remission (CR) was 39% with a disease-free survival (DFS) of 34% and a relapse risk of 64%.[205] Compared with patients with de novo AML undergoing autologous transplantation on similar protocols, the DFS was lower and the relapse risk higher in MDS. DFS was somewhat better for patients who had not yet progressed to AML. Patients younger than 40 had a DFS of 39%, compared with 25% for those over 40, and transplant-related mortality was higher in the older patients, 39%, vs. 17% in the younger patients.

In most published studies, marrow was used as the source of engrafting cells. Peripheral blood stem cell transplantation (PBSCT) is associated with higher harvest yields and shorter duration of aplasia, and PBSCT is replacing BMT as the modality of choice.[206] Polyclonal (and presumed normal) progenitors can be obtained in PBSC harvests in MDS patients after CR induction with chemotherapy, especially early in the disease course.[203, 204] A European randomized study of autologous PBSCT vs a second course of intensive chemotherapy should help determine the best consolidation strategy for the high-risk MDS or MDS-AML patient who is in CR after induction chemotherapy. Lower transplant-related morbidity and mortality would justify use of high-dose chemotherapy followed by autologous PBSCT in patients with early or lower-risk disease. The issue of purging is unsettled: the one published study using purged marrow cells reported very prolonged times to engraftment.[202]

Differentiation Therapy or Low-Dose Chemotherapy

Interest in the use of lower-dose nonmyeloablative chemotherapy in MDS has been stimulated by the observation that certain drugs at modest, nontoxic concentrations produce differentiation of myeloid cell lines and primary leukemic cells in vitro.[207, 208] Differentiation therapy has been successful in acute promyelocytic leukemia. In MDS, many agents have been studied, including low-dose cytarabine (ara-C), all-*trans*-retinoic acid (tretinoin), *cis*- retinoic acid (CRA), hexamethylene bisacetamide (HMBA), 5-azacytadine (5-AZA), phenylbutyrate (PB), and vitamin D derivatives.[209, 210]

The initial success of "low-dose" cytarabine clinical efficacy in phase II trials has not been confirmed, and responses appear to have been due to myeloablation as opposed to differentiation.[211] There was no positive impact on survival induction, and treatment was associated with toxicity in later trials, including a randomized protocol comparing low-dose cytarabine with supportive care alone.[212] Retinoids, including both the *cis*- and *trans*- forms of retinoic acid, have resulted in only occasional and transient hematologic improvement in MDS and neither can be recommended for the treatment of MDS.[213, 214] HMBA failed to show benefit in a clinical trial but caused myelosuppression.[215]

5-AZA inhibits DNA methyltransferase activity, resulting in nonspecific demethylation of some transcriptional control elements for previously silenced genes and differentiation of leukemic cell lines.[207] 5-AZA has been extensively studied in MDS patients: 5-AZA produced hematologic responses in over 40% of patients in some phase II studies, but CR rates were lower, 11% or less.[216, 217] A randomized comparison of 5-AZA and supportive care in a cohort of 191 patients is ongoing; preliminary data have suggested increased hematologic response and improved quality of life in patients receiving the drug, but analysis of survival benefit and impact on natural history is confounded by the crossover design of the study.[218, 219] Toxicity appears less than with conventional chemotherapy, although significant myelosuppression and increased frequency of transfusion during the treatment phase with 5-AZA implicate a primary effect of clonal suppression rather than induction of differentiation.

Phenylbutyrate has myeloid differentiation activity in vitro and little direct cytotoxicity.[220] A small phase I/II study reported increase in ANC in 63% of MDS patients and disappearance of peripheral myeloblasts in three patients with AML, inspiring the initiation of larger current studies.[221] Initial trials with vitamin D$_3$ were disappointing, but a more recent trial using calcitriol in low-to-intermediate risk MDS reported improved blood counts in 11 of 19 patients.[222] Additional derivatives of vitamin D with more potent differentiative qualities await clinical trial. Interferons have also been investigated but with little evidence of efficacy: of a total of 66 patients with low- and high-risk MDS treated with IFN-α at doses varying from 0.5 mU three times a week to 3 mU/m²/day in six studies, the mean response rate was 29% with a CR rate of 10%.[210, 223–225]

In the older patient, where curative therapy is not the intent and quality-of-life issues are primary, low-dose or oral chemotherapy may occasionally be useful to alleviate bone pain or other symptoms, particularly in CMML or RAEB-T. Options include oral low-dose etoposide (VP-16) or hydroxyurea.[226] In a randomized comparison of hydroxyurea and etoposide in CMML, the overall response rate favored hydroxyurea (60% vs. 36%), by the definition of improvement in this study.[227] Similarly, low-dose therapy for RAEB-T or "smoldering" AML progressing from MDS can achieve cycloreduction, potentially with less risk and discomfort than with high dose chemotherapy, alleviating cytopenias and transfusion-dependence in a few patients.

Anti-apoptosis and Immunosuppressive Therapies

As discussed in the pathophysiology section above, there may be overlap between the clinically and morphologically defined syndromes of aplastic anemia and MDS, with immune destruction and apoptosis playing some role in the generation of cytopenias in both. Immunomodulating or anti-apoptosis therapies that have been tested in MDS include corticosteroids, ATG, cyclosporine, amifostine, and IFN-α. Initial results hold promise for their use in alleviating cytopenias.

Bagby and co-workers reported in 1980 that prednisone alone improved depressed blood counts in a minority of patients with MDS and that the response could be predicted by in vitro enhancement of marrow colony-forming unit—granulocyte macrophase (CFU_{GM}) growth by cortisol.[228] In a separate study of patients with concurrent autoimmune diseases, 6 out of 27 patients with MDS showed improvement in cytopenias with prednisone.[229] Low response rates and infectious complications associated with their chronic use make corticosteroids unattractive agents for MDS. Androgenic steroids have also been studied; the largest controlled trial reported no benefit and evidence for more rapid progression to leukemia in the treatment arm, although other, noncontrolled studies have not noted an unexpectedly high rate of transformation.[230] In selected patients with isolated anemia and hypocellular marrows, a trial of androgens may be indicated in an attempt to avoid transfusions.[231]

Interest in investigating alternative immunosuppressive therapies in MDS was stimulated by the observations that some patients with hypocellular MDS, often initially diagnosed as aplastic anemia, responded to ATG or cyclosporine.[232] A larger trial has been reported from the National Institutes of Health (NIH), which has now been extended and updated since publication.[233] Sixteen out of 42 patients with MDS (excluding RAEB-T and CMML) who were treated with ATG at 40 mg/kg/day for 4 days became transfusion-independent, the rate being highest (61%) for patients with RA, although patients with RAEB also responded (32%). Neutrophil and platelet counts also improved in patients who became transfusion-independent for RBCs. Responses occurred even in patients with hypercellular marrows but were more frequent in those with hypocellular marrows. No patient with RARS responded, but improvements were seen even in patients with intermediate-2 or high-risk IPSS disease. Previously detectable cytogenetic abnormalities persisted despite increased blood counts, suggesting that ATG treatment resulted in more effective hematopoiesis, not a return to hematopoiesis derived from residual normal progenitor or stem cells. In a few well-studied patients, response correlated with a loss of cytotoxic lymphocyte activity against autologous CFU_{GM}.[63] Toxicity of ATG therapy was largely fever and rigors associated with infusions, with fewer than 15% of patients developing serum sickness. A Czech group has reported that cytopenias improved in 14 out of 17 RA patients treated with cyclosporine at 5 to 6 mg/kg/day, with subsequent adjustment of doses to maintain blood levels between 100 and 300 ng/mL. Nine of the 17 patients had hypocellular marrows; of the three nonresponders, one had a hypocellular marrow.[61] An ongoing U.S. study has reported similar results with cyclosporine alone.[62]

Amifostine is a phosphorylated organic thiol that is metabolized to intermediates with antioxidant activities.[234] Amifostine may also function to suppress inflammatory cytokine release or to protect cells from oxidant stress after exposure to cytokines such as TNF-α.[139] In vitro the drug has been shown to rescue cells from apoptosis-inducing stresses such as radiation and chemotherapy. Incubation with amifostine improved colony growth of MDS marrow cells in culture.[221] In an American study, 15 of 18 MDS patients treated with amifostine had single or multilineage hematologic responses; the granulocyte responses abated between courses of treatment, and the persistence of cytogenetic changes in responders confirmed the in vitro observations of differentiation or improved survival of the abnormal MDS clone.[235] One third of patients had a clinically significant reduction in RBC transfusion requirements. Of five patients with excess bone marrow myeloblasts, three experienced a rise in blast percentage during study treatment, and two progressed to AML, a worrisome observation. Nonetheless, amifostine is now being investigated in larger phase II trials.

CONCLUSIONS

Laboratory investigators and clinicians are still some distance away from understanding the underlying pathophysiology of MDS and thus handicapped in the design of rational, specific treatments. Recent progress in clinically relevant subtyping of AML based on molecular analyses should also be possible in MDS, and will open new avenues for biologic inquiry, allow more accurate prognosis, and spur development of specific therapies. Epidemiologic studies may allow prevention or early detection through directed screening. Currently, use of the IPSS along with considerations such as patient age, willingness to participate in experimental protocols, and the availability of an allogeneic transplantation donor must guide treatment decisions.

REFERENCES

1. Bennett JM, Catovsky D, Daniel MT, et al: The French-American-British (FAB) Co-operative Group: Proposals for the classification of the myelodysplastic syndromes. Br J Haematol 1982; 51:189.
2. Greenberg P, Cox C, LeBeau MM, et al: International scoring system for evaluating prognosis in myelodysplastic syndromes. Blood 1997; 89:2079.
3. Rhoads CP, Barker WH: Refractory anemia. JAMA 1938; 110:794.
4. Bjorkman SE: Chronic refractory anemia with sideroblastic bone marrow: A study of four cases. Blood 1956; 11:250.
5. Hamilton-Patterson JL: Pre leukaemic anaemia. Acta Haematol 1949; 2:302.
6. Crosby WH, Feinstein FE, Heilmeyer L, et al: XII. Hypoplastic-aplastic anemia. Blood 1957; 12:193.
7. Hayhoe FGJ, Quaglino D: Refractory sideroblastic anaemia and erythraemic myelosis: Possible relationship and cytochemical observations. Br J Haematol 1960; 6:381.
8. Dameshek W: Sideroblastic anemia: Is this a malignancy? Br J Haematol 1965; 2:52.
9. Dreyfus B, Rochant H, Salmon C, et al: Anémies refractaires, états préleucémiques at anomalies enzymatiques multiples. C R Acad Sa III 1968; 266:1627.
10. Saarni MI, Linman JW: Myelomonocytic leukemia: Disorderly proliferation of all marrow cells. Cancer 1971; 27:1221.
11. Saarni M, Linman J: Preleukemia: Hematologic syndrome preceding acute leukemia. Am J Med 1973; 55:38.
12. Bennett JM, Catovsky D, Daniel MT, et al: Proposals for the classification of the acute leukaemias. Br J Haematol 1976; 33:451.

13. Tricot GJ: Minimal diagnostic criteria for the myelodysplastic syndrome in clinical practice. Leuk Res 1992; 16:5.
14. Kouides PA, Bennett JM: Morphology and classification of the myelodysplastic syndromes and their pathologic variants. Semin Hematol 1996; 33:95.
15. Verhoef GE, Pittaluga S, De Wolf-Peters C, et al: FAB classification of myelodysplastic syndromes: Merits and controversies. Ann Hematol 1995; 71:3.
16. Williamson PJ, Kruger AR, Reynolds PJ, et al: Establishing the incidence of myelodysplastic syndrome. Br J Haematol 1994; 87:743.
17. Aul C, Gattermann N, Schneider W: Age-related incidence and other epidemiological aspects of myelodysplastic syndromes. Br J Haematol 1992; 82:358.
18. Tuncer MA, Pagliuca A, Hisconmez G, et al: Primary myelodysplastic syndrome in children: The clinical experience in 33 cases. Br J Haematol 1992; 82:347.
19. Paul B, Reid MM, Davison EV, et al: Familial myelodysplasia: Progressive disease associated with emergence of monosomy 7. Br J Haematol 1987; 65:321.
20. Shannon KM, Turhan AG, Chang SSY, et al: Familial bone marrow monosomy 7: Evidence that the predisposing locus is not on the long arm of chromosome 7. J Clin Invest 1989; 84:984.
21. Aksoy M, Dincol K, Erdem S, et al: Acute leukemia due to chronic exposure to benzene. Am J Med 1972; 52:160.
22. Rinsky RA, Smith AB, Hornung R, et al: Benzene and leukemia: An epidemiologic risk assessment. N Engl J Med 1987; 316:1044.
23. Brandt L, Nilsson PG, Mitelman F: Occupational exposure to petroleum products in men with acute non-lymphocytic leukaemia. BMJ 1978; 1:553.
24. Farrow A, Jacobs A, West RR: Myelodysplasia, chemical exposure, and other environmental factors. Leukemia 1989; 3:33.
25. West RR, Stafford DA, Farrow A, et al: Occupational and environmental exposures and myelodysplasia: A case-controlled study. Leuk Res 1995; 19:127.
26. Ido M, Nagata C, Kawakami N, et al: A case-control study of myelodysplastic syndromes among Japanese men and women. Leuk Res 1996; 20:727.
27. Coiffier B, Adeleine P, Viala JJ, et al: Dysmyelopoietic syndromes. A search for prognostic factors in 193 patients. Cancer 1983; 52:83.
28. Pedersen-Bjergaard J, Larsen SO, Struck J, et al: Risk of therapy-related leukaemia and preleukaemia after Hodgkin's disease: Relation to age, cumulative dose of alkylating agents, and time from chemotherapy. Lancet 1987; 2:83.
29. Michels SD, McKenna RW, Arthur DC, et al: Therapy-related acute myeloid leukemia and myelodysplastic syndrome: A clinical and morphologic study of 65 cases. Blood 1985; 65:1364.
30. Felix CA: Secondary leukemias induced by topoisomerase-targeted drugs. Biochim Biophys Acta 1998; 1400:233.
31. Sterkers Y, Preudhomme C, Lai JL, et al: Acute myeloid leukemia and myelodysplastic syndromes following essential thrombocythemia treated with hydroxyurea: High proportion of cases with 17p deletion. Blood 1998; 91:616.
32. Orchard JA, Bolam S, Oscier DG: Association of myelodysplastic changes with purine analogues. Br J Haematol 1998; 100:677.
33. Stone RM: Myelodysplastic syndrome: After autologous transplantation for lymphoma: The price of progress? Blood 1994; 83:3437.
34. Heim S: Cytogenetic findings in primary and secondary MDS. Leuk Res 1992; 16:43.
35. Fohlmeister I, Fischer R, Modder B, et al: Aplastic anaemia and the hypocellular myelodysplastic syndrome: Histomorphological, diagnostic, and prognostic features. J Clin Pathol 1985; 38:1218.
36. Longacre TA, Smoller BR: Leukemia cutis. Analysis of 50 biopsy-proven cases with an emphasis on occurrence in myelodysplastic syndromes. Am J Clin Pathol 1993; 100:276.
37. Peto TEA, Pippard MJ, Weatherall DJ: Iron overload in mild sideroblastic anaemias. Lancet 1983; 1:375.
38. Weintraub LR, Conrad ME, Crosby WH: Regulation of intestinal absorption of iron by the rate of cytopoiesis. Br J Haematol 1965; 11:432.
39. Juneja SK, Imbert M, Jouault H, et al: Haematological features of primary myelodysplastic syndromes (PMDS) at initial presentation: A study of 118 cases. J Clin Pathol 1983; 36:1129.
40. Pomeroy C, Oken MM, Rydell RE, et al: Infection in the myelodysplastic syndromes. Am J Med 1991; 90:338.
41. Najean Y, Lecompte T: Chronic pure thrombocytopenia in elderly patients. An aspect of the myelodysplastic syndrome. Cancer 1989; 64:2506.
42. Rao AK, Walsh PN: Acquired qualitative platelet disorders. Clin Haematol 1983; 12:201.
43. Tulliez M, Testa U, Rochant H, et al: Reticulocytosis, hypochromia, and microcytosis: An unusual presentation of the preleukemic syndrome. Blood 1982; 59:293.
44. Kornberg A, Goldfarb A: Preleukemia manifested by hemolytic anemia with pyruvate-kinase deficiency. Arch Intern Med 1986; 146:785.
45. Pintado T, Maldonado J: Ultrastructure of platelet aggregation in refractory anemia and myelomonocytic leukemia. Mayo Clin Proc 1976; 51:443.
46. Dunn DE, Tanawattanacharoen P, Boccuni P, et al: Paroxysmal nocturnal hemoglobinuria cells in patients with bone marrow failure syndromes. Ann Intern Med 1999; 131:401.
47. Tricot G, De Wolf-Peeters C, Vlietinck R, et al: Bone marrow histology in myelodysplastic syndromes. Br J Haematol 1984; 58:217.
48. Seo IS, Li CY, Yam LT: Myelodysplastic syndrome: Diagnostic implications of cytochemical and immunocytochemical studies. Mayo Clin Proc 1993; 68:47.
49. Knapp RH, Dewald GW, Pierre RV: Cytogenetic

studies in 174 consecutive patients with preleukemic or myelodysplastic syndromes. Mayo Clin Proc 1985; 60:507.
50. Yunis JJ, Lobell M, Arnesen MA, et al: Refined chromosome study helps define prognostic subgroups in most patients with primary myelodysplastic syndrome and acute myelogenous leukaemia. Br J Haematol 1988; 68:189.
51. LeBeau MM, Albain KS, Larson RA, et al: Clinical and cytogenetic correlations in 63 patients with therapy-related myelodysplastic syndromes and acute nonlymphocytic leukemia: Further evidence for characteristic abnormalities of chromosomes No. 5 and 7. J Clin Oncol 1986; 4:325.
52. White AD, Culligan DJ, Hoy TG, et al: Extended cytogenetic follow-up of patients with myelodysplastic syndrome. Br J Haematol 1992; 81:499.
53. Jennings CD, Foon KA: Recent advances in flow cytometry: Application to the diagnosis of hematologic malignancy, Blood 1997; 90:2863.
54. Maschek H, Kaloutsi V, Rodriguez-Kaiser M, et al: Hypoplastic myelodysplastic syndrome: Incidence, morphology, cytogenetics, and prognosis. Ann Hematol 1993; 66:117.
55. Yoshida Y, Oguma S, Uchino H, et al: Refractory myelodysplastic anaemias with hypocellular bone marrow. J Clin Pathol 1988; 41:763.
56. Tuzuner N, Cox C, Rowe JM, et al: Hypocellular myelodysplastic syndromes (MDS): New proposals. Br J Haematol 1995; 91:612.
57. de Planque MM, Kluin-Nelemans HC, van Krieken HJM, et al: Evolution of acquired severe aplastic anaemia to myelodysplasia and subsequent leukaemia in adults. Br J Haematol 1988; 70:55.
58. Tichelli A, Gratwohl A, Wursch A, et al: Late haematological complications in severe aplastic anaemia. Br J Haematol 1988; 69:413.
59. Speck B, Tichelli A, Gratwohl A, et al: Treatment of severe aplastic anemia: A 12-year follow-up of patients after bone marrow transplantation or after therapy with antilymphocyte globulin. In Shahidi NT (ed): Aplastic Anemia and Other Bone Marrow Failure Syndromes. London, Springer-Verlag, 1990, p 96.
60. Rosenfeld SJ, Young NS: Aplastic anemia treated by immunosuppression is a chronic relapsing illness but prognosis is unaffected by relapse (abstract). Blood 1997; 90 (suppl 1):435a.
61. Jonasova A, Neuwirtova R, Cermak J, et al: Cyclosporin A therapy in hypoplastic MDS patients and certain refractory anaemias without hypoplastic bone marrow. Br J Haematol 1998; 200:304.
62. List AF, Glinsmann-Gibson B, Spier C, et al: In vitro and in vivo response to cyclosporin-A in myelodysplastic syndromes: Identification of a hypocellular subset responsive to immune suppression (abstract). Blood 1992; 80 (suppl 1):28a.
63. Molldrem JJ, Jiang YZ, Stetler-Stevenson M, et al: Haematological response of patients with myelodysplastic syndrome to antithymocyte globulin is associated with a loss of lymphocyte-medicated inhibition of CFU-GM and alterations in T-cell receptor Vβ profiles. Br J Haematol 1998; 102:1314.
64. Young NS: The problem of clonality in aplastic anemia. Dr. Dameshek's riddle, restated. Blood 1992; 79:1385.
65. Lambertenghi-Deliliers G, Orazi A, Luksch R, et al: Myelodysplastic syndrome with increased marrow fibrosis: A distinct clinico-pathological entity. Br J Haematol 1991; 78:161.
66. Verhoef GE, De Wolf-Peeters C, Ferrant A, et al: Myelodysplastic syndromes with bone marrow fibrosis: A myelodysplastic disorder with proliferative features. Ann Hematol 1991; 63:235.
67. Lange BJ, Kobrinsky N, Barnard DR, et al: Distinctive demography, biology, and outcome of acute myeloid leukemia and myelodysplastic syndrome in children with Down syndrome: Children's Cancer Group Studies 2861 and 2891. Blood 1998; 91:608.
68. Harris CE, Biggs JC, Concannon AJ, et al: Peripheral blood and bone marrow findings in patients with acquired immunodeficiency syndrome. Pathology 1990; 22:206.
69. Kaloutsi V, Kohlmeyer U, Maschek H, et al: Comparison of bone marrow and hematologic findings in patients with human immunodeficiency virus infection and those with myelodysplastic syndromes and infectious diseases. Am J Clin Pathol 1994; 101:123.
70. Geary CG, Catovsky D, Wiltshaw E, et al: Chronic myelomonocytic leukemia. Br J Haematol 1975; 30:289.
71. Miescher PA, Farquet JJ: Chronic myelomonocytic leukemia in adults. Semin Hematol 1974; 11:129.
72. Ribera J-M, Cervantes F, Rozman C: A multivariate analysis of prognostic factors in chronic myelomonocytic leukaemia according to the FAB criteria. Br J Haematol 1987; 65:307.
73. Bennett JM, Catovsky D, Daniel MT, et al: The chronic myeloid leukemias: Guidelines for distinguishing chronic granulocytic, atypical chronic myeloid, and chronic myelomonocytic leukemia. Proposals by the French-American-British Cooperative Leukemia Group Br J Haematol 1994; 87:746.
74. Sokal G, Michaux JL, Van den Berghe H, et al: A new hematologic syndrome with a distinct karyotype: The 5q-chromosome. Blood 1975; 46:519.
75. Boultwood J, Lewis S, Wainscoat JS: The 5q-syndrome. Blood 1994; 84:3253.
76. Foucar K, McKenna RW, Bloomfield CD, et al: Therapy-related leukemia: A panmyelosis. Cancer 1979; 43:1285.
77. Anderson JE, Appelbaum FR, Fisher LD, et al: Allogeneic bone marrow transplantation for 93 patients with myelodysplastic syndrome. Blood 1993; 82:677.
78. Appelbaum FR, Anderson J: Allogeneic bone marrow transplantation for myelodysplastic syndrome: Outcomes analysis according to IPSS score. Leukemia 1998; 12 (suppl):S25.
79. Raskind WH, Tirumali N, Jacobson R, et al: Evi-

dence for a multistep pathogenesis of a myelodysplastic syndrome. Blood 1984; 63:1318.
80. Jacobs A, Clark RE: Pathogenesis and clinical variations in the myelodysplastic syndromes. Clin Haematol 1986; 15:925.
81. Temin HM: Evolution of cancer genes as a mutation-driven process. Cancer Res 1988; 48:1697.
82. Dameshek W: Riddle: What do aplastic anemia, paroxysmal nocturnal hemoglobinuria (PNH) and "hypoplastic" leukemia have in common? Blood 1967; 30:251.
83. Raskind WH, Fialkow PJ: The use of cell markers in the study of human hematopoietic neoplasia. Adv Cancer Res 1987; 49:127.
84. Busque L, Gilliland DG: X-inactivation analysis in the 1990s: Promise and potential problems. Leukemia 1998; 12:128.
85. Hotta T: Clonality in hematopoietic disorders. Int J Hematol 1997; 66:403.
86. Prchal JT, Throckmorton DW, Carroll AJ, et al: A common progenitor for human myeloid and lymphoid cells. Nature 1978; 274:590.
87. Abkowitz JL, Fialkow PJ, Niebrugge DJ, et al: Pancytopenia as a clonal disorder of a multipotent hematopoietic stem cell. J Clin Invest 1984; 73:258.
88. Busque L, Zhu J, DeHart D, et al: An expression based clonality assay at the human androgen receptor locus (HUMARA) on chromosome X. Nucl Acids Res 1994; 22:697.
89. Janssen JWG, Buschle M, Layton M, et al: Clonal analysis of myelodysplastic syndromes: Evidence of multipotent stem cell origin. Blood 1989; 73:248.
90. Weimar IS, Bourhis J-H, de Gast GC, et al: Clonality in myelodysplastic syndromes. Leuk Lymphoma 1994; 13:215.
91. Lawrence HJ, Broudy VC, Magenis RE, et al: Cytogenetic evidence for involvement of B lymphocytes in acquired sideroblastic anemia. Blood 1987; 70:1003.
92. van Lom K, Hagemeijer A, Smit E, et al: Cytogenetic clonality analysis in myelodysplastic syndrome: Monosomy 7 can be demonstrated in the myeloid and in the lymphoid lineage. Leukemia 1995; 9:1818.
93. Kroef MJ, Bolk MJ, Muus P, et al: Mosaicism of the 5q deletion as assessed by interphase FISH is a common phenomenon in MDS and restricted to myeloid cells. Leukemia 1997; 11:519.
94. Van Kamp H, Fibbe WE, Jansen RP, et al: Clonal involvement of granulocytes and monocytes, but not of T and B lymphocytes and natural killer cells in patients with myelodysplasia: Analysis by X-linked restriction fragment polymorphisms and polymerase chain reaction of the phosphogycerate kinase gene. Blood 1992; 80:1774.
95. Saitoh K, Miura I, Takahashi N, et al: Fluorescence in situ hybridization of progenitor cells obtained by fluorescence-activated cell sorting for the detection of cells affected by chromosome abnormality trisomy 8 in patients with myelodysplastic syndromes. Blood 1998; 92:2886.
96. Asano H, Ohashi H, Ichihara M, et al: Evidence for nonclonal hematopoietic progenitor cell populations in bone marrow of patients with myelodysplastic syndromes. Blood 1994; 84:588.
97. Delforge M, Demuynck H, Verhoef G, et al: Patients with high-risk myelodysplastic syndrome can have polyclonal or clonal haemopoiesis in complete haematological remission. Br J Haematol 1998; 102:486.
98. Mach-Pascual S, Legare RD, Lu D, et al: Predictive value of clonality assays in patients with non-Hodgkin's lymphoma undergoing autologous bone marrow transplant: A single institution study. Blood 1998; 91:4496.
99. Traweek ST, Slovak ML, Nademanee AP, et al: Clonal karyotypic hematopoietic cell abnormalities occurring after autologous bone marrow transplantation for Hodgkin's disease and non-Hodgkin's lymphoma. Blood 1994; 84:957.
100. Gale RE, Bunch C, Moir DJ, et al: Demonstration of developing myelodysplasia/acute myeloid leukaemia in haematologically normal patients after high-dose chemotherapy and autologous bone marrow transplantation using X-chromosome inactivation patterns. Br J Haematol 1996; 93:53.
101. Busque L, Mio R, Mattioli J, et al: Nonrandom x-inactivation patterns in normal females: Lyonization ratios vary with age. Blood 1996; 88:59.
102. Gale RE, Fielding AK, Harrison CN, et al: Acquired skewing of X-chromosome inactivation patterns in myeloid cells of the elderly suggests stochastic clonal loss with age. Br J Haematol 1997;98:512.
103. Abkowitz JL, Taboada M, Shelton GH, et al: An X chromosome gene regulates hematopoietic stem cell kinetics. Proc Natl Acad Sci U S A 1998; 95:3862.
104. Mecucci C: Molecular features of primary MDS with cytogenetic changes. Leuk Res 1998; 22:293.
105. Pederson-Bjergaard J, Rowley JD: The balanced and the unbalanced chromosome aberrations of acute myeloid leukemia may develop in different ways and may contribute differently to malignant transformation. Blood 1994; 83:2780.
106. Clurman B, Groudine M: Tumour-suppressor genes. Killer in search of a motive? Nature 1997; 389:122.
107. Nimer SD, Golde DW: The 5q-abnormality. Blood 1987; 70:1705.
108. Nagarajan L, Zavadil J, Claxton D, et al: Consistent loss of the D5S89 locus mapping telomeric to the interleukin gene cluster and centromeric to EGR-1 in patients with 5q-chromosome. Blood 1994; 83:199.
109. Horrigan SK, Westbrook CA, Kim AH, et al: Polymerase chain reaction-based diagnosis of del (5q) in acute myeloid leukemia and myelodysplastic syndrome identifies a minimal deletion interval. Blood 1996; 88:2665.
110. Boultwood J, Fidler C: Chromosomal deletions in myelodysplasia. Leuk Lymphoma 1995; 17:71.
111. Willman CL, Sever CE, Pallavicini MG, et al: Deletion of IRF-1, mapping to chromosome

111. 5q31.1, in human leukemia and preleukemic myelodysplasia. Science 1993; 259:968.
112. Harada H, Takahashi E, Itoh S, et al: Structure and regulation of the human interferon regulatory factor 1 (IRF-1) and IRF-2 genes: Implications for a gene network in the interferon system. Mol Cell Biol 1994; 14:1500.
113. Boultwood J, Fidler C, Lewis S, et al: Allelic loss of IRF1 in myelodysplasia and acute myeloid leukemia: Retention of IRF1 on the 5q- chromosome in some patients with the 5q-syndrome. Blood 1993; 82:2611.
114. Johnson EJ, Scherer SW, Osborne L, et al: Molecular definition of a narrow interval at 7q22.1 associated with myelodysplasia. Blood 1996; 87:3579.
115. Rowley JD, Reshmi S, Sobulo O, et al: All patients with the T (11;16)(q23;p13.3) that involves MLL and CBP have treatment-related hematologic disorders. Blood 1997; 90:535.
116. Taki T, Sako M, Tsuchida M, et al: The t(11;16)(q23;p13) translocation in myelodysplastic syndrome fuses the MLL gene to the CBP gene. Blood 1997; 89:3945.
117. Jotterland Bellomo M, Parlier V, Muhlematter D, et al: Three new cases of chromosome 3 rearrangement in bands q21 and q26 with abnormal thrombopoiesis bring further evidence to the existence of a 3q21q26 syndrome. Cancer Genet Cytogenet 1992; 59:138.
118. Nucifora G, Begy CR, Erickson P, et al: The 3;21 translocation in myelodysplasia results in a fusion transcript between the AML1 gene and the gene for EAP, a highly conserved protein associated with the Epstein-Barr virus small RNA EBER 1. Proc Natl Acad Sci U S A 1993; 90:7784.
119. Golub TR, Barker GF, Lovett M, et al: Fusion of PDGF receptor beta to a novel ets-like gene, tel, in chronic myelomonocytic leukemia with t(5;12) chromosomal translocation. Cell 1994; 77:307.
120. Golub TR: TEL gene rearrangement in myeloid malignancy. Hematol Oncol North Am 1997; 11:1207.
121. Gallagher A, Darley RL, Padua R: The molecular basis of myelodysplastic syndromes. Haematologica 1997; 82:191.
122. Janssen JWG, Steenvoorden AGM, Lyons J, et al: RAS gene mutations in acute and chronic myelocytic leukemia, chronic myeloproliferative disorders, and myelodysplastic syndromes. Proc Natl Acad Sci U S A 1987; 84:9228.
123. Pedersen-Bjergaard J, Janssen JWG, Lyons J, et al: Point mutations of the ras protooncogenes and chromosome aberrations in acute nonlymphocytic leukemia and preleukemia related to therapy with alkylating agents. Cancer Res 1988; 48:1812.
124. Bar-Eli M, Ahuja H, Gonzalez-Cadavid N, et al: Analysis of N-RAS exon-1 mutations in myelodysplastic syndromes by polymerase chain reaction and direct sequencing. Blood 1989; 73:281.
125. Padua RA, Carter G, Hughes D, et al: RAS mutations in myelodysplasia detected by amplification, oligonucleotide hybridization, and transformation. Leukemia 1988; 2:503.
126. Hirai H, Okada M, Mizoguchi H, et al: Relationship between an activated N-ras oncogene and chromosomal abnormality during leukemic progression from myelodysplastic syndrome. Blood 1988; 71:256.
127. Van Kamp H, de Pijper C, Verlaan-de Vries M, et al: Longitudinal analysis of point mutations of the N-ras proto-oncogene in patients with myelodysplasia using archived blood smears. Blood 1992; 79:1266.
128. Mitani K, Hangaishi A, Imamura N, et al: No concomitant occurence of the N-ras and p53 gene mutations in myelodysplastic syndromes. Leukemia 1997; 11:863.
129. O'Marcaigh AS, Shannon KM: Role of the NF1 gene in leukemogenesis and myeloid growth control. J Pediatr Hematol Oncol 1997; 19:551.
130. Kitagawa M, Yamaguchi S, Takahashi M, et al: Localization of Fas and Fas ligand in bone marrow cells demonstrating myelodysplasia. Leukemia 1998; 12:486.
131. Raza A, Gezer S, Mundle S, et al: Apoptosis in bone marrow biopsy samples involving stromal and hematopoietic cells in 50 patients with myelodysplastic syndromes. Blood 1995; 86:268.
132. Rajapaksa R, Ginzton N, Rott LS, et al: Altered oncoprotein expression and apoptosis in myelodysplastic syndrome marrow cells. Blood 1996; 88:4275.
133. Parker JE, Fishlock KL, Mijovic A, et al: "Low-risk" myelodysplastic syndrome is associated with excessive apoptosis and an increased ratio of pr versus anti-apoptotic bcl-2-related proteins. Br J Haematol 1998; 103:1075.
134. Horikawa K, Nakakuma H, Kawaguchi T, et al: Apoptosis resistance of blood cells from patients with paroxysmal nocturnal hemoglobinuria, aplastic anemia, and myelodysplastic syndrome. Blood 1997; 90:2716.
135. Bouscary D, De Vos J, Guesnu M, et al: Fas/Apo-1 (CD95) expression and apoptosis in patients with myelodysplastic syndromes. Leukemia 1997; 11:839.
136. Hamblin T: Immunologic abnormalities in myelodysplastic syndromes. Hematol Oncol North Am 1992; 6:571.
137. Maciejewski J, Selleri C, Anderson S, et al: Fas antigen expression on CD34+ human marrow cells is induced by interferon-gamma and tumor necrosis factor-alpha and potentiates cytokine-mediated hematopoietic suppression in vitro. Blood 1995; 85:3183.
138. Kitagawa M, Saito I, Kuwata T, et al: Overexpression of tumor necrosis factor (TNF)-α and interferon (INF)-gamma by bone marrow cells from patients with myelodysplastic syndromes. Leukemia 1997; 11:2049.
139. Peddie CM, Wolf CR, McLellan LI, et al: Oxidative DNA damage in CD34+ myelodysplastic cells is associated with intracellular redox changes and elevated plasma tumour necrosis factor-alpha concentration. Br J Haematol 1997; 99:625.
140. Knox SJ, Greenberg BR, Anderson RW, et al:

Studies of T-lymphocytes in preleukemic disorders and acute nonlymphocytic leukemia: In vitro radiosensitivity, mitogenic responsiveness, colony formation, and enumeration of lymphocytic subpopulations. Blood 1983; 61:449.
141. Zoumbos N, Gascon P, Trost S, et al: Circulating activated suppressor T lymphocytes in aplastic anemia. N Engl J Med 1985; 312:257.
142. Hokland P, Kerndrup G, Griffin JD, et al: Analysis of leukocyte differentiation antigens in blood and bone marrow from preleukemia (refractory anemia) patients using monoclonal antibodies. Blood 1986; 67:898.
143. Gersuk G, Lee JW, Beckham CA, et al: Fas (CD95) receptor and fas-ligand expression in bone marrow cells from patients with myelodysplastic syndrome. Blood 1996; 88:1122.
144. Cazzola M, Bergamaschi G, Huebers HA, et al: Pathophysiological classification of acquired bone marrow failure based on quantitative assessment of erythroid function. Eur J Haematol 1987; 38:426.
145. Boivin P, Galand G, Hakim J, et al: Acquired erythroenzymopathies in blood disorders: Study of 200 cases. Br J Haematol 1975; 31:531.
146. Valentine WN, Konrad PN, Paglia DE: Dyserythropoiesis, refractory anemia, and "preleukemia:" metabolic features of the erythrocytes. Blood 1973; 41:857.
147. Juneja SK, Imbert M, Sigaux F, et al: Prevalence and distribution of ringed sideroblasts in primary myelodysplastic syndromes. J Clin Pathol 1983; 36:566.
148. May A, De Souza P, Barnes K, et al: Erythroblast iron metabolism in sideroblastic marrows. Br J Haematol 1982; 52:611.
149. Simon M, Beaumont C, Briere J, et al: Is the HLA-linked haemochromatosis allele implicated in idiopathic refractory sideroblastic anaemia? Br J Haematol 1985; 60:75.
150. Aoki Y: Multiple enzymatic defects in mitochondria in hematological cells of patients with primary sideroblastic anemia. J Clin Invest 1980; 66:43.
151. May A, Bishop DF: The molecular biology and pyridoxine-responsiveness of X-linked sideroblastic anemia. Haematologica 1998; 83:56.
152. Rasi V, Lintula R: Platelet function in the myelodysplastic syndromes. Scand J Haematol 1986; 36 (suppl 45):71.
153. Maldonado J: Platelet granulopathy. Mayo Clin Proc 1976; 51:452.
154. Boogaerts MA, Nelissen V, Roelant C, et al: Blood neutrophil function in primary meylodysplastic syndromes. Br J Haematol 1983; 55:217.
155. Cech P, Markert M, Perrin LH: Partial myeloperoxidase deficiency in preleukemia. Blut 1983; 47:21.
156. Nakaseko C, Takayoshi A, Wakita H: Signalling defect in FMLP-induced neutrophil respiratory burst in myelodysplastic syndrome. Br J Haematol 1996; 95:482.
157. Hamblin T: Clinical features of MDS. Leuk Res 1992; 16:89.
158. Tricot G, Vlietinck R, Boogaerts MA, et al: Prognostic factors in the myelodysplastic syndromes: Importance of initial data on peripheral blood counts, bone marrow cytology, trephine biopsy and chromosomal analysis. Br J Haematol 1985; 60:19.
159. Sanz GF, Sanz MA, Vallespi T, et al: Two regression models and a scoring system for predicting survival and planning treatment in myelodysplastic syndromes: A multivariate analysis of prognostic factors in 370 patients. Blood 1989; 74:395.
160. Kerkhofs H, Hermans J, Haak HL, et al: Utility of the FAB classification for myelodysplastic syndromes: Investigation of prognostic factors in 237 cases. Br J Haematol 1987; 65:73.
161. Mufti GJ, Stevens JR, Oscier DG, et al: Myelodysplastic syndromes: A scoring system with prognostic significance. Br J Haematol 1985; 59:425.
162. Grimwade D, Walker H, Oliver F, et al: The importance of cytogenetics on outcome in AML: Analysis of 1,612 patients entered into the MRC AML 10 trial. Blood 1998; 92:2322.
163. Yunis JJ, Rydell RE, Oken MM, et al: Refined chromosome analysis as an independent prognostic indicator in de novo myelodysplastic syndromes. Blood 1986; 67:1721.
164. Morel P, Hebbar M, Lai JL, et al: Cytogenetic analysis has strong predictive value in de novo myelodysplastic syndromes and can be incorporated in a new scoring system. Leukemia 1993; 7:1315.
165. Dewald GW, Davis MP, Pierre RV, et al: Clinical characteristics and prognosis of 50 patients with a myeloproliferative syndrome and deletion of part of the long arm of chromosome 5. Blood 1985; 66:189.
166. Jacobs RH, Cornbleet MA, Vardiman JW, et al: Prognostic implications of morphology and karyotype in primary myelodysplastic syndromes. Blood 1986; 67:1765.
167. Wattel E, Lai JL, Hebbar M, et al: De novo myelodysplastic syndrome with deletion of the long arm of chromosome 20: A subtype of MDS with distinct hematological and prognostic features? Leuk Res 1993; 17:921.
168. Greenberg PL: Biologic and clinical implications of marrow culture studies in the myelodysplastic syndromes. Semin Hematol 1996; 33:163.
169. Greenberg PL, Mara B: The preleukemic syndrome: Correlation of in vitro parameters of granulopoiesis with clinical features. Am J Med 1979; 66:951.
170. Soligo DA, Oriani A, Annalaro C, et al: CD34 immunohistochemistry of bone marrow biopsies: Prognostic significance in primary myelodysplastic syndromes. Am J Hematol 1994; 46:9.
171. Pedersen-Bjergaard J, Philip P, Pedersen NT, et al: Acute nonlymphocytic leukemia, preleukemia, and acute myeloproliferative syndrome secondary

to treatment of other malignant diseases. Cancer 1984; 54:452.
172. Bennett JM, Moloney WC, Greene MH, et al: Acute myeloid leukemia and other myelopathic disorders following treatment with alkylating agents. Hematol Pathol 1987; 1:99.
173. Ley TJ, Griffith P, Nienhuis AW: Transfusion haemosiderosis and chelation therapy. Clin Haematol 1982; 11:437.
174. Olivieri NF, Nathan DG, MacMillan JH, et al: Survival in medically treated patients with homozygous beta-thalassemia. N Engl J Med 1994; 331:574.
175. Jacobs A, Janowska-Wieczorek A, Caro J, et al: Circulating erythropoietin in patients with myelodysplastic syndromes. Br J Haematol 1989; 73:36.
176. Hellström-Lindberg E: Efficacy of erythropoietin in the myelodysplastic syndromes: A meta-analysis of 205 patients from 17 studies. Br J Haematol 1995; 89:67.
177. Negrin RS, Haeuber DH, Nagler A, et al: Treatment of myelodysplastic syndromes with recombinant human granulocyte colony-stimulating factor. Ann Intern Med 1989; 110:976.
178. Negrin RS, Greenberg PL: Therapy of hematopoietic disorders with recombinant colony-stimulating factors. Adv Pharmacol 1992; 23:263.
179. Hoelzer D, Ganser A, Volkers B, et al: In vitro and in vivo action of recombinant human GM-CSF (rhGM-CSF) in patients with myelodysplastic syndromes. Blood Cells 1988; 14:551.
180. Vadhan-Raj S, Broxmeyer HE, Spitzer G, et al: Stimulation of nonclonal hematopoiesis and suppression of the neoplastic clone after treatment with recombinant human granulocyte-macrophage colony–stimulating factor in a patient with therapy-related myelodysplastic syndrome. Blood 1989; 74:1491.
181. Willemze R, van der Lely N, Zwierzina H, et al: A randomized phase-I/II multicenter trial of recombinant human granulocyte-macrophage colony–stimulating factor (GM-CSF) therapy for patients with myelodysplastic syndromes and a relatively low risk of acute leukemia. Ann Hematol 1992; 64:173.
182. Greenberg P, Taylor K, Larson R, et al: Phase III randomized multicenter trial of G-CSF vs. observation for myelodysplastic syndromes (MDS) (abstract). Blood 1993; 82:196a.
183. Negrin RS, Stein R, Vardiman J, et al: Treatment of the anemia of myelodysplastic syndromes using recombinant human granulocyte colony–stimulating factor in combination with erythropoietin. Blood 1993; 82:737.
184. Negrin RS, Stein R, Doherty K, et al: Maintenance treatment of the anemia of myelodysplastic syndromes with recombinant human granulocyte colony–stimulating factor and erythropoietin: Evidence for in vivo synergy. Blood 1996; 87:4076.
185. Hellstrom-Lindberg E, Ahlgren T, Beguin Y, et al: Treatment of anemia in myelodysplastic syndromes with granulocyte colony–stimulating factor plus erythropoietin: Results from a randomized phase II study and long-term follow-up of 71 patients. Blood 1998; 92:68.
186. Hellstrom-Lindberg E, Negrin R, Stein R, et al: Erythroid response to treatment with G-CSF plus erythtopoietin for the anaemia of patients with myelodysplastic syndromes: Proposal for a predictive model. Br J Haematol 1997; 99:344.
187. Appelbaum FR, Anderson J: Bone marrow transplantation for myelodysplasia in adults and children: When and who? Leuk Res 1998; 22 (suppl 1):S35.
188. Runde V, de Witte T, Arnold R, et al: Bone marrow transplantation from HLA-identical siblings as first-line treatment in patients with myelodysplastic syndromes: Early transplantation is associated with improved outcome. Chronic Leukemia Working Party of the European Group for Blood and Marrow Transplantation. Bone Marrow Transplant 1998; 21:255.
189. Arnold R, de Witte T, Van Biezen A, et al: Unrelated bone marrow transplantation in patients with myelodysplastic syndromes and secondary acute myeloid leukemia: An EBMT survey. European Blood and Marrow Transplantation Group. Bone Marrow Transplant 1998; 21:1213.
190. Ballan KK, Gilliland DG, Guinan EC, et al: Bone marrow transplantation for therapy-related myelodysplasia: Comparison with primary myelodysplasia. Bone Marrow Transplant 1997; 20:737.
191. O'Donnell MR, Long GD, Parker PM, et al: Busulfan/cyclophosphamide as conditioning regimen for allogeneic bone marrow transplantation for myelodysplasia. J Clin Oncol 1995; 13:2973.
192. Slavin S, Nagler A, Naparstek E, et al: Nonmyeloablative stem cell transplantation and cell therapy as an alternative to conventional bone marrow transplantation with lethal cytoreduction for the treatment of malignant and nonmalignant hematologic diseases. Blood 1998; 91:756.
193. Childs R, Bahceci E, Clave E, et al: Non-myeloablative allogeneic peripheral blood stem cell transplants (PBSCT) for malignant diseases reduces transplant-related mortality (TRM) (abstract). Blood 1998; 92 (suppl 1):137a.
194. Leith CP, Kopecky KJ, Godwin J, et al: Acute myeloid leukemia in the elderly: Assessment of multidrug resistance (MDR1) and cytogenetics distinguishes biologic subgroups with remarkably distinct responses to standard chemotherapy. A Southwest Oncology Group study. Blood 1997; 89:3323.
195. Head DR: Revised classification of acute myeloid leukemia. Leukemia 1996; 10:1826.
196. Bernasconi C, Alessandrino EP, Bernasconi P, et al: Randomized clinical study comparing aggressive chemotherapy with or without G-CSF support for high-risk myelodysplastic syndromes or secondary acute myeloid leukaemia evolving from MDS. Br J Haematol 1998; 102:678.
197. Godwin JE, Kopecky KJ, Head DR, et al: A double-blind placebo-controlled trial of granulocyte colony–stimulating factor in elderly patients with previously untreated acute myeloid leukemia:

197. [continued] A Southwest Oncology Group study (9031). Blood 1998; 91:3607.
198. Estey E, Thall P, Beran M, et al: Effect of diagnosis: Refractory anemia with excess blasts, refractory anemia with excess blasts in transformation, or acute myeloid leukemia (AML) on outcome of AML-type chemotherapy. Blood 1997; 90:2969.
199. Beran M, Kantarjian H, O'Brien S, et al: Topotecan, a topoisomerase I inhibitor, is active in the treatment of myelodysplastic syndrome and chronic myelomonocytic leukemia. Blood 1996; 88:2473.
200. Parker JE, Pagliuca A, Mijovic A, et al: Fludarabine, cytarabine, G-CSF and idarubicin (FLAG-IDA) for the treatment of poor-risk myelodysplastic syndromes and acute myeloid leukemia. Br J Haematol 1997; 99:939.
201. Bernstein SH, Brunetto VL, Davey FR, et al: Acute myeloid leukemia–type chemotherapy for newly diagnosed patients without antecedent cytopenias having myelodysplastic syndrome as defined by French-American-British criteria: A Cancer and Leukemia Group B Study. J Clin Oncol 1996; 14:2486.
202. Laporte JP, Isnard F, Lesage S, et al: Autologous bone marrow transplantation with marrow purged by mafosfamide in seven patients with myelodysplastic syndromes in transformation (AML-MDS): A pilot study. Leukemia 1993; 7:2030.
203. Carella AM, Dejana A, Lerma E, et al: In vivo mobilization of karyotypically normal peripheral blood progenitor cells in high-risk MDS, a secondary or therapy-related acute myelogenous leukaemia. Br J Haematol 1996; 95:127.
204. Delforge M, Demuynck H, Vandenberghe P, et al: Polyclonal primitive hematopoietic progenitors can be detected in mobilized peripheral blood from patients with high-risk myelodysplastic syndromes. Blood 1995; 86:3660.
205. de Witte T, Van Biezen A, Hermans J, et al: Autologous bone marrow transplantation for patients with myelodysplastic syndrome (MDS) or acute myeloid leukemia following MDS. Blood 1997; 90:3853.
206. Demuynck H, Delforge M, Verhoef GE, et al: Feasibility of peripheral blood progenitor cell harvest and transplantation in patients with poor-risk myelodysplastic syndromes. Br J Haematol 1996; 92:351.
207. Christman JK, Mendelsohn N, Herzog D, et al: Effect of 5-azacytidine on differentiation and DNA methylation in human promyelocytic leukemia cells (HL-60) Cancer Res 1983; 43:763.
208. Griffin J, Munroe D, Major P, et al: Induction of differentiation of human myeloid leukemia cells by inhibitors of DNA synthesis. Exp Hematol 1982; 10:774.
209. Santini V, Ferrini PR: Differentiation therapy of myelodysplastic syndromes: Fact or fiction? Br J Haematol 1998; 102:1124.
210. Cheson BD: Standard and low-dose chemotherapy for the treatment of myelodysplastic syndromes. Leuk Res 1998; 22 (suppl 1):S17.
211. Griffin JD, Spriggs DR, Wisch JS: Treatment of preleukemic syndromes with continuous intravenous infusion of low dose cytosine arabinoside. J Clin Oncol 1985; 3:982.
212. Miller KB, Kim K, Morrison FS, et al: The evaluation of low-dose cytarabine in the treatment of myelodysplastic syndromes: A phase-III intergroup study. Ann Hematol 1992; 65:162.
213. Koeffler HP, Heitjan D, Mertelsmann R, et al: Randomized study of 13-*cis* retinoic acid *v* placebo in the myelodysplastic disorders. Blood 1988; 71:703.
214. Clark RE, Jacobs A, Lush CJ, et al: Effect of 13-cis-retinoic acid on survival of patients with myelodysplastic syndrome. Lancet 1986; 2:763.
215. Rowinsky EK, Conley BA, Jones RJ, et al: Hexamethylene bisacetamide in myelodysplastic syndrome: Effect of five-day exposure to maximal therapeutic concentrations. Leukemia 1992; 6:526.
216. Wijermans PW, Krulder JW, Huijgens PC, et al: Continuous infusion of low-dose 5-AZA-2'-deoxycytidine in elderly patients with high-risk myelodysplastic syndrome. Leukemia 1997; 11:1.
217. Silverman LR, Holland JF, Weinberg RS, et al: Effects of treatment with 5-azacytidine on the in vivo and in vitro hematopoiesis in patients with myelodysplastic syndromes. Leukemia 1993; 7 (suppl 1):21.
218. Silverman LR, Demakos EP, Peterson B, et al: A randomized controlled trial of subcutaneous azacitidine (aza c) in patients with the myelodysplastic syndrome (MDS): A study of Cancer and Leukemia Group B (CALGB) (abstract). Proc Am Soc Clin Oncol 1998; 17:14a.
219. Kornblith AB, Herndon, II, Silverman LR, et al: The impact of 5-azacytidine on the quality of life of patients with the myelodysplastic syndrome (MDS) treated in a randomized phase III trial of the Cancer and Leukemia Group B (CALGB) (abstract). Proc Am Soc Clin Oncol 1998; 17:49a.
220. Gore SD, Samid D, Weng LJ: Impact of the putative differentiating agents sodium phenylbutyrate and sodium phenylacetate on proliferation, differentiation, and apoptosis of primary neoplastic myeloid cells. Clin Cancer Res 1997; 3:1755.
221. List A: Hematopoietic stimulation by amifostine and sodium phenylbutarate: What is the potential in MDS? Leuk Res 1998; 1 (suppl):7.
222. Mellibovsky L, Diez A, Perez-Vila E, et al: Vitamin D treatment in myelodysplastic syndromes. Br J Haematol 1998; 100:516.
223. Galvani D, Nethersell A, Bottomley J: Treatment of myelodysplasia with interferon. Leukemia 1987; 1:786.
224. Galvani DW, Nethersell ABW, Cawley JC: Alpha-interferon in myelodysplasia: Clinical observations and effects on NK cells. Leuk Res 1988; 12:257.
225. Petti MC, Lagagliata R, Avvisati G, et al: Treatment of high-risk myelodysplastic syndromes with lymphoblastoid alpha-interferon. Br J Haematol 1996; 95:364.
226. Doll DC, Kasper LM, Taetle R, et al: Treatment

227. Wattel E, Guerci A, Hecquet B, et al: A randomized trial of hydroxyurea versus VP16 in adult chronic myelomonocytic leukemia. Groupe Français des Myélodysplasies and European CMML Group. Blood 1996; 88:2480.
228. Bagby GC, Gabourel JD, Linman JW: Gluticocorticoid therapy in the preleukemic syndrome (hemopoietic dysplasia). Ann Intern Med 1980; 92:55.
229. Enright H, Jacob HS, Vercellotti G, et al: Paraneoplastic autoimmune phenomena in patients with myelodysplastic syndromes: Response to immunosuppressive therapy. Br J Haematol 1995; 91:403.
230. Najean Y, Pecking A: Refractory anaemia with excess of myeloblasts in the bone marrow: A clinical trial of androgens in 90 patients. Br J Haematol 1977; 37:25.
231. Riccardi A, Giordano M, Girino M, et al: Refractory cytopenias: Clinical course according to bone marrow cytology and cellularity. Blut 1987; 54:153.
232. Biesma DH, van den Tweel JG, Verdonck LF: Immunosuppressive therapy for hypoplastic myelodysplastic syndrome. Cancer 1997; 79:1548.
233. Molldrem J, Caples M, Mavroudis D, et al: Antithymocyte globulin (ATG) abrogates cytopenias in patients with myelodysplastic syndrome. Br J Haematol 1997; 99:699.
234. Kurbacher CM, Mallmann PK: Chemoprotection in anticancer therapy: The emerging role of amifostine (WR-2721). Anticancer Res 1998; 18:2203.
235. List AF, Brasfield F, Heaton R, et al: Stimulation of hematopoiesis by amifostine in patients with myelodysplastic syndrome. Blood 1997; 90:3364.
236. Fenaux P, Morel P, Rosse C, et al: Prognostic factors in adult de novo myelodysplastic syndromes treated by intensive chemotherapy. Br J Haematol 1991; 77:497.
237. Ganser A, Heil G, Kolbe K, et al: Aggressive chemotherapy combined with G-CSF and maintenance therapy with interleukin-2 for patients with advances myelodysplastic syndrome, subacute or secondary acute myeloid leukemia—initial results. Ann Hematol 1993; 66:123.
238. Preisler HD, Raza A, Barcos M, et al: High-dose cytosine arabinoside in the treatment of preleukemic disorders: A Leukemia Intergroup study. Am J Hematol 1986; 23:131.

4

Paroxysmal Nocturnal Hemoglobinuria

Daniel E. Dunn, M.D., Ph.D.
Johnson M. Liu, M.D.
Neal S. Young, M.D.

HISTORY

In 1866, William Gull described the first recorded case of "intermittent haematinuria" in a 33-year-old leather-dyer[1]: "burgundy-wine colour[ed]" urine was often observed in the morning, changing within "an hour or two . . . to pale straw colour." "No blood corpuscles [were] to be seen," and Gull erroneously identified the urine pigment as "prismatic crystals of haematin." Sixteen years later the German physician Paul Strübing[2] correctly attributed the pigmentation to hemoglobin in his report of a patient who "voided dark, hemoglobinous urine only in the morning." He carefully described how the patient's plasma turned red after an especially severe attack and construed this as evidence that erythrocytes were disintegrating in the blood vessels and not in the kidney or urine. Strübing was the first to recognize that these symptoms were part of a new disease entity, for which the Dutch physician Enneking[3] in 1928 introduced the term "paroxysmal nocturnal hemoglobinuria." As early as the 1930s, Ham in the United States and Dacie in England showed that in paroxysmal nocturnal hemoglobinuria (PNH) it is the red blood cells that are defective, and that slight acidification of the plasma in vitro results in increased hemolysis, a finding that for decades served as the confirmatory laboratory test in the diagnosis of the disease.[4, 5] Beginning in the late 1950s, an increasing number of molecules were found to be deficient on the PNH cell surface: acetylcholinesterase first, followed by leukocyte alkaline phosphatase, and the decay-accelerating factor (DAF).[6–8] The realization that these proteins and many others are all attached to the cell membrane by a particular glycolipid anchor (glycosylphosphatidylinositol [GPI]) provided a major insight into the molecular lesion in PNH. In 1970 Oni et al.[9] demonstrated that the defective erythrocytes in PNH were all derived from a common ancestor, using classic glucose-6-phosphate dehydrogenase (G6PD) isoenzyme analyses in heterozygous female patients; this placed PNH in the family of clonal hematologic disorders such as chronic myelogenous leukemia (CML), polycythemia vera (PCV), essential thrombocytosis, or myelofibrosis. Two decades later, Kinoshita and coworkers identified the gene which, when mutated, results in the GPI-anchored protein [GPI-AP]–deficient phenotype[10–12]: PIG-A. This gene is necessary for the first step in the biosynthesis of the GPI anchor moiety. Localization of this gene to the X chromosome explained how a single somatic mutational event was sufficient to result in complete loss of GPI-AP expression in affected hematopoietic cells. The clinical association of PNH with aplastic anemia (AA) was first described by Dacie and Lewis in the 1960s.[13, 14] The precise pathophysiologic basis for this association remains incompletely elucidated to this day and data bearing on this association will be a major focus of this chapter.

CASE DEFINITION

At first, the case definition of PNH relied on the finding of intermittent hemoglobinous urine, predominantly in the mornings. With the advent of Ham's test, it became possible to diagnose PNH in nonclassic cases in which hemoglobinuria might not necessarily be apparent; the case definition thus evolved to include any patient with one or more of the three clinical manifestations of PNH—hemolysis, thrombosis, or bone marrow failure—coupled with a positive Ham's test. While the Ham's test is specific, it is not very sensitive, in particular in patients receiving red blood cell transfusions. Recently, flow cytometric techniques have been used to quantitate the GPI-AP–deficient leukocyte counterparts of PNH red blood cells. The current case definition of PNH thus consists of clinical evidence of hemolysis, thrombosis, or bone marrow failure, in conjunction with flow cytometric evidence of a discrete population of GPI-AP–deficient leukocytes. GPI-AP–deficient erythrocytes are *not* required as no such cells may be detectable in *either* PNH patients who have lysed all affected erythrocytes or in hypoplastic patients who are entirely dependent on red blood cell transfusions. The wider application of flow cytometric methods for detection of PNH-phenotype leukocytes in this latter population, including patients with myelodysplastic syndromes (MDS), as well as classic AA, is likely to result in a significant increase in the diagnosis of PNH.

EPIDEMIOLOGY

PNH may present at almost any age, from the second to the eighth decade of life; the median age at diagnosis is about 40 years. The disease is always acquired, never inherited. Males and females are equally affected. The prevalence of PNH has been estimated[15, 16] at roughly 1 in 100,000 but may soon be found to be an underestimate, in light of newly available diagnostic techniques with significantly enhanced sensitivity compared with Ham's test (see below). PNH may be more common in the Orient, although no precise epidemiologic study has been published. The rate of thrombotic complication, however, is apparently quite different in these two populations: approximately one third of PNH patients of European or Indian descent eventually suffer a major thrombotic event,[17–19] whereas fewer than 10% of PNH patients from the Far East experience thrombosis.[20, 21] Conversely, Asian PNH patients are more likely to develop clinically evident bone marrow aplasia[22]: pediatric patients also seem skewed more toward developing aplasia rather than thrombosis.[23] The only known risk factor for PNH is a history of AA or MDS.

CLINICAL MANIFESTATIONS

Most of the symptoms of PNH are directly attributable to the three major pathologic processes of the disease—hemolysis, thrombosis, and pancytopenia. Thus PNH patients will often suffer from the predictable symptoms of anemia such as fatigue or dyspnea on exertion. During hemolytic paroxysms, the patient may note jaundice. Dark-colored urine is a relatively uncommon, if dramatic, symptom, especially now that sophisticated laboratory techniques permit earlier diagnosis of PNH. Thrombotic events, most commonly in the splanchnic, hepatic, or cerebral venous systems, may give rise to symptoms of abdominal pain or swelling, headache, or focal neurologic deficits. Neutropenia may manifest as fever, aphthous oral ulcers, or myriad infectious processes. Thrombocytopenia may come to the patient's attention as petechiae, easy bruising, nose or gum bleeding, or oral blood blisters. PNH patients will also occasionally complain of pressure sensations in the chest, dysphagia, or impotence, especially during hemolytic crises. Intravascular hemolysis has been hypothesized to lead to nitric oxide sequestration by free hemoglobin in the plasma, thus antagonizing relaxation of smooth muscle in the esophagus or the walls of vessels supplying the penis.[16]

The various signs of PNH on physical examination follow from the underlying hemolysis, thrombosis, or pancytopenia. These include pallor, jaundice, hepatomegaly, ascites, splenomegaly (if the splenic vein has thrombosed), focal neurologic findings or papilledema,[24, 25] petechiae, purpura, aphthous ulcers with or without blood, and retinal hemorrhages—none of which are specific for PNH.

Other than the obligatory presence of a GPI-deficient subpopulation of leukocytes or erythrocytes, or both, in the blood (determined by flow cytometry or Ham's test), the laboratory findings in PNH are diverse and inconstant. The numbers and morphology of circulating erythrocytes, platelets, and leukocytes may be entirely unremarkable.

If a patient is anemic due primarily to hemolysis, reticulocytosis and polychromasia will be evident on the blood smear; if the anemia is due primarily to bone marrow failure, reticulocytopenia and macrocytosis should be apparent. The characteristic macrocytosis of AA may not be present, however, if the patient is entirely dependent on red blood cell transfusions.

Platelet counts in the range of 50 to 100 ×

10^9/L are common; such minor depressions in the platelet count are of no clinical consequence but may represent a modest degree of bone marrow failure. Platelet counts of less than 50×10^9/L are indicative of progression to the full AA-PNH overlap syndrome. Neutropenia is seen only in the overlap syndrome with AA.

The bone marrow morphology is also highly variable. In PNH cases dominated by hemolysis, the marrow is generally hypercellular with more erythroid than myeloid forms. Dys- and megaloblastic erythropoiesis may be evident. In PNH-AA cases, the bone marrow will be hypo- or even acellular. The residual elements may be either myeloid, lymphoid, or mast cells, as is characteristic in AA. Dysplastic morphology is common in erythroid cells, less so in other lineages. If uninuclear or micromegakaryocytes or dysplastic granulocytes are present, then a diagnosis of PNH-MDS is warranted.

Bone marrow chromosomal analysis in PNH is almost always normal, notwithstanding the bias in the PNH literature to report cytogenetically abnormal cases.[26–34]

Additional laboratory findings may include evidence of intravascular hemolysis such as the presence of plasma hemoglobin, low haptoglobin, hemoglobinuria (not hematuria), urine hemosiderin, and depressed iron indices—secondary to urinary iron loss—such as serum iron or ferritin (iron-binding capacity will be elevated.) Other markers of hemolysis not specific for intravascular destruction include elevated lactate dehydrogenase (LDH), and high levels of unconjugated bilirubin. The direct Coombs' test should not be positive.

In PNH-AA, following multiple red blood cell transfusions, the ferritin may be markedly elevated due to iron overload. In cases of PNH complicated by the Budd-Chiari syndrome, laboratory values consistent with liver failure may develop, such as low albumin or prolonged prothrombin and activated partial thromboplastin times.

A highly characteristic radiographic sign of PNH can be seen on magnetic resonance imaging (MRI) of the kidneys: a signal void in the kidney cortex reflects excess iron accumulation in the cells of the proximal convoluted tubule, where hemoglobin (and hence iron) is first reclaimed from the glomerular filtrate. If thrombosis is suspected in a PNH patient, computed tomography (CT) with intravenous contrast, MRI, or ultrasound of the suspected abdominal vasculature will often be diagnostic; suspected thrombosis of the cerebral sinuses is best evaluated by MRI.

The diagnosis of PNH may be overlooked unless in the presence of a history of classic episodes of hemoglobinuria or of AA. Many patients thus report years of symptoms antedating their formal diagnosis that, in retrospect, were obviously secondary to PNH. PNH should therefore be considered in all undiagnosed clinical cases of hemolytic anemia, cytopenias, or thrombophilia, especially the Budd-Chiari syndrome, and flow cytometric analyses should be performed to determine if the patient's blood harbors a GPI-AP–deficient subpopulation of leukocytes. If only the Ham's test is available, its insensitivity may result in missed or delayed diagnosis in many cases. The acidified serum lysis test is highly specific, and is positive in only one other hematologic condition (congenital dyserythropoietic anemia, type II [CDA-II], also known as hereditary erythroblastic multinuclearity with a positive acidified serum test [HEMPAS]). There are no human diseases other than PNH known to result in a population of blood cells globally deficient in GPI-AP.

PATHOPHYSIOLOGY

The mechanism by which a defect in GPI anchor biosynthesis results in the hemolysis of affected red blood cells in PNH patients has been fully elucidated. Likely the same biochemical lesion in platelets is responsible for the thrombotic diathesis of PNH. The next section details our current understanding of the molecular basis of these two major clinical manifestations of PNH. How the biology of GPI-APs might explain the clinical association of PNH with aplasia is discussed subsequently.

The Glycosylphosphatidylinositol Anchor

Proteins are associated with cell membranes via several mechanisms (Fig. 4–1A). Integral membrane proteins maintain intimate contact with the inner aliphatic chains of the phospholipid bilayer membrane through their own hydrophobic amino acid sequences in one or more transmembrane segments. Hydrophobicity is sometimes enhanced by acylation of amino acid side chains with the fatty acids myristate or palmitate. Knowledge of a new class of over 50 extracellular membrane proteins has emerged over the past 15 years; these proteins are distinguished by their attachment to the cell membrane by a phosphatidylinositol anchor linked covalently by a short oligosaccharide to the mature protein's C-terminal[35] (Fig. 4–1B). The GPI anchor is now recognized as a common mechanism by which entirely extracellular proteins are anchored in the outer leaflet of the eukar-

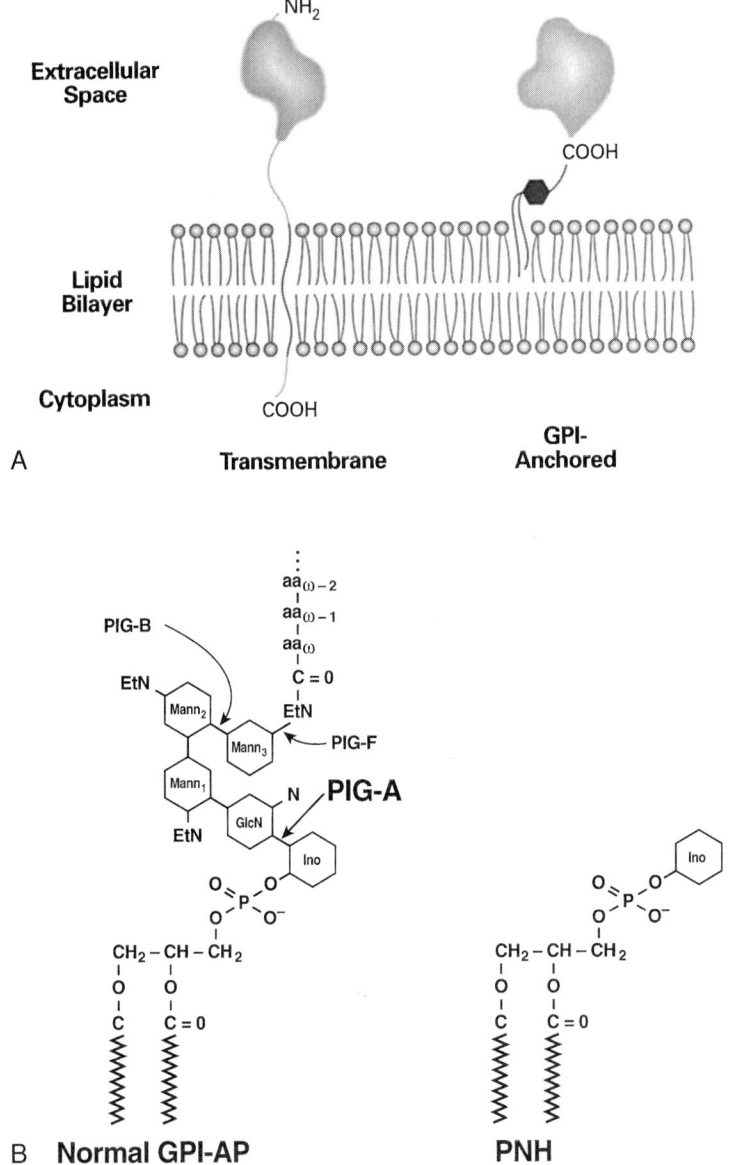

Figure 4–1 (A) Structural differences between classic transmembrane proteins and glycosylphosphatidylinositol (GPI)-anchored proteins. Note that the entire mature polypeptide component of a GPI-anchored protein is extracellular and there is no obvious mechanism by which ligand engagement transduces a signal across the cell membrane lipid bilayer. **(B)** Structure of GPI-anchored proteins (GPI-AP). An oligosaccharide consisting of inositol (Ino), glucosamine (GlcN), and three mannoses ($Mann_{1-3}$), plus a linking ethanolamine (EtN), bridge the terminal amino acid of a given protein (aa_ω) by an EtN to the alkyl-acyl glycerol moiety, which anchors the resultant GPI-AP in the cell membrane. In paroxysmal nocturnal hemoglobinuria (PNH), somatic mutations in the *PIG-A* gene (located on the X chromosome) result in defective GPI anchor biosynthesis. Cell surface expression of all proteins dependent on this mode of membrane anchoring is lost in the progeny of affected hematopoietic stem cells.

yotic cell membrane. The unique biophysical features conferred by the GPI anchor to this class of proteins[36, 37] are partly understood, but the functional advantage of these specific properties is largely unknown. For example, GPI-linked proteins in general may show greater lateral mobility than their transmembrane counterparts, and endocytosis by some cells may take place via membrane domains rich in GPI-APs.[38–41]

The discovery of the GPI-linked proteins began with the isolation of bacterial phospholipases in the 1960s. One of these enzymes, phosphatidylinositol-specific phospholipase C (PI-PLC), was found to release alkaline phosphatase from the plasma membrane of intact cells.[42] The structure of the GPI moiety was subsequently further elucidated by work on trypanosomes, whose major surface protein is GPI-anchored: variant surface glycoprotein[43] (VSG); it has been hypothesized that shedding of antigenic VSG proteins from the parasite cell surface, perhaps by release of an endogenous trypanosomal phospholipase, may permit the organism to evade humoral attack by the host immune system.

The fundamental structure of the GPI anchor is remarkably similar in a wide variety of mammalian, yeast, and parasitic cells and consists of three parts (see Fig. 4–1):

1. An inositol phospholipid, which forms the main connection to the cell membrane and is sensitive to PI-PLC digestion. An additional acyl group can be affixed to the inositol moiety during the biosynthesis of the anchor; in this case, GPI-AP will not be released from a cell after PI-PLC digestion (PI-PLC treatment is therefore not an absolute means of proving the presence of a GPI anchor[44]).
2. A glycan core, consisting of a molecule of glucosamine and three mannose residues.
3. A phosphoethanolamine (PE) molecule affixed to the terminal mannose. This molecule connects the GPI anchor to the protein by an amide bond between the amine moiety of PE and the mature protein's C-terminal (the so-called ω amino acid) carboxyl group.

GPI-APs share a common and unique pathway of biosynthesis. Synthesis begins in the endoplasmic reticulum (ER) and is probably completed in the Golgi apparatus.[45] The nascent form of a typical polypeptide destined to become GPI-anchored contains a specific hydrophobic c-terminal signal peptide, which is removed during its processing in the ER, in a transamidation reaction, leading to covalent attachment to the GPI moiety. The GPI anchor is presynthesized independently in the ER. Curiously, for certain proteins, for example, LFA-3 (CD58) or NCAM (CD56), two mature molecular species are produced, one transmembrane and one GPI-anchored, as a result of either gene duplication or alternative splicing.

Information on the biosynthetic pathway comes mostly from complementation studies with somatic cell lines. Through somatic fusion of defective cells and by analyzing the products for the presence or absence of GPI anchor intermediates, several different complementation groups have been characterized.[46–48] Cells from three complementation classes (A, C, H) share the same phenotype, in that defective cells from each of these classes are unable to attach N-acetylglucosamine to phosphatidylinositol,[49, 50] the first step in GPI anchor biosynthesis. Other complementation groups exhibit defects in later stages of the biosynthesis of the GPI anchor, such as deacetylation of N-acetylglucosamine after addition to phosphatidylinositol, or attachment of subsequent mannose or phosphoethanolamine moieties. Biochemical studies of GPI-AP–deficient cells from PNH patients revealed that it was the first step in GPI anchor biosynthesis that was defective. Thus it was possible that acquired mutations in either the PIG-A, -C, or -H genes were responsible for PNH.

The PIG-A Gene

The first experimental evidence of the clonal nature of PNH came from the study of red blood cells from two female patients from Africa, using a classic G6PD heterozygosity approach.[9] Since in most PNH patients deficient expression of GPI-AP can be demonstrated on a subset of erythrocytes, leukocytes, and lymphocytes (but not on nonhematopoietic cells), PNH was inferred to be a clonal disorder arising at the level of the hematopoietic stem cell (HSC).[51] In vitro studies have confirmed that hematopoietic progenitor cells from PNH patients give rise to progeny with a PNH phenotype.[52, 53] Cell fusion experiments, utilizing GPI-AP(−) Epstein-Barr virus (EBV)–transformed lymphoblastoid cell lines [LCLs] from PNH patients,[54, 55] established that the genetic defect in PNH patients maps uniformly to complementation group A.[56]

The gene responsible for the PNH phenotype is PIG-A.[10-12] PIG-A was isolated by employing an expression cloning strategy in class A-mutant LCLs. The gene[57, 58] is organized in six exons extending over 17 kb, and the 1455-nucleotide coding sequence yields a 484–amino acid protein product[59] with a predicted molecular weight of 54 kD. PIG-A has been mapped to the short arm of the X chromosome (Xp22.1)[11, 58] and this location explained how a single, somatically acquired mutation could result in complete loss of GPI-linked protein expression on the surface of the progeny of the mutant PNH stem cell.[10, 60]

Erythrocytes derived from a PIG-A–mutant HSC will be deficient in expression of GPI-APs, two of which are membrane inhibitor of reactive lysis (MIRL or CD59) and DAF (or CD55); both proteins are involved in the antagonism of the assembly of activated complement components on the surface of erythrocytes and platelets. Thus, during transient endotoxemia, as may occur at night or in the context of an infection, low levels of complement may become activated, leading to lysis of GPI-AP–deficient erythrocytes and presentation with paroxysmal hemoglobinuria or, if the hemolysis is more indolent, symptoms of anemia. The in vitro recapitulation of this process is the acidified serum lysis or Ham's test which for decades has served as the confirmatory laboratory test for PNH. The sugar-water or sucrose hemolysis test is an alternative in vitro technique for complement activation; it may be more sensitive than the Ham's test in PNH, but is also less specific.

The origin of PIG-A mutations in HSCs is unknown. Neither PNH nor acquired AA is familial, which argues against a constitutional mutator phenotype. No case of congenital PNH due to an inherited PIG-A mutation[61] has ever been described; the experience with knock-out mice suggests that such a genotype is lethal in utero,[62] even in females. The location of *PIG-A* mutations, collated from a large number of PNH patients, is essentially random,[63–66] and almost every patient's mutation is unique.[67] The most common type of mutation is insertion or deletion of one or two nucleotides, introducing a frame shift and thereby giving rise to a severely dysfunctional gene product. Mutations in splice sites, the second most frequent type, result in deletion of one or more exons. It has been hypothesized that *PIG-A* mutations arise in the HSCs of PNH patients no more frequently than in the HSCs of healthy subjects, but that in PNH patients such GPI-AP–deficient HSC clones undergo selective expansion[68, 69] (see below).

The thrombotic diathesis in PNH is believed also to arise as a direct consequence of GPI-AP deficiency on the surface of affected platelets and perhaps also of deficient erythrocytes. Because affected platelets from PNH patients lack DAF (CD55) and MIRL (CD59), excess complement will accumulate on their surface during periods of intravascular complement activation. Such platelets would not necessarily lyse but could rather undergo activation. Activated platelets become hyperaggregable, shed procoagulant microvesicles, and express elevated factor Va binding sites, thereby promoting prothombinase complex (VaXa) formation.[70–74] Similar microvesicle shedding by complement-laden erythrocytes might contribute to the thrombotic diathesis in PNH as well.[75] Finally, the cellular receptor for urokinase-type plasminogen activator (uPAR or CD87) is known to be GPI-anchored.[76] Inflammatory cells that participate in thrombus resorption or fibrinolysis might thus be defective in PNH.

PAROXYSMAL NOCTURNAL HEMOGLOBINURIA AND BONE MARROW FAILURE

The central etiologic dilemma in PNH is why a *PIG-A*–mutant HSC expands dramatically to account, in most cases, for the bulk of hematopoiesis, without inevitable progression to complete replacement of wild-type (GPI-AP(+)) hematopoiesis, polycythemia, or leukemia. The reciprocal question might alternatively be posed: depending on estimates of HSC number and the expected mutation rate, why does not everyone develop PNH? The key to answering these questions may lie in Lewis and Dacie's association of PNH with bone marrow failure and especially AA.[13, 14] Only about a third of patients with PNH will have received a formal diagnosis of AA prior to their physician's recognition of PNH; another third, however, subsequent to their diagnosis of PNH, eventually fulfill the criteria for severe or moderate AA over the ensuing years to decades. Even the remaining "hemolytic" PNH patients have evidence of bone marrow failure by in vitro assays of hematopoiesis (see below). In this section clinical, experimental, and theoretical observations and considerations on PNH patients, *PIG-A* mutations, and HSC biology are discussed, and a Darwinian model of *PIG-A*–mutant HSC evolution in the context of selection by the processes underlying bone marrow aplasia is proposed.

Observations on Paroxysmal Nocturnal Hemoglobinuria: Clinical Behavior and Studies With Patient Samples

Inferences from observation of hematopoiesis in vivo and in vitro have been useful in providing insights into the basic pathologic processes at work in PNH. First, PNH is a clonal disease[9] and the ontogenic stage of the genetic lesion is at or before the pluripotent hematopoietic progenitor: in many PNH patients, every lymphoid and myeloid lineage harbors GPI-AP(−) cells: T cells, B cells, natural killer (NK) cells, granulocytes, monocytes, platelets, and erythrocytes.[77] The advantage conferred by the *PIG-A*-defective genotype, whether intrinsic or extrinsic, must occur at the level of *stem* cell biology, although it is possible that selection may also be applied at the level of more mature progenitors. (But progenitors, by definition, do not self-renew and therefore are not capable of making an enduring contribution to hematopoiesis.) Second, the natural history of PNH is neither inexorable expansion of the mutant clone nor inevitable progression to leukemia. Rather, evolution to bone marrow failure is the second leading cause of death in PNH patients (after thrombosis).[17] Moreover, in one longitudinal study of PNH patients that survived at least 10 years, 15% had a spontaneous remission.[17] Serial measurements of the percent of neutrophils deficient in GPI-AP expression in our patients have revealed very little change over almost 2 years of periodic cytofluorimetric monitoring. Even when PNH patients develop cytogenetic abnormalities and are thus considered to have evolved into MDS, this cytogenetically abnormal clone does not inevitably coincide with the GPI-AP(−) clone.[26–28, 78, 79]

Bone marrow transplantation (BMT) appears to cure PNH—but only if preceded by a cytotoxic regimen. Simple infusion of syngeneic bone marrow is generally not effective[80–86] (Table 4–1).

TABLE 4–1 Summary of Outcomes of Syngeneic Marrow Transplants in PNH

Fefer[84] (Ann Int Med, 1976)	Recovery, late relapse PNH
Hershko[86] (Lancet, 1979)	Recurrent PNH
Jehn[85] (Klin Woch, 1983)	Persistent PNH
Kolb[82] (BMT, 1989)	Persistent PNH
Kawahara[80, 87] (Am J Hematol, 1992)*	1. Transient recurrent Ham(+); later thromboses with Ham(−)
	2. Recurrent hemolysis, persistent Ham(+)
Endo[83] (Blood, 1996)	Recurrent PNH

*Patient #1 has been reported twice.[80, 87]

Nonablative transplants from identical twins have been attempted only when PNH has evolved to bone marrow failure, but hematologic improvement, if achieved, is rarely permanent. In one recently reported case, a patient experienced a clinical remission for 10 years before symptoms recurred,[81] and the *PIG-A* mutation that was identified at relapse was different from that found at diagnosis a decade earlier.[81] This case suggests that *PIG-A*-mutant HSCs may undergo clonal "exhaustion" (as likely do normal HSCs), and expansion of a *PIG-A*-mutant HSC clone to a clinically evident level may be a very slow process, perhaps requiring years. Furthermore, since the twin donor did not develop PNH or molecular evidence of the post-transplant *PIG-A* mutation, host pathologic changes can be inferred as necessary for selection of *PIG-A* mutant HSCs. The preparative regimen used in transplants in PNH patients is usually high-dose cyclophosphamide, but relapse after such transplants is rare.[87, 88] High-dose cyclophosphamide, without infusion of allogeneic HSCs, appears to be therapeutic in AA[89] without stem cell rescue. This regimen has been applied in PNH; two PNH patients treated at the National Institutes of Health (NIH), however, showed no increase in the percentages of their GPI-AP(+) neutrophils after recovery of their counts (unpublished observations). Treatment of cases of PNH-AA with conventional antithymocyte globulin (ATG) or cyclosporine or both, (CsA), while frequently improving blood counts, does not necessarily result in an increased proportion of normal [GPI-AP(+)] hematopoiesis (unpublished observations). At least two explanations may be offered to explain failure of the *PIG-A*-mutant contribution to regress. First, multiple inhibitory processes may suppress hematopoiesis in PNH-AA, only one of which depends upon GPI-AP expression by the target HSCs; the process reversed by ATG and CsA would then necessarily be GPI-AP *in*dependent (an example of a latter such mechanism might be interferon-γ [IFN-γ] or tumor necrosis factor-α [TNF-α]–mediated marrow suppression).[90, 91] Alternatively, at the level of normal stem cell biology, in the absence of pathologic inhibition of hematopoiesis, *PIG-A* mutations in the stem cells may be entirely neutral, and the relative levels of mutant and wild-type hematopoiesis *prior* to and after therapy would then be expected to remain unchanged. This second explanation is consistent with the natural history of untreated PNH only if either the driving disease process frequently "burns out" at some point short of complete HSC replacement or if the intensity of the pathologic inhibition varies inversely with the level of hematopoiesis contributed by GPI-AP(+) HSCs. While the period of time over which we have followed GPI-AP(−) cell to normal cell ratios in PNH patients has been relatively short, retrospective cross-sectional data from our AA patients support these inferences, as patients with AA-PNH analyzed at longer follow-up intervals, up to 12 years, do not inevitably have higher fractions of *PIG-A*-mutant hematopoiesis than patients studied much earlier in their course.

Laboratory Studies

A component of bone marrow failure is evident in most cases of PNH, either clinically, as manifested by bone marrow hypocellularity or thrombocytopenia,[22, 92] or experimentally, as reflected by in vitro colony assays performed on cells from even hypercellular bone marrow aspirates.[52, 93–96] Individual patients with PNH represent a convenient source of hematopoietic progenitors that are chimeric with regard to the presence of *PIG-A* mutations but which have arisen from an identical genetic background and presumably in comparable microenvironments. Fluorescent-activated cell sorting [FACS] has been utilized to separate wild-type GPI-AP(+) progenitors from *PIG-A*-mutant GPI-AP(−) progenitors. When such progenitors have been assayed in various in vitro assays of hematopoiesis such as colony formation (colony-forming unit—granulocyte-macrophase [CFU$_{GM}$ or blast-forming unit—erythroid (BFU-E), or the long-term culture–initiating cell [LTCIC] assay, no significant difference in clonogenicity between these two subpopulations has been observed.[97] As mentioned above, however, the overall levels of colony formation, whether primary or secondary, are typically low in even hypercellular cases of PNH[52, 93–96] compared with normal controls.

If expansion of *PIG-A*-mutant HSC clone(s) in cases of PNH represents a selective adaptation of the bone marrow to external stress,[68, 69, 98] then why is the growth of isolated GPI-AP(−) progenitors impaired? And, when the proportion of hematopoiesis contributed by *PIG-A* mutant clone(s) exceeds 80% or 90% (as is common in cases of "hemolytic" PNH), why is any diminution in progenitor cell numbers observed with unsorted bone marrow samples? Several conceptual and methodologic considerations may account for the data. First, over a 2-week in vitro assay, the difference in growth between *PIG-A*-mutant and wild-type progenitors may fall below the level of precision of typical colony-forming experiments (20% to 30%); a small difference compounded over a year or more, however, could easily result ultimately in dramatic expansion of a mutant clone. Second, the equivalent poor growth of GPI-AP(−) and GPI-AP(+) progenitors in vitro may reflect a balance of two unrelated phenomena: *PIG-A* mutations may actually confer a modest disadvantage in vivo which may be exacerbated in vitro (for example, the folate receptor is GPI-anchored); the poor growth of GPI-AP(+) progenitors in vitro, on the other hand, may represent the residual effect of their in vivo inhibition. Finally, it is possible that *PIG-A*-mutations may indirectly result in aberrant or delayed expression of differentiation markers; in such a case, comparison of progenitor numbers per GPI-AP(+) or GP-AP(−) CD34+ cell, despite being derived from the same bone marrow sample, would not be appropriate.

The relative growth of human GPI-AP(+) and GPI-AP(−) hematopoietic cells has also been examined in a surrogate in vivo assay system, the SCID (severe combined immunodeficiency disease) mouse.[99] "Engraftment" of intravenously injected BM samples from PNH patients in these partially immunodeficient mice (SCID mice actually possess *augmented* NK cell activity) was variable from donor to donor, but whatever human cells did engraft were found consistently to be GPI-AP(−). The authors inferred from these results that *PIG-A*-mutant HSCs from PNH patients possessed an undefined intrinsic growth advantage, which they postulated was due either to the *PIG-A* mutation itself or additional mutation(s) acquired by the *PIG-A*-mutant clone. The results with normal bone marrow samples in this study, however, differ from other published studies of human hematopoiesis in immunodeficient mice[100–102] as the investigators were unable to obtain engraftment of BM inocula from healthy subjects, and the human cells that did engraft from the PNH patients did not retain any CD34 expression. SCID/NOD mice, which are NK cell–deficient, are required in order to obtain optimal engraftment of control normal adult bone marrow.[100] Thus the failure of BM inocula from normal subjects to engraft in SCID mice could be due solely to active destruction by NK cells shortly after the intravenous injection and not to any intrinsic growth disadvantage of *PIG-A*-normal progenitors. Were the interaction of mouse NK cells with human hematopoietic targets dependent on target GPI-AP expression, PNH bone marrow would show a selective advantage in SCID mice.

In growth experiments utilizing sorted GPI-AP(+) and GPI-AP(−) cells derived from patients, there is an implicit assumption that the only differences between the two populations relate to *PIG-A* gene function. Ideally, one would experimentally impose *PIG-A*-mutant or–wild-type status upon an otherwise homogeneous collection of primitive hematopoietic progenitors and then compare the behavior of such cells in assays of hematopoiesis.

The effects of experimentally manipulating *PIG-A* expression have been examined in cells other than hematopoietic progenitors, EBV-transformed B LCLs using cloned *PIG-A*-mutant, GPI-AP(−) LCLs from PNH patients.[54, 55] The first report[103] compared the relative sensitivities of the parental GPI-AP(−) LCL with its *PIG-A*-transfected GPI-AP(+) daughter line with regard to various modes of programmed cell death. With two independent GPI-AP(−) LCLs, reconstitution of *PIG-A* function appeared to result in restoration of susceptibility to apoptosis induced by either serum deprivation or gamma irradiation. Control transfection of the GPI-AP(−) LCL with an irrelevant vector was not described.[103] The second report of such experiments utilized two independent *PIG-A*-expression vectors (one retroviral, the other EBV-based), as well as control vectors, and came to a different conclusion: restoration of PIG-A function produced no consistent effect on sensitivity to apoptosis.[104] If PIG-A gene product dysfunction rendered HSCs resistant to apoptosis, expansion of the PNH clone would be due to an intrinsic advantage. However, such a result would be inconsistent with the rarity of PNH, especially after mutagenic stress such as chemotherapy. Also lacking is a mechanism by which *PIG-A* mutations would somehow influence the apoptotic process, as none of the myriad members of the expanding list of apoptosis-triggering cell surface molecules expressed by hematopoietic cells is known to be GPI-anchored. (There is, however, one recently reported example of an apparent GPI-anchored death transducer in nonhematopoietic cell lineages.[105]) A recently described "decoy" death receptor with significant homology to the other members of the death receptor family, termed DcR1, has been found to be GPI-anchored,[106] but loss of expression of DcR5 by a *PIG-A*-mutant cell should increase susceptibility to apoptosis. Alternatively, an inactive *PIG-A* gene product might directly or indirectly affect biochemical pathways supplementary to the biosynthesis of the GPI anchor. The PIG-A gene product might participate in glycosylation of intracellular proteins involved in signal transduction analogous to the recently described post-translational modification of the cytoplasmic estrogen receptor by covalent attachment of an *N*-acetylglucosamine.[107] For another example, ceramide is known to cotraffic with GPI-AP in polarized epithelial cells to the basolateral membrane.[108] If impaired synthesis of the GPI moiety were to result in altered ceramide trafficking, then membrane ceramide content would be diminished in *PIG-A*-mutant cells, influencing signal transduction.[109–114]

Apoptosis resistance of primary cells from PNH patients has been investigated.[103, 104, 115] While neutrophils and more primitive (CD34+) hematopoietic cells from PNH patients undergo less apoptosis than similar cells from healthy persons, it does not appear that such resistance can be attributed to PIG-A dysfunction. The degree of resistance to apoptosis of neutrophils from different PNH patients did not correlate with the proportion of GPI-deficient neutrophils[104, 115] thus two PNH patients with, for example, 10% vs. 90% GPI-AP(−) granulocytes exhibited equivalent degrees of resistance to apoptosis compared with controls. Second, the apoptosis resistance seen with neutrophils and CD34+ cells from PNH patients is also seen in AA and MDS patients without PNH.[115] In vitro apoptosis resistance of hematopoietic cells from bone marrow failure patients may reflect an underlying pathologic process common to PNH, AA, and MDS. Resistance to apoptosis could be secondary to an accelerated cell cycle or to appropriate compensatory elevations in plasma concentrations of hematopoietic growth factors. Regardless of the precise mechanism, it is likely that only the most resistant cells manage to survive under the conditions that produce bone marrow failure.

Genetically Engineered Murine Models

Cloning of the *PIG-A* gene made possible the development of knock-out murine models, in which the direct effects of PIG-A gene product dysfunction on hematopoiesis in vivo could be studied in isolation. The uniform conclusion from studies of knock-out chimeric murine hematopoiesis is that a nonfunctioning *PIG-A* gene confers no intrinsic advantage to affected hematopoietic clones under physiologic conditions,[62, 116, 117] and instead chimeric mice tend to show a trend of decreasing *PIG-A*-mutant hematopoietic contribution over months of follow-up.[117] In vivo murine studies were initially performed with C57BL/6 blastocysts injected with 129/Sv PIG-A–knock-out embryonic stem cells (ESCs); thus the mutant and wild-type contributions differed by more than the targeted disruption in PIG-A (germline incorporation of unconditional *PIG-A* mutations proved fatal in utero, thus preventing generation of an inbred PIG-A–knock-out mouse strain.) One of the initial eight PIG-A–knock-out chimeric mice did develop a delayed dramatic expansion of GPI-AP(−) erythrocytes at age 10 months and eventually died of unknown causes.[62] Whether this isolated instance of clonal expansion was related to the disrupted *PIG-A* gene or due to either an acquired mutation in the knock-out ESC line or the resultant mouse is unknown. Subsequent studies have therefore utilized F1 animals derived from inbred mice with modified *PIG-A* genes flanked by lox recombination sites crossed with mice transgenic for the Cre recombinase.[117] Again, no tendency for mutant HSCs to expand in such systems was observed[118, 119]: the *PIG-A*-mutant contribution to the circulating red and white blood cell populations diminished gradually over time.[118] Caution should be exercised in extrapolating these results from mice to humans: the homologue(s) of a given human GPI-AP may not, in fact, be GPI-anchored in the mouse or such homologues may be GPI-anchored in both species but subserve fundamentally different physiologic (or pathologic) functions in humans vs. mice. For example, expression of CD24 (a GPI-AP in both species) is largely restricted in humans to the lymphocyte lineage, while in mice it is present on diverse lineages, ranging from ESCs to terminally differentiated erythrocytes. It remains to be seen in knock-out mice whether, under conditions of experimental hematopoietic stress, *PIG-A*-mutant hematopoiesis is favored.

An Immune Model of Paroxysmal Nocturnal Hemoglobinuria Pathogenesis

To be consistent with the observations presented above, a model of PNH pathogenesis must posit both *PIG-A* mutations in the HSC pool and extrinsic selection of HSCs which is dependent, at least in part, on some aspect of normal PIG-A function, most probably GPI-AP biosynthesis. Genetic stability in PNH patients may be normal[120] or increased as a presumed direct result of the underlying attack on the bone marrow.[121] We have estimated in normal clonogenic progenitors a 10^{-6} mutation rate in the hypoxanthine-guanine phosphoribosyltransferase (*hgpt*) gene (unpublished observations.) Using this conservative figure and an estimate of the number of human HSCs (extrapolated from mice) of 300,000 or greater, a human, on average, would have greater than a 1 in 4 chance of harboring at least one *PIG-A* mutant HSC. Empirical evidence of *PIG-A* mutations in mature myeloid cells has recently been reported in healthy humans.[122] Araten et al. sorted CD55(−), CD59(−) granulocytes (defined by granularity and expression of CD11b) from healthy subjects and in over half of the subjects obtained mutant *PIG-A* sequences that were considered likely to result in an inactive gene product. In one person, the mutation introduced a new restriction endonuclease site; this permitted independent confirmation of the *PIG-A*-mutant clone 5 months later by repeat sorting followed by gene amplification and restriction endonuclease digestion. The range of frequency of CD55(−), CD59(−) granulocytes in five normal subjects was 10 to $60/10^6$. While this study could not directly address whether the *PIG-A* mutation was present in the HSC pool, it is likely that at least some of the cells arose from mutant primitive progenitors. Thus most healthy persons appear to harbor minor *PIG-A*-mutant hematopoietic clones.

The mechanism by which profound selection of *PIG-A*-mutant precursors takes place in PNH is unknown. Iatrogenic immunoselection of *PIG-A*-mutant lymphocytes in humans has been documented by investigators under artificial circumstances involving medical therapy.[123–125] Each group studied the unintended consequences of administering CAMPATH-1H (a humanized monoclonal antibody to CDw52, which is, coincidentally, GPI-anchored) to patients with either non-Hodgkin's lymphoma, rheumatoid arthritis, or chronic lymphocytic lymphoma. Patients in each of these disease categories were observed to develop a major population of GPI-AP(−) lymphocytes after several courses of CAMPATH-1H and over a relatively short time period of 1 to 2 months. The basis for the GPI-AP(−) phenotype in the emergent lymphocyte subpopulation was shown in several cases to be due to *PIG-A* mutations. Thus immune-mediated attack, here humoral, was adequate to drive expansion of variant cells that are negative for the targeted immune epitope; in the case of GPI-anchored targets, mutations in *PIG-A* would appear to be the genetic events most likely to accomplish this.

No case of AA or PNH, however, has ever been related to autoantibodies against GPI-AP on HSCs. It has been proposed that the mere stress of repopulating a depleted (aplastic) bone marrow by a handful of surviving HSCs might be sufficient pressure to select for the *PIG-A*-mutant genotype. In order to address whether nonspecific myelosuppression is sufficient to select for significant expansion of *PIG-A*-mutant progenitors, we examined GPI-AP expression in peripheral blood samples from several cohorts of patients whose hematopoietic progenitor pool had undergone contraction as a result of medical therapy.[126] PNH did not develop in patients who had received multiple cycles of cytotoxic chemotherapy (N = 18), nor in patients who had undergone allogeneic BMT (N = 28). These figures are very different from the frequency at which PNH is observed in bone marrow failure patients: 25 of 115 AA patients and 9 of 39 MDS patients seen at the NIH (22%). Thus the mechanism of myelosuppression would appear to be critical to emergence of the PNH clone.

The clinical association of the rare diseases of PNH and AA (or MDS) is clearly an important clue to the underlying pathologic process. Collective clinical and laboratory data strongly implicate an (auto-) immune pathogenesis in AA. An activated CD8+ T lymphocyte appears to be the proximal cell responsible for the destruction of primitive hematopoietic cells.[127] Laboratory studies show that multiple parameters of T cell activation are elevated in AA patients (IFN-γ messenger RNA expression in bone marrow;[128], HLA-DR and interleukin-2 receptor expression by CD8+ cells[129]), and bone marrow function in patients improves after immunosuppression[130, 131] (see section on therapy and Chapter 1). Moreover, syngeneic bone marrow transplants (using an identical twin) will often fail in AA unless preceded by immunosuppressive conditioning.[82, 83]

To account for the association of PNH with AA, several mechanisms can be hypothesized in which GPI-AP–deficient HSCs might escape cytotoxic attack:

- A peptide derived from a GPI-AP expressed by stem cells may serve as an autoantigen in some or all cases of AA, or perhaps only in those that progress to PNH (Fig. 4–2). How-

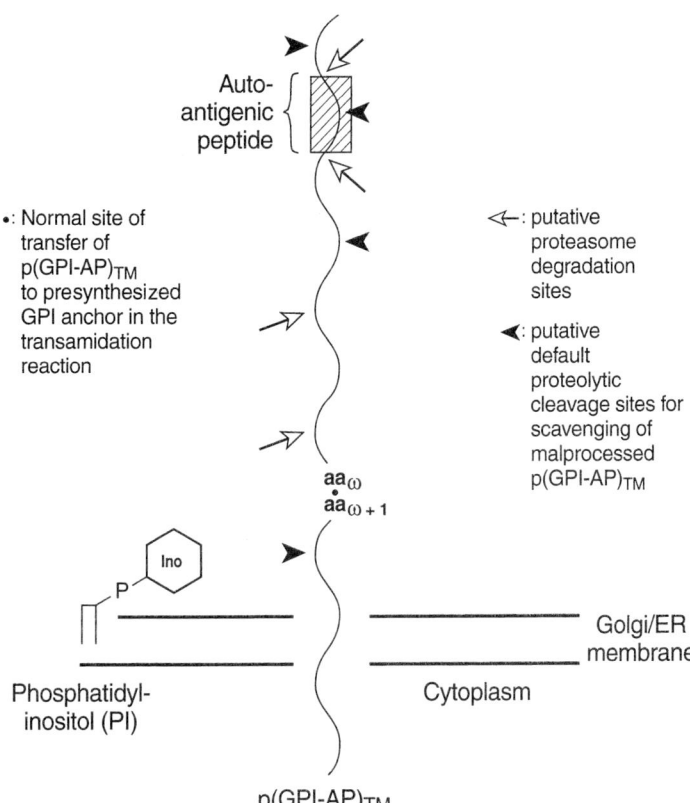

Figure 4–2 *PIG-A* mutation and antigenic peptide presentation. A mature glycosylphosphatidylinositol-anchored protein (GPI-AP) is generated in a transamidation reaction when the first ω amino acids (aa$_\omega$) (after the signal peptide) of the transmembrane precursor polypeptide of a GPI-AP [p(GPI-AP)$_{TM}$] are transferred to the presynthesized GPI anchor. If no fully assembled GPI anchor is available to accept aa$_\omega$ in the transamidation reaction, then p(GPI-AP)$_{TM}$ will be shunted to proteolytic scavenge pathways, including degradation in the endoplasmic reticulum and in autophagocytic lysosomes.[182] It is possible that cleavage through this default pathway might prevent generation of a full-length (putative) autoantigenic peptide derived from a properly processed GPI-AP species. Thus, if a peptide from a GPI-AP was a hematopoietic stem cell (HSC) autoantigen in aplastic anemia, *PIG-A*-mutant HSC would enjoy a survival advantage. (see also Fig. 4–1.) Ino, inositol; ER, endoplasmic reticulum.

ever, since both GPI(+) *and* GPI(−) cells synthesize the polypeptide precursors [p(GPI-AP)$_{TM}$] of mature GPI-AP,[132] it would be necessary to postulate that in *PIG-A*-mutant cells the proper (auto-) antigenic peptide fragment is inefficiently generated or malprocessed (see Fig. 4–2).

- Receptors on HSCs for secreted CD8+ T cell products might be GPI-anchored (Fig. 4–3). However, no such examples are known and GPI-APs play no role in the action of IFN-γ, TNF-α, perforin, granzymes, or Fas ligand. (A GPI-anchored TGF-β-binding protein of unknown signal-transducing capacity has been described in endometrium and keratinocytes.[133–135]) GPI-AP can transduce signals to the interior of the cell, at least in response to cross-linking by antibodies.[136] Less common are examples of natural ligands which employ GPI-anchored receptors, on any cell type, for signal transduction. The three best characterized of such ligands are ciliated neurotrophic factor (CNTF), neurturin (NTN), and glial cell line–derived neurotrophic factor (GDNF). Intracellular signals of all three of these factors are transduced by heterodimers consisting of a factor-specific, GPI-anchored receptor coupled noncovalently with a transmembrane partner.[137–144] While the target tissue of all three is neural, it is interesting to note that HSCs do in fact express gp130 (the partner for the GPI-anchored CNTF receptor) as a heterodimer with either the IL-6 or leukemic inhibitory factor receptor (neither of which is GPI-anchored). Thus if some undiscovered GPI-anchored partner for gp130 is expressed by HSCs, then inability to respond to its ligand could alter the behavior such a *PIG-A*-mutant stem cell and confer advantage.

- A cytopathic stem cell–tropic virus (Fig. 4–4, top) may either usurp a GPI-AP for entry into HSC (non-stem cell-tropic examples include echo- and coxsackieviruses[145–147]), or a noncytopathic virus may encode for a viral GPI-AP[148, 149] (vGPI-AP) that proves to be the immunodominant antigen (Fig. 4–4, bottom). In the latter case, *PIG-A*-mutant HSCs would fail to elicit what ultimately would be a deleterious immune response, and their expansion would thus be favored. A cytopathic viral model, however, would not account for the long-term clinical improvements frequently observed after treatment of uncomplicated AA with immunosuppression or BMT.

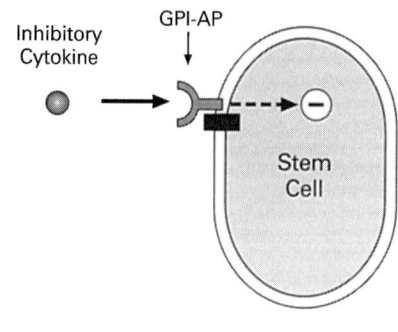

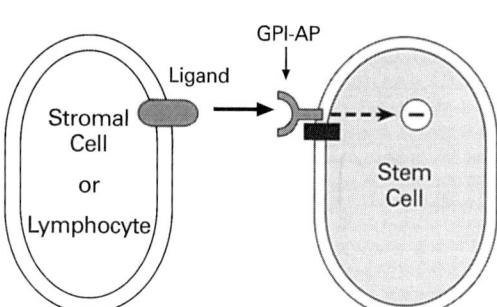

Figure 4–3 Model in which a glycosylphosphatidyl-inositol-anchored protein (GPI-AP) may serve as a receptor for a hematoinhibitory ligand. Top: A GPI-AP may serve as a receptor (or coreceptor) for a hematoinhibitory cytokine such as transforming growth factor-β (TGF-β) or some other uncharacterized factor. Signal transduction by the GPI-anchored receptor may require cis-interaction with a transmembrane coreceptor, depicted as a rectangle (analogous to the interaction in neural cells between gp130, which is a transmembrane protein, and the receptor for ciliated neurotrophic factor [CNTFRc], which is GPI-anchored. Bottom: The external inhibitory signal need not be soluble but may be cell-associated. The cell delivering the negative signal could be a stromal cell, lymphocyte (see also Fig. 4–5), or some other uncharacterized cell.

- Expression of one or more GPI-APs by the HSCs may be necessary for optimal attack on normal HSCs by the T cells that mediate AA (Fig. 4–5). Plausible mechanisms that could account for such targeting would include the following:
  - Some direct or indirect consequence of *PIG-A* mutations attenuates the transduction of apoptosis signals to HSCs by immune effectors. This possibility has been discussed earlier in this chapter (see also the bottom of Fig. 4–5).

- A GPI-anchored member of the "costimulatory" family[150–157] of molecules might exist (Fig. 4–5, top) and be expressed on HSCs in either health or disease. Such molecules, however, are important primarily in the afferent phase of an immune response, not the effector phase. Thus after establishment of autoimmunity in AA, which presumably develops at a time when a patient is greater than 99% GPI(+), both wild-type [GPI-AP(+)] and *PIG-A*-mutant [GPI-AP(−)] HSC targets should be equally susceptible to attack by activated T cells, unless periodic "repriming" with signal 1 (antigen or autoantigen) plus signal 2 (costimulator) is necessary for the long-term maintenance of autoimmunity.
- GPI-anchored ligands for T cell surface ad-

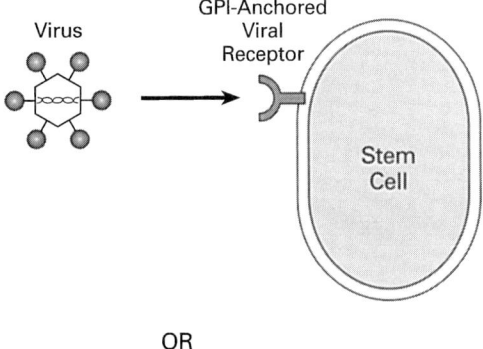

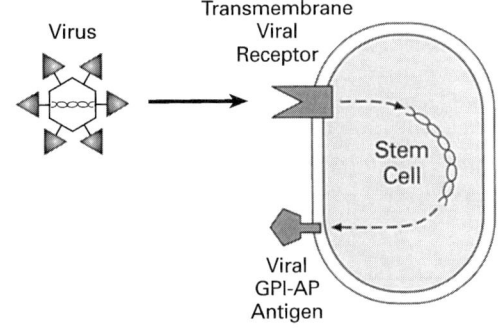

Figure 4–4 Two viral models for selection of *PIG-A*-mutant hematopoietic stem cell (HSC). Top: The viral receptor is glycosylphosphatidylinositol (GPI)-anchored. Bottom: The viral receptor is not GPI-anchored, but the virus encodes for a GPI-anchored molecule, which happens also to be the dominant antigen against which the immune response is directed. This latter model would allow for survival (and clonal expansion) of the infected HSC only in the event that the virus was noncytopathic.

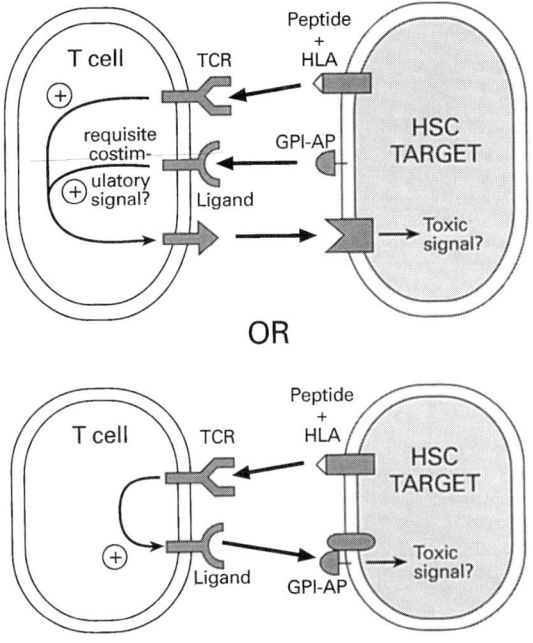

Figure 4–5 T lymphocyte–mediated selection of *PIG-A*-mutant hematopoietic stem cells (HSC). T cell receptor (TCR) engagement by an antigenic complex of (auto-)peptide plus HLA is presumably necessary (but may not be sufficient) for T cell activation. Top: Expression of an uncharacterized glycosylphosphatidylinositol (GPI)-anchored protein on the target HSC may be necessary for delivery of the immunotoxic signal. A transmembrane *cis*-associating partner for the GPI-AP (*shaded ellipse*) may be required for transduction of the inhibitory signal. Bottom: Complete activation of the pathogenic T cells in aplastic anemia may depend on costimulation by an accessory molecule which, on HSC, may be GPI-anchored.

hesion molecules may play an important role in T cell attack on HSCs (Fig. 4–5, bottom). Three GPI-APs, CD58 (LFA-3), CD48, and CD59, serve as ligands of varying avidity for CD2,[158–160] a signal-transducing molecule present on the surface of all T cells (and NK cells). The functional importance of interactions between CD2 and any of these three ligands, however, has yet to be demonstrated. For example, using EBV-transformed LCLs (which do express CD48, CD58, and CD59) as immunologic targets, Hollander et al.[161] demonstrated that a GPI-AP(−) daughter line was equally susceptible to cell-mediated killing in three different assays of killing: the classical cytolytic (CD8+) T lymphocytes (CTL) assay, the NK assay, and the antibody-dependent cellular cytotoxicity (ADCC) assay.

On the other hand, some in vitro data suggest that circulating lymphocytes from PNH patients may exert GPI-dependent selection (Fig. 4–6). These experiments originated from the observation that *PIG-A*-mutant LCLs are very difficult to obtain from EBV transformations of peripheral blood leukocytes (PBLs) from PNH patients, even in patients with readily demonstrable GPI-AP(−) B cell subpopulations on analysis of fresh blood. The EBV receptor on B cells, CD21, is *not* GPI-anchored. These findings suggested that *PIG-A*-mutant LCLs were actually at a disadvantage as measured by cell proliferation or viral transformation. Because almost everyone has been naturally exposed to EBV and thus normal PBLs contain a population of T cells capable of destroying EBV-transformed B cells, it is necessary when establishing LCL lines to include CsA in the primary culture of PBLs with EBV supernatant. However, when CsA was deliberately omitted from EBV transformations of PNH PBLs, allowing expression of endogenous anti-EBV immunity, a discrete population of *PIG-A*-mutant lymphocytes emerged (Fig. 4–6). This phenomenon has been seen in about half of the PNH patients we have examined. These data are consistent with a relative survival advantage for the GPI-AP(−) phenotype under certain types of immune attack. Precisely which effector population mediates this GPI-dependent selection and which receptor-ligand interactions are involved have yet to be determined. These results can be reconciled with those of Hollander et al.[161] by taking into account that the target of immune attack in our system is not a fully transformed latently infected B cell blast (which is known to be resistant to certain modes of programmed cell death[162]), but rather a B cell at an earlier stage of EBV infection, which may not yet have acquired the apoptosis-resistant phenotype of established LCL; furthermore, effectors in our system were derived from PNH patients, who may harbor fundamentally skewed, deranged, or hyperactive immune cell populations.

A working model accommodating much of the data discussed above can be proposed in which the *PIG-A* mutation protects affected HSCs from the cytotoxic autoimmune attack that characterizes

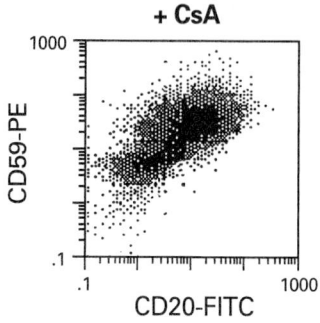 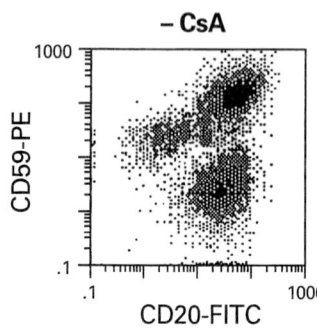

Figure 4–6 Autologous T cells from paroxysmal nocturnal hemoglobinuria (PNH) patients preferentially suppress Ebstein-Barr virus (EBV) transformation and expansion of glycosylphosphatidylinositol-anchored protein (GPI-AP) (+) B cell clones. Left: The result when an unfractionated peripheral blood mononuclear cell (PBMC) culture from a PNH patient is transformed with EBV under standard conditions. Cyclosporine (CsA) is included in such routine transformations in order to inhibit the EBV-immune T cells present in the peripheral blood leukocytes of 95% of the population, which would otherwise destroy nascent EBV-infected B cell clones in vitro. CD20 (abscissa) is a marker for B cells. CD59 (ordinate) is a GPI-anchored antigen present on cells of all hematopoietic lineages, including B cells. Essentially all of the CD20(+) cells are GPI-AP(+) in the transformation in which CsA was included (left). The reason why GPI-AP(−) B cells (from PNH patients) are not efficiently transformed under these standard conditions is not known. The CD20(−)/dim cells are T cells. Right: The result when PBMCs from the same PNH patient are EBV-transformed in the absence of CsA. A GPI-AP(−) B cell population (bottom right) has been selected, presumably by uninhibited T cells.

AA (Fig. 4–7). Protection could be conferred by loss of expression of one or more GPI-APs by mutant HSCs, as this is the only known molecular consequence of *PIG-A* gene dysfunction. Future efforts need to focus on identifying the precise GPI-anchored molecules on HSCs involved, as well as their cognate ligands secreted by or expressed on the surface of pathogenic lymphocytes (see Fig. 4–6). Characterization of these molecules should then facilitate development of novel and, presumably, more narrowly targeted therapeutic approaches than currently available, as discussed below.

NATURAL HISTORY AND TREATMENT

Three large-scale analyses of the clinical course and prognostic factors in PNH have been published, comprising 460 patients.[17, 18, 22] All used the Ham's test for definitive diagnosis. Median survival ranged from 10 to 15 years after diagnosis[15, 17, 18, 22, 163]; approximately one fourth of patients will survive 25 years. Symptoms attributable to PNH may, in retrospect, precede diagnosis by as long as a decade. Approximately one third of deaths in the European studies were related to thrombotic complications,[17, 18] compared to fewer than 10% in the Japanese study.[22] Conversely, hemorrhage (from thrombocytopenia due to AA) was the largest single cause of death among Japanese[22] (39%), but only 15% to 25% of Europeans died of this complication.[17, 18] Of those patients presenting with thrombosis, 60% died within 4 years.[18] Transformation to leukemia occurs in fewer than 3% of patients.[15, 17, 18, 22] A curious prognostic feature noted in the French study[18] was that an antecedent history of AA was associated with a 2.5-fold lower relative risk of death.

The replacement of Ham's test with the more sensitive flow cytometric techniques recently introduced for the detection of GPI-AP will doubtless result in more diagnoses of PNH, in milder cases, at earlier time points, and in a broader spectrum of patients (including, especially, MDS[126]). The net impact on time of survival post diagnosis is difficult to predict; lead-time bias should lengthen the apparent median survival, while increased representation of previously occult MDS-PNH cases conversely may shorten it.

Treatment of Hemolysis

Laboratory evidence of hemolysis in different PNH patients may range from mild biochemical abnormalities such as a low haptoglobin or elevated LDH, to profound anemia (hemoglobin less than 50 g/L) with marked reticulocytosis. Accordingly, hemolysis in PNH patients should be treated only if there is a clinical indication such as physical impairment or a coexisting medical condition exacerbated by anemia (such as coronary artery disease). Since normal red blood cells in the circulation of a PNH patient are not subject to the same pathologic destruction as the patient's own GPI-AP–deficient erythrocytes, transfusion is very effective in managing anemia. PNH patients can lose considerable quantities of iron in the urine due to intravascular hemolysis; iron levels should therefore be monitored and, when low, iron should be supplemented by the oral or, if necessary, parenteral route. With evolution to AA, however, secondary hemochromatosis can eventually develop, generally after transfusion of 50 units of red blood cells, and require iron chelation therapy. Folate deficiency due to the potentially high level of erythropoietic turnover is theoretically possible but rarely observed.

Chronic, alternate-day corticosteroid regimens have been advocated[164, 165] for the amelioration of anemia, based largely on a study in which 7 of 19

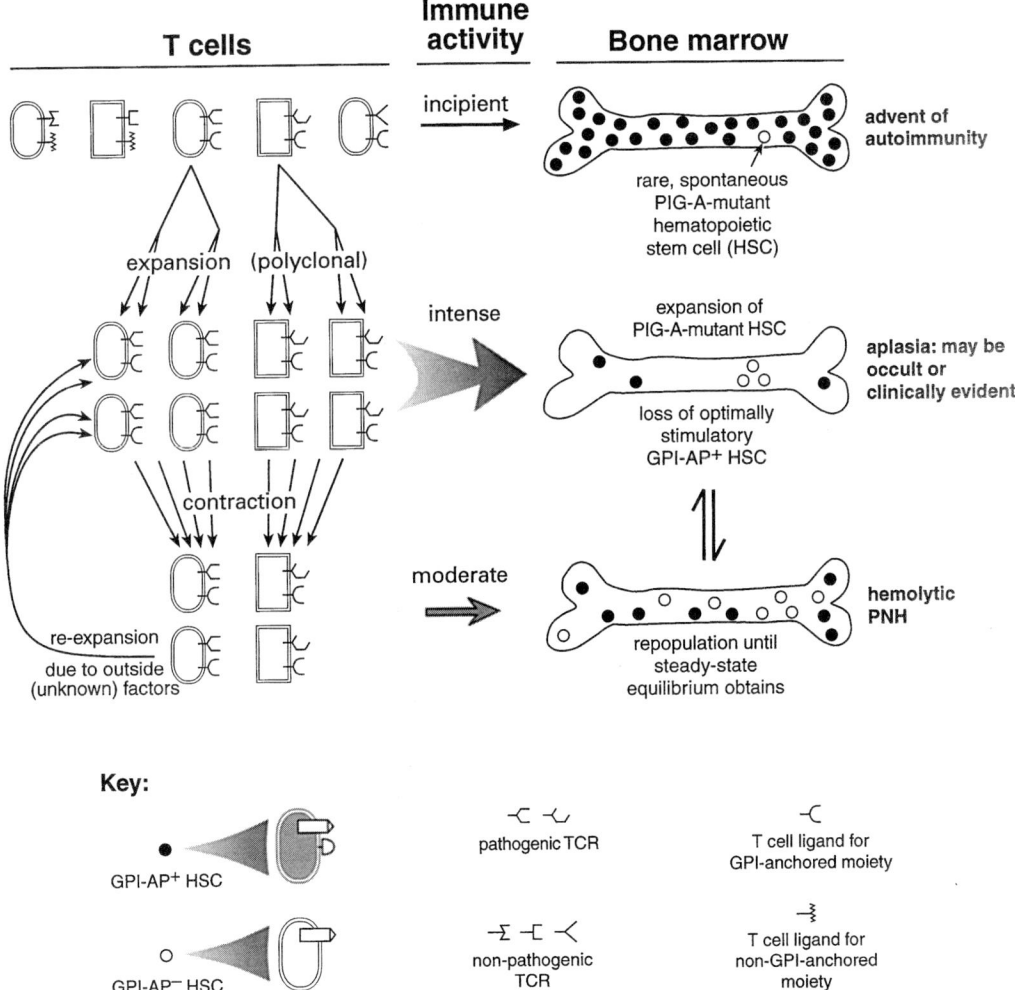

Figure 4–7 A model of immune selection favoring expansion of *PIG-A*-mutant hematopoiesis. Multiple T cell clones may pathologically target normal hematopoietic stem cells (HSCs). If these T cells require target expression of glycosylphosphatidylinositol (GPI)-anchored costimulatory, adhesion, or death signal–transducing molecules for optimal attack or sustained (poly-)clonal expansion, outgrowth of even rare *PIG-A*-mutant HSCs will occur. The self-renewal capacity of stem cells will permit non-neoplastic mutant clones to support hematopoiesis for prolonged periods. Epigenetic events such as intercurrent illnesses, especially infections, may transiently reexpand the pathologic T cells or modulate their requirement for "costimulation."

Thai patients[164] became red blood cell transfusion–independent. No data on the effects of corticosteroids on long-term survival have been published. An alternate-day regimen (15 to 30 mg of prednisone every other day) was recommended in order to avoid the well-known long-term sequelae. Short-term use of higher doses (1 mg/kg/day) during hemolytic crises, theoretically, might decrease the incidence of associated thrombotic episodes.[16] Androgens have also been reported to mitigate the need for red blood cell transfusions in individual cases.[166, 167]

Thrombolytic and Anticoagulation Therapy

Life-threatening thromboses, in particular the Budd-Chiari syndrome and cerebral thrombosis, must be treated aggressively—if diagnosed within the first few 3 to 4 days—using thrombolytic agents,[168] unless there is evidence of hemorrhage[169] or other contraindications. Once a patient manifests a thrombotic diathesis, an unproven but common practice is to recommend life-long anticoagulation, initially with heparin, then orally with warfarin sodium. The actual efficacy of warfarin prophylaxis against the thrombotic process in PNH, which is presumed to be related to GPI-AP deficiency on affected platelets, is unknown. Unfortunately, the first thrombotic event often proves fatal[17] and a strategy of expectant management will be too late for some patients.

Amelioration of Impaired Hematopoiesis

The overlap of PNH and AA comes to medical attention in three chronologically distinct fashions. First, a patient presenting with pancytopenia may have a Ham's test or flow cytometry performed in the course of the initial workup; in this case, the diagnosis of AA and PNH will be concurrent. Second, a predominantly "hemolytic" PNH patient may be found after months or years of observation to develop absolute reticulocytopenia (less than 60,000/μL), thrombocytopenia, or neutropenia, in any combination. (Even during the hemolytic phase of PNH, evidence of impaired hematopoiesis may be demonstrable in vitro.[52, 93–96]) Finally, an AA (or MDS) patient may be diagnosed with PNH by Ham's test or flow cytometry months or years after presentation with marrow failure. Unfortunately, it is common for neither test to have been performed at the time of initial diagnosis with AA, and AA patients do not exhibit a positive Ham's test if heavily transfused with normal red blood cells. Of note, our current experience with 35 prospectively followed AA patients is that all patients ultimately destined to develop PNH (n = 5) had flow cytometric evidence of GPI-AP(−) granulocytes at the time of initial diagnosis with AA.[126] However, the therapeutic approach to hypoplastic PNH is essentially the same as for AA,[170] regardless of the sequence of diagnoses (see below).

The treatments for the life-threatening cytopenic complications of PNH include immunosuppression with ATG and CsA, or BMT (see below). The response rates[23, 171–173] reported for ATG or CsA are generally 50% or greater; our own unpublished experience with ATG plus CsA indicates improvement in 80% to 90% of cases of AA-PNH and MDS-PNH.[126] ATG administration may have added toxicity in PNH patients. Intravascular immune complex formation between equine antibodies and the human target leukocytes, or between horse proteins and the patient's antibodies produced in response to ATG, can result in complement activation and lysis of GPI-AP(−) red blood cells. In patients with a high percentage of PNH erythrocytes, fever, rigors, hypotension, massive hemolysis, or renal failure can occur during ATG infusion, analogous to a major transfusion reaction.[172] Intravenous steroids may temper this reaction, but they are administered as prophylaxis against serum sickness in all cases.[131] Slowing the rate of infusion of ATG may also lessen the intensity of the reaction. Aggressive hydration and transfusion support should be given during ATG administration. Despite salutary effects on hematopoiesis, however, immunosuppressive therapies do not eradicate the GPI-AP–deficient hematopoietic clones,[174, 175] nor does the proportion of normal hematopoiesis inevitably improve.[176] Accordingly, even responding patients remain at risk for future episodes of hemolysis or thrombosis.

Bone Marrow Transplantation

BMT offers the only curative therapy for PNH. Unfortunately, fully engrafted patients may develop acute or chronic graft-versus-host disease (GvHD) and attendant infections and thus some "cured" patients eventually die not from PNH but from complications of the procedure. The decision to proceed with transplant, therefore, must involve careful weighing of the potential benefits and risks of an irreversible intervention.

As discussed above, it is clear from rare cases of PNH in which a syngeneic (identical twin) donor was available that aggressive conditioning is necessary for consistent, durable replacement of the patient's mutant HSCs[80–83] (see Table 4–1). Preparative regimens typically consist of high-dose cyclophosphamide plus additional immunosuppressive or myeloablative components such as procarbazine, busulfan, ATG, or total body irradiation.[82, 87, 177, 178] Relapse of PNH after allogeneic marrow transplantation preceded by cyclophosphamide plus busulfan[87] or cyclophosphamide alone[88] has been reported but is rare (relapse in one patient was associated with a post-transplant course of IFN-α therapy for hepatitis).

Only two groups have published results with more than a few HLA-identical sibling bone marrow transplants in PNH,[80, 87, 178] and in only the publication from Seattle is it clear that all of the PNH transplant cases were reported. Six out of six (95% confidence interval: 54% to 100%) of the HLA-identical siblings transplanted there were alive at 2 to 19 years follow-up, although one of these patients had biochemical evidence of PNH post BMT, despite a preparative regimen which included busulfan.[87] Four of these six patients developed chronic GvHD. A report from Boston[177] describes four PNH transplant patients, all of whom were alive and well with full donor chimerism at follow-up (1 to 60 months). One PNH patient treated with two consecutive haploidentical-related transplants (from first her father, then her brother) died of pulmonary hemorrhage at 39 days after the first transplant without evidence of engraftment.[87]

The current consensus indications for BMT in PNH are the development of either serious aplastic or thrombotic complications. Unfortunately, delaying BMT until after the first thrombosis may be too late, as this event is often permanently disabling or fatal.[17] On the other hand, Budd-Chiari syndrome has been shown to resolve in at least one PNH case after BMT.[178] Hemolysis as the sole clinical manifestation of PNH is not considered sufficient indication to warrant BMT. Because children with PNH appear to have a worse prognosis,[23] tolerate better the rigors of transplantation, and have a greater potential survival benefit, early transplant has been suggested in the pediatric population.[23]

Future Therapies

Alternative therapies for PNH need to be investigated. Further characterization of the thrombotic diathesis should ultimately provide a molecular basis for the design of rational antithrombotic therapies, both for PNH and other thrombophilic syndromes as well. To control hemolysis, inhibition of intravascular complement activation offers a more specific approach than corticosteroids. Protein therapy[179] with DAF or CD59 could replace these critical molecules on the red blood cell surface and protect them from lysis[180]; transfer of GPI-AP has been effected in vitro[116] and in vivo.[181] Stem cell minitransplant, consisting of a less toxic preparative regimen of fludarabine, high-dose cyclophosphamide, and ATG, may be found to provide a more favorable risk-benefit ratio than traditional BMT in PNH, especially if a graft-versus-autoimmunity effect is shown to exist. Finally, various biologic response modifiers such as IL-10, CTLA4-Ig, humanized anti-CD25, soluble TNF receptor, mycophenolate, and others to be developed might be found to reverse the pathologic changes underlying the expansion of *PIG-A*-mutant stem cell clones.

SUMMARY

PNH is an acquired clonal disorder in which *PIG-A*-mutant clones of hematopoietic stem cells undergo massive but non-neoplastic expansion. The only known consequence of *PIG-A* gene dysfunction is loss of GPI-AP expression by the mutant HSC and its progeny. In erythrocytes, this defect results in episodes of intravascular hemolysis when complement is activated in the context of inflammation; in platelets, the defect is believed to favor thrombus formation. On the other hand, *PIG-A* mutations do not appear to directly give rise to the bone marrow aplasia that frequently accompanies PNH. More likely is that the underlying pathophysiologic process of AA confers on *PIG-A*-mutant stem cells a relative survival advantage. Clarifying the molecular basis for this "unnatural" selection process will impact on our understanding not only of PNH, AA, and other autoimmune syndromes but also of the unique biology of GPI-APs as well as the adaptive physiology of HSCs.

REFERENCES

1. Gull WW: A case of intermittent haematinuria with remarks. Guys Hosp Rep 1866; 12:381–392.
2. Strübing P: Paroxymale Hämoglobinurie. Dtsch Med Wochenschr 1882; 8:1.
3. Enneking J: Eine neue Form interittierender Hämoglobinurie (Haemoglobinuria paroxymalis nocturna). Klin Wochenschr 1928; 7: 2045–2047.
4. Ham TH, Dingle JH: Studies on the destruction of red blood cells. II. Chronic hemolytic anemia with paroxysmal nocturnal hemoglobinuria: Certain immunological aspects of the hemolytic mechanism with special reference to serum complement. J Clin Invest 1938; 18:657.
5. Dacie JV, Israels MCG, Wilkinson JF: Paroxysmal nocturnal haemoglobinuria of the Marchiafava type. Lancet 1938; 234:479–485.
6. DeSandre G, Giotto G, Mastella G: L'acetilcol-

inesterasi eritrocitaria: II. Rapporticon le malattie emolitiche. Acta Med Patavina 1956; 16:310–315.
7. Lewis SM, Dacie JV: Neutrophil (leucocyte) alkaline phosphatase in paroxysmal nocturnal haemoglobinuria. Br J Haematol 1965; 11:549–556.
8. Pangburn MK, Schreiber RD, Muller-Eberhard HJ: Deficiency of an erythrocyte membrane protein with complement regulatory activity in paroxysmal nocturnal hemoglobinuria. Proc Nat Acad Sci USA 1983; 80:5430–5434.
9. Oni SB, Osunkoya BO, Luzzatto L: Paroxysmal nocturnal hemoglobinuria: Evidence for monoclonal origin of abnormal red cells: Blood 1970; 36:145–152.
10. Miyata T, Takeda J, Iida Y, et al: The cloning of PIG-A, a component in the early step of GPI-anchor biosynthesis. Science 1993; 259:1318–1320.
11. Takeda J, Miyata T, Kawagoe K, T, et al: Deficiency of the GPI anchor caused by a somatic mutation of the PIG-A gene in paroxysmal nocturnal hemoglobinuria. Cell 1993; 73:703–711.
12. Miyata-T, Yamada N, Iida Y, et al: Abnormalities of PIG-A transcripts in granulocytes from patients with paroxysmal nocturnal hemoglobinuria. N Engl J Med 1994; 330:249–255.
13. Lewis SM, Dacie JV: The aplastic anaemia—paroxysmal nocturnal haemoglobinuria syndrome. Br J Haematol 1967; 13:236–251.
14. Dacie JV, Lewis SM: Paroxysmal nocturnal haemoglobinuria: Variation in clinical severity and association with bone-marrow hypoplasia. Br J Haematol 1961; 7:442–457.
15. Rosse WF, Young NS, Gongora-Biachi R: Hypoproliferative disorders of stem cells. Rev Invest Clin 1997; 49 (suppl 1):83–88.
16. Rosse WF: Paroxysmal nocturnal hemoglobinuria as a molecular disease. Medicine (Baltimore) 1997; 76:63–93.
17. Hillmen P, Lewis SM, Bessler M, et al: Natural history of paroxysmal nocturnal hemoglobinuria. N Engl J Med 1995; 333:1253–1258.
18. Socié G, Mary JY, de Gramont A, et al: Paroxysmal nocturnal haemoglobinuria: Long-term follow-up and prognostic factors. Lancet 1996; 348:573–577.
19. Koduri PR, Gowrishankar S: Paroxysmal nocturnal haemoglobinuria in Indians. Acta Haematol 1992; 88:126–128.
20. Dunn P, Shih LY, Liaw SJ: Paroxysmal nocturnal hemoglobinuria: Analysis of 40 cases. J Formos Med Assoc 1991; 90:831–835.
21. Kruatrachue M, Wasi P, Na-Nakorn S: Paroxysmal nocturnal haemoglobinuria in Thailand with special reference to an association with aplastic anaemia. Br J Haematol 1978; 39:267–276.
22. Fujioka S, Asai T: Prognostic features of paroxysmal nocturnal hemoglobinuria in Japan. Nippon Ketsueki Gakkai Zasshi 1989; 52:1386–1394.
23. Ware RE, Hall SE, Rosse WF: Paroxysmal nocturnal hemoglobinuria with onset in childhood and adolescence. N Engl J Med 1991; 325:991–996.
24. Hauser D, Barzilai N, Zalish M, et al: Bilateral papilledema with retinal hemorrhages in association with cerebral venous sinus thrombosis and paroxysmal nocturnal hemoglobinuria. Am J Ophthalmol 1996; 122:592–593.
25. Aktan S, Kansu T, Kansu E, et al: Papilledema in paroxysmal nocturnal hemoglobinuria. J Clin Neuroophthalmol 1984; 4:47–48.
26. Van Kamp H, Smit JW, Van den Berg E, et al: Myelodysplasia following paroxysmal nocturnal haemoglobinuria: Evidence for the emergence of a separate clone. Br J Haematol 1994; 87:399–400.
27. Longo L, Bessler M, Beris P, et al: Myelodysplasia in a patient with pre-existing paroxysmal nocturnal haemoglobinuria: A clonal disease originating from within a clonal disease. Br J Haematol 1994; 87:401–403.
28. Jin JY, Tooze JA, Marsh JCW, et al: Myelodysplasia following aplastic anaemia–paroxysmal nocturnal haemoglobinuria syndrome after treatment with immmunosuppression and G-CSF: Evidence for the emergence of a separate clone. Br J Haematol 1996; 94:510–512.
29. Nagakura S, Kawaguchi T, Fujimoto K, et al: Sequential development of myelodysplasia and paroxysmal nocturnal hemoglobinuria in a patient with preceding aplastic anemia. Int J Hematol 1997; 65:187–189.
30. Kuriya S, Dan K, Nomura T: Cytogenetic studies of paroxysmal nocturnal haemoglobinuria. Nippon Ketsueki Gakkai Zasshi 1981; 44:839–844.
31. Iwanaga M, Furukawa K, Amenomori T, et al: Paroxysmal nocturnal haemoglobinuria clones in patients with myelodysplastic syndromes. Br J Haematol 1998; 102:465–474.
32. Viniou N, Michali E, Meletis J, et al: Trisomy 8 in a patient who responded to therapy with all-trans-retinoic acid and developed paroxysmal nocturnal haemoglobinuria. Br J Haematol 1997; 97:135–136.
33. Zaccaria A, Barbieri D, Castoldi GL, et al: Normal bone marrow karyotype in paroxysmal nocturnal hemoglobinuria—a cooperative European study. Cancer Genet Cytogenet 1983; 9:211–215.
34. Krause JR: Paroxysmal nocturnal hemoglobinuria and acute non-lymphocytic leukemia. A report of three cases exhibiting different cytologic types. Cancer 1983; 51:2078–2082.
35. Cross GAM: Glycolipid anchoring of plasma membrane proteins. Annu Rev Cell Biol 1990; 6:1–39.
36. Friedrichson T, Kurzchalia TV: Microdomains of GPI-anchored proteins in living cells revealed by crosslinking. Nature 1998; 394:802–805.
37. Varma R, Mayor S: GPI-anchored proteins are organized in submicron domains at the cell surface. Nature 1998; 394:798–801.
38. Low MG, Saltiel AR: Structural and functional roles of glycosyl-phosphatidylinositol in membranes. Science 1988; 239:268–275.
39. Anderson RG, Kamen BA, Rothberg KG, et al: Potocytosis: Sequestration and transport of small molecules by caveolae. Science 1992; 255:410–411.

40. Schnitzer JE, McIntosh DP, Dvorak AM, et al: P. Separation of caveolae from associated microdomains of GPI-anchored proteins. Science 1995; 269:1435–1439.
41. Schubert J, Ostendorf T, Schmidt RE: Biology of GPI anchors and pathogenesis of paroxysmal nocturnal hemoglobinuria. Immunol Today 1994; 15:299–301.
42. Low MG, Finean JB: Release of alkaline phosphatase from membranes by a phosphatidylinositol-specific phospholipase C. Biochem J 1977; 167:281–284.
43. Ferguson MA, Low MG, Cross GA: Glycosyl-sn-1,2-dimyristylphosphatidylinositol is covalently linked to *Trypanosoma brucei* variant surface glycoprotein. J Biol Chem 1985; 260:14547–14555.
44. Rosenberry TL: A chemical modification that makes glycoinositol phospholipids resistant to phospholipase C cleavage: Fatty acid acylation of inositol. Cell Biol Int Rep 1991; 15:1133–1150.
45. Udenfriend S, Kodukula K: How glycosylphosphatidylinositol-anchored membrane proteins are made. Annu Rev Biochem 1995; 64:563–591.
46. Stevens VL, Raetz CR: Defective glycosyl phosphatidylinositol biosynthesis in extracts of three Thy-1 negative lymphoma cell mutants. J Biol Chem 1991; 266:10039–10042.
47. Puoti A, Desponds C, Fankhauser C, et al: Characterization of glycophospholipid intermediate in the biosynthesis of glycophosphatidylinositol anchors accumulating in the Thy-1-negative lymphoma line SIA-b. J Biol Chem 1991; 266:21051–21059.
48. DeGasperi R, Thomas LJ, Sugiyama E, et al: Correction of a defect in mammalian GPI anchor biosynthesis by a transfected yeast gene. Science 1990; 250:988–991.
49. Hillmen P, Bessler M, Mason PJ, et al: Specific defect in *N*-acetylglucosamine incorporation in the biosynthesis of the glycosylphosphatidylinositol anchor in cloned cell lines from patients with paroxysmal nocturnal hemoglobinuria. Proc Natl Acad Sci USA 1993; 90:5272–5276.
50. Takahashi M, Takeda J, Hirose S, et al: Deficient biosynthesis of *N*-acetylglucosaminyl-phosphatidylinositol, the first intermediate of glycosyl phosphatidylinositol anchor biosynthesis, in cell lines established from patients with paroxysmal nocturnal hemoglobinuria. J Exp Med 1993; 177:517–522.
51. Josten KM, Tooze JA, Borthwick-Clarke C, et al: Acquired aplastic anemia and paroxysmal nocturnal hemoglobinuria: Studies on clonality. Blood 1991; 78:3162–3167.
52. Rotoli B, Robledo R, Luzzatto L: Decreased number of circulating BFU-Es in paroxysmal nocturnal hemoglobinuria. Blood 1982; 60:157–159.
53. Rotoli B, Robledo R, Scarpato N, et al: Two populations of erythroid cell progenitors in paroxysmal nocturnal hemoglobinuria. Blood 1984; 64:847–851.
54. Ueda E, Nishimura J-I, Kitani T, et al: Deficient surface expression of glycosylphosphatidylinositol-anchored proteins in B cell lines established from patients with paroxysmal nocturnal hemoglobinuria. Int Immunol 1992; 4:1263–1271.
55. Hillmen P, Bessler M, Crawford DH, et al: Production and characterization of lymphoblastoid cell lines with the paroxysmal nocturnal hemoglobinuria phenotype. Blood 1939; 80:193–199.
56. Bessler M, Mason PJ, Hillmen P, et al: Paroxysmal nocturnal haemoglobinuria (PNH) is caused by somatic mutations in the PIG-A gene. EMBO J 1994; 13:110–117.
57. Iida Y, Takeda J, Miyata T, et al: Characterization of genomic PIG-A gene: A gene for glycosylphosphatidylinositol-anchor biosynthesis and paroxysmal nocturnal hemoglobinuria. Blood 1994; 83:3126–3131.
58. Bessler M, Hillman P, Longo L, Luzzatto L, et al: Genomic organisation of the X-linked gene (PIG-A) that is mutated in paroxysmal nocturnal haemoglobinuria and of a related pseudogene mapped to 12q21. Hum Mol Genet 1994; 3:751–757.
59. Watanabe R, Inoue N, Westfall B, et al: The first step of glycosylphosphatidylinositol biosynthesis is mediated by a complex of PIG-A, PIG-H, PIG-C and GPI1. EMBO J 1998; 17:877–885.
60. Ware RE, Howard TA, Kamitani T, et al: Chromosomal assignment of genes involved in glycosylphosphatidylinositol anchor biosynthesis: Implications for the pathogenesis of paroxysmal nocturnal hemoglobinuria. Blood 1994; 83:3753–3757.
61. Yamashina M, Ueda E, Kinoshita T, et al: Inherited complete deficiency of 20-kilodalton homologous restriction factor (CD59) as a cause of paroxysmal nocturnal hemoglobinuria. N Engl J Med 1990; 323:1184–1189.
62. Kawagoe K, Kitamura D, Okabe M, et al: Glycosylphosphatidylinositol-anchor–deficient mice: Implications for clonal dominance of mutant cells in paroxysmal nocturnal hemoglobinuria. Blood 1996; 87:3600–3606.
63. Nafa K, Mason PJ, Hillmen P, et al: Mutations in the PIG-A gene causing paroxysmal nocturnal hemoglobinuria are mainly of the frameshift type. Blood 1995; 86:4650–4655.
64. Yamada N, Miyata T, Maeda K, et al: Somatic mutations of the PIG-A gene found in Japanese patients with paroxysmal nocturnal hemoglobinuria. Blood 1995; 85:885–892.
65. Pramoonjago P, Wanachiwanawin W, Chinprasertsak S, et al: Somatic mutations of PIG-A in Thai patients with paroxysmal nocturnal hemoglobinuria. Blood 1995; 86:1736–1739.
66. Nafa K, Bessler M, Castro-Malaspina H, et al: The spectrum of somatic mutations in the PIG-A gene in paroxysmal nocturnal hemoglobinuria includes large deletions and small duplications. Blood Cells Mol Dis 1998; 24:370–384.
67. Rosse WF, Ware RE: The molecular basis of paroxysmal nocturnal hemoglobinuria. Blood 1995; 86:3277–3286.
68. Rotoli B, Luzzatto L: Paroxysmal nocturnal hemoglobinuria. Semin Hematol 1989; 26:201–207.
69. Young NS: The problem of clonality in aplastic

anemia. Dr. Dameshek's riddle, restated. Blood 1992; 79:1385–1392.
70. Sims PJ, Wiedmer T: The response of human platelets to activated components of the complement system. Immunol Today 1991; 12:338–342.
71. Wiedmer T, Hall SE, Ortel TL, et al: Complement-induced vesiculation and exposure of membrane prothrombinase sites in platelets of paroxysmal nocturnal hemoglobinuria. Blood 1993; 82:1192–1196.
72. Wiedmer T, Sims PJ: Participation of protein kinases in complement C5b-9–induced shedding of platelet plasma membrane vesicles. Blood 1991; 78:2880–2886.
73. Gilbert GE, Sims PJ, Wiedmer T, et al: Platelet-derived microparticles express high affinity receptors for factor VIII. J Biol Chem 1991; 266:17261–17268.
74. Wiedmer T, Esmon CT, Sims PJ: Complement proteins C5b-9 stimulate procoagulant activity through platelet prothrombinase. Blood 1986; 68:875–880.
75. Ninomiya H, Kawashima Y, Hasegawa Y, et al: Complement-induced procoagulant alteration of red blood cell membranes with microvesicle formation in paroxysmal nocturnal haemoglobinuria (PNH): Implication for thrombogenesis in PNH. Br J Haematol 1999; 106(1):224–231.
76. Wei Y, Lukashev M, Simon DI, et al: Regulation of integrin function by the urokinase receptor. Science 1996; 273:1551–1555.
77. Rotoli B, Bessler M, Alfinito F, et al: Membrane proteins in paroxysmal nocturnal haemoglobinuria. Blood Rev 1993; 7:75–86.
78. Nishimura J, Inoue N, Azenishi Y, et al: Analysis of PIG-A gene in a patient who developed reciprocal translocation of chromosome 12 and paroxysmal nocturnal hemoglobinuria during follow-up of aplastic anemia. Am J Hematol 1996; 51:229–233.
79. Viniou N, Michali E, Meletis J, et al: Trisomy 8 in a patient who responded to therapy with all-trans-retinoic acid and developed paroxysmal nocturnal haemoglobinuria. Br J Haematol 1997; 97:135–136.
80. Szer J, Deeg HJ, Witherspoon RP, et al: Long-term survival after marrow transplantation for paroxysmal nocturnal hemoglobinuria with aplastic anemia. Ann Intern Med 1984; 102:193–195.
81. Nafa K, Bessler M, Deeg HJ, et al: New somatic mutation in the PIG-A gene emerges at relapse of paroxysmal nocturnal hemoglobinuria. Blood 1998; 92:3422–3427.
82. Kolb HJ, Holler E, Bender GC, et al: Myeloablative conditioning for marrow transplantation in myelodysplastic syndromes and paroxysmal nocturnal haemoglobinuria. Bone Marrow Transplant 1989; 41:29–34.
83. Endo M, Beatty PG, Vreeke TM, et al: Syngeneic bone marrow transplantation without conditioning in a patient with paroxysmal nocturnal hemoglobinuria: In vivo evidence that the mutant stem cells have a survival advantage. Blood 1996; 88:742–750.

84. Fefer A, Freeman H, Storb R, et al: Paroxysmal nocturnal hemoglobinuria and marrow failure treated by infusion of marrow from an identical twin. Ann Intern Med 1976; 84:692–695.
85. Jehn U, Sauer H, Kolb HJ, et al: Bone marrow transplantation in adults in acute leukemia, aplastic anemia, and paroxysmal nocturnal hemoglobinuria Results of the medical clinic lli of LMU (Ludwig-Maximilians University) Munich. Klin Wochenschr 1983; 61:321–328.
86. Hershko C, Ho WG, Gale RP, et al: Cure of aplastic anemia in paroxysmal nocturnal hæmoglobinuria by marrow transfusion from identical twin: Failure of peripheral-leucocyte transfusion to correct marrow aplasia. Lancet 1979; 1:945–947.
87. Kawahara K, Witherspoon RP, Storb R: Marrow transplantation for paroxysmal nocturnal hemoglobinuria. Am J Hematol 1992; 39:283–288.
88. de Souza MH, Abdelhay E, Silva ML, et al: Late marrow allograft rejection following alpha-interferon therapy for hepatitis in a patient with paroxysmal nocturnal hemoglobinuria. Bone Marrow Transplant 1992; 9:495–497.
89. Brodsky RA, Sensenbrenner LL, Jones RJ: Complete remission in severe aplastic anemia after high-dose cyclophosphamide without bone marrow transplantation. Blood 1996; 87:491–494.
90. Selleri C, Maciejewski JP, Sato T, et al: Interferon-γ constitutively expressed in the stromal microenviroment of human marrow cultures mediates potent hematopoietic inhibition. Blood 1996; 87:4149–4157.
91. Selleri C, Sato T, Anderson S, et al: Interferon-γ and tumor necrosis factor-α suppress both early and late stages of hematopoiesis and induce programmed cell death. J Cell Physiol 1995; 165:538–546.
92. Dacie JV: Paroxysmal nocturnal haemoglobinuria. Proc R Soc Med 1963; 56:587–596.
93. Moore JG, Humphries RK, Frank MM, et al: Characterization of the hematopoietic defect in paroxysmal nocturnal hemoglobinuria. Exp Hematol 1986; 14:222–229.
94. Rickard KA, Brown RD, Wilkinson T, et al: The colony forming cell in the myeloproliferative disorders and aplastic anaemia. Scand J Haematol 1979; 22:121–128.
95. Issaragrisil S, Piankijagum A, Chinprasertsuk S, et al: Growth of mixed erythroid-granulocytic colonies in culture derived from bone marrow of patients with paroxysmal nocturnal hemoglobinuria without addition of exogenous stimulator. Exp Hematol 1986; 14:861–866.
96. Tumen J, Kline LB, Fay JW, et al: Complement sensitivity of paroxysmal nocturnal hemoglobinuria bone marrow cells. Blood 1980; 55:1040–1046.
97. Maciejewski JP, Sloand EM, Sato T, et al: Impaired hematopoiesis in paroxysmal nocturnal hemoglobinuria/aplastic anemia is not associated with a selective proliferative defect in the glyco-

sylphosphatidylinositol-anchored protein-deficient clone. Blood 1997; 89:1173–1181.
98. Luzzatto L, Bessler M, Rotoli B: Somatic mutations in paroxysmal nocturnal hemoglobinuria: A blessing in disguise. Cell 1997; 88:1–4.
99. Iwamoto N, Kawaguchi T, Horikawa K, et al: Preferential hematopoiesis by paroxysmal nocturnal hemoglobinuria clone engrafted in SCID mice. Blood 1996; 87:4944–4948.
100. Hogan CJ, Shpall EJ, McNiece I, et al: Multilineage engraftment in NOD/LtSz-scid/scid mice from mobilized human CD34+ peripheral blood progenitor cells. Biol Blood Marrow Transplant 1997; 3:236–246.
101. Larochelle A, Vormoor J, Lapidot T, et al: Engraftment of immune-deficient mice with primitive hematopoietic cells from β-thalassemia and sickle cell anemia patients: Implications for evaluating human gene therapy protocols. Hum Mol Genet 1995; 4:163–172.
102. Vormoor J, Lapidot T, Pflumio F, et al: Immature human cord blood progenitors engraft and proliferate to high levels in severe combined immunodeficient mice. Blood 1994; 83:2489–2497.
103. Brodsky RA, Vala MS, Barber JP, et al: Resistance to apoptosis caused by PIG-A gene mutations in paroxysmal nocturnal hemoglobinuria. Proc Natl Acad Sci USA 1997; 94:8756–8760.
104. Ware RE, Nishimura J, Moody MA, et al: The PIG-A mutation and absence of glycosylphosphatidylinositol-linked proteins do not confer resistance to apoptosis in paroxysmal nocturnal hemoglobinuria. Blood 1998; 92:2541–2550.
105. Gonzalez AD, Kaya M, Shi W, et al: OCI-5/GPC3, a glypican encoded by a gene that is mutated in the Simpson-Golabi-Behmel overgrowth syndrome, induces apoptosis in a cell line–specific manner. J Cell Biol 1998; 141:1407–1414.
106. Pan G, Ni J, Wei YF, et al: An antagonist decoy receptor and a death domain-containing receptor for TRAIL. Science 1997; 277:815–818.
107. Jiang MS, Hart GW: A subpopulation of estrogen receptors are modified by O-linked N-acetylglucosamine. J Biol Chem 1997; 272:2421–2428.
108. Mays RW, Siemers KA, Fritz BA, et al: Hierarchy of mechanisms involved in generating Na/K-ATPase polarity in MDCK epithelial cells. J Cell Biol 1995; 130:1105–1115.
109. Casaccia-Bonnefil P, Carter BD, Dobrowsky RT, et al: Death of oligodendrocytes mediated by the interaction of nerve growth factor with its receptor p75. Nature 1996; 383:716–719.
110. Cuvillier O, Pirianov G, Kleuser B, et al: Suppression of ceramide-mediated programmed cell death by sphingosine-1-phosphate. Nature 1996; 381:800–803.
111. De Maria R, Lenti L, Malisan F, et al: Requirement for GD3 ganglioside in CD95- and ceramide-induced apoptosis. Science 1997; 277:1652–1655.
112. Hannun YA: Functions of ceramide in coordinating cellular responses to stress. Science 1996; 274:1855–1859.
113. Pronk GJ, Ramer K, Amiri P, et al: Requirement of an ICE-like protease for induction of apoptosis and ceramide generation by REAPER. Science 1996; 271:808–810.
114. Verheij M, Bose R, Lin XH, et al: Requirement for ceramide-initiated SAPK/JNK signalling in stress-induced apoptosis. Nature 1996; 380:75–79.
115. Horikawa K, Nakakuma H, Kawaguchi T, et al: Apoptosis resistance of blood cells from patients with paroxysmal nocturnal hemoglobinuria, aplastic anemia, and myelodysplastic syndrome. Blood 1997; 90:2716–2722.
116. Dunn DE, Yu J, Nagarajan S, et al: A knock-out model of paroxysmal nocturnal hemoglobinuria: Pig-a(-) hematopoiesis is reconstituted following intercellular transfer of GPI-anchored proteins. Proc Natl Acad Sci USA 1996; 93:7938–7943.
117. Rosti V, Tremml G, Soares V, et al: Murine embryonic stem cells without pig-a gene activity are competent for hematopoiesis with the PNH phenotype but not for clonal expansion. J Clin Invest 1997; 100:1028–1036.
118. Tremml G, Dominguez C, Rosti V, et al: Increased sensitivity to complement and a decreased red blood cell life span in mice mosaic for a nonfunctional piga gene. Blood 1999; 94:2945–2954.
119. Dunn DE, Ware RE, Parker CJ, et al: Research directions in paroxysmal nocturnal hemoglobinuria. Immunol Today 1999; 20:168–171.
120. Purow DB, Howard TA, Marcus SJ, et al: Genetic instability as the etiology of acquired somatic piga mutations in paroxysmal nocturnal hemoglobinuria. Blood Cells Molec Dis 1999; 25:81–91.
121. Hattori H, Machii T, Ueda E, et al: Increased frequency of somatic mutations at glycophorin A loci in patients with aplastic anaemia, myelodysplastic syndrome and paroxysmal nocturnal haemoglobinuria. Br J Haematol 1997; 98: 384–391.
122. Araten DJ, Nafa K, Pakdeesuwan K, Luzzatto L: Clonal populations of hematopoietic cells with paroxysmal nocturnal hemoglobinuria genotype and phenotype are present in normal individuals. Proc Natl Acad Sci USA 1999; 96:5209–5214.
123. Hertenstein B, Wagner B, Bunjes D, et al: Emergence of CD52-, phosphatidylinositolglycan-anchor–deficient T lymphocytes after in vivo application of Campath-1H for refractory B-cell non-Hodgkin lymphoma. Blood 1995; 86: 1487–1492.
124. Taylor VC, Sims M, Brett S, et al: Antibody selection against CD52 produces a paroxysmal nocturnal haemoglobinuria phenotype in human lymphocytes by a novel mechanism. Biochem J 1997; 322(pt 3): 919–925.
125. Rawstron AC, Rollinson SJ, Richards S, et al: The PNH phenotype cells that emerge in most patients after CAMPATH-1H therapy are present prior to treatment. Br J Haematol 1999; 107(1):148–153.
126. Dunn DE, Tanawattanacharoen P, Boccuni P, et al: Paroxysmal nocturnal hemoglobinuria cells in patients with bone marrow failure syndromes. Ann Intern Med 1999; 131:401–408.
127. Young NS, Maciejewski JP: The pathophysiology

of acquired aplastic anemia. N Engl J Med 1997; 336: 1365–1372.
128. Nisticò A, Young NS: Interferon-γ gene expression in the bone marrow of patients with aplastic anemia. Ann Intern Med 1994; 120: 463–469.
129. Zoumbos N, Gascon P, Trost S, et al: Circulating activated suppressor T lymphocytes in aplastic anemia. N Engl J Med 1985; 312: 257–265.
130. Frickhofen N, Kaltwasser JP, Schrezenmeier H, et al: Treatment of aplastic anemia with antithymocyte globulin and methylprednisolone with or without cyclosporine. N Engl J Med 1991; 324: 1297–1304.
131. Rosenfeld SE, Kimball J., Vining D, et al: Intensive immunosuppression with antithymocyte globulin and cyclosporine as treatment for severe acquired aplastic anemia. Blood 1995; 85: 3058–3065.
132. Brodbeck WG, Liu D, Sperry J, et al: Localization of classical and alternative pathway regulatory activity within the decay-accelerating factor. J Immunol 1996; 156: 2528–2533.
133. Tam BY, Germain L, Philip A: TGF-beta receptor expression on human keratinocytes: A 150 kDa GPI-anchored TGF-beta 1 binding protein forms a heteromeric complex with type I and type II receptors. J Cell Biochem 1998; 70: 573–586.
134. Dumont N, O'Connor-McCourt MD, Philip A: Transforming growth factor-beta receptors on human endometrial cells: Identification of the type I, II, and III receptors and glycosyl-phosphatidylinositol anchored TGF-beta binding proteins. Mol Cell Endocrinol 1995; 111: 57–66.
135. Nishimura J, Smith CA, Phillips KL, et al: Paroxysmal nocturnal hemoglobinuria: Molecular pathogenesis and molecular therapeutic approaches. Hematopathol Mol Hematol 1998; 11: 119–146.
136. Robinson PJ: Phosphatidyinositol membrane anchors and T-cell activation. Immunol Today 1991; 12: 35–41.
137. Nomoto S, Ito S, Yang LX, et al: Molecular cloning and expression analysis of GFR alpha-3, a novel cDNA related to GDNFR alpha and NTNR alpha. Biochem Biophys Res Commun 1998; 244: 849–853.
138. Buj-Bello A, Adu J, Pinon LG, et al: Neurturin responsiveness requires a GPI-linked receptor and the Ret receptor tyrosine kinase. Nature 1997; 387: 721–724.
139. Klein RD, Sherman D, Ho WH, et al: A GPI-linked protein that interacts with Ret to form a candidate neurturin receptor. Nature 1997; 387: 717–721.
140. Treanor JJ, Goodman L, de Sauvage F, et al: Characterization of a multicomponent receptor for GDNF. Nature 1996; 382: 80–83.
141. Jing S, Wen D, Yu Y, et al: GDNF-induced activation of the ret protein tyrosine kinase is mediated by GDNFR-alpha, a novel receptor for GDNF. Cell 1996; 85: 1113–1124.
142. Zhang XG, Gu JJ, Lu Zy, et al: Ciliary neurotropic factor, interleukin 11, leukemia inhibitory factor, and oncostatin M are growth factors for human myeloma cell lines using the interleukin 6 signal transducer gp 130. J Exp Med 1994; 179: 1337–1342.
143. Davis S, Aldrich TH, Stahl N, et al: LIFR beta and gp 130 as heterodimerizing signal transducers of the tripartite CNTF receptor. Science 1993; 260: 1805–1808.
144. Davis S, Aldrich TH, Ip NY, et al: Released form of CNTF receptor alpha component as a soluble mediator of CNTF responses. Science 1993; 259: 1736–1739.
145. Shafren DR, Bates RC, Agrez MV, et al: Coxsackieviruses B1, B3 and B5 use decay accelerating factor as a receptor for cell attachment. J Virol 1995; 69: 3873–3877.
146. Ward T, Pipkin PA, Clarkson NA, et al: Decay-accelerating factor CD55 is identified as the receptor for echovirus 7 using CELICS a rapid immuno-focal cloning method. EMBO J 1994; 13: 5070–5074.
147. Bergelson JM, Chan M, Solomon KR, et al: Decay-accelerating factor (CD55) a glycosylphosphatidylinositol-anchored complement regulatory protein is a receptor for several echoviruses. Proc Natl Acad Sci U S A 1994; 91: 6245–6248.
148. Albrecht JC, Nicholas J, Cameron KR, et al: Herpesvirus saimiri has a gene specifying a homologue of the cellular membrane glycoprotein CD59. Virology 1992; 190: 527–530.
149. Rother RP, Rollins SA, Fodor WL, et al: Inhibition of complement-mediated cytolysis by the terminal complement inhibitor of herpesvirus saimiri. J Virol 1994; 68: 730–737.
150. Vanderlugt CL, Begolka WS, Neville KL, et al: The functional significance of epitope spreading and its regulation by co-stimulatory molecules. Immunol. Rev 1998; 164:63–72: 63–72.
151. Greenfield EA, Nguyen KA, Kuchroo VK: CD28/B7 costimulation: A review. Crit Rev Immunol 1998; 18: 389–418.
152. Sayegh MH, Turka LA: The role of T-cell co-stimulatory activation pathways in transplant rejection. N Engl J Med 1998; 338: 1813–1821.
153. Lu P, Wang YL, Linsley PS: Regulation of self-tolerance by CD80/CD86 interactions. Curr Opin Immunol 1997; 9: 858–862.
154. Thompson CB, Allison JP: The emerging role of CTLA-4 as an immune attenuator. Immunity 1997; 7: 445–450.
155. Daikh D, Wofsy D, Imboden JB: The CD28-B7 co-stimulatory pathway and its role in autoimmune disease. J Leuk Biol 1997; 62: 156–162.
156. Boussiotis VA, Freeman GJ, Gribben JG, et al: The role of B7-1/B7-2: CD28/CLTA-4 pathways in the prevention of anergy, induction of productive immunity and down-regulation of the immune response. Immunol Rev 1996; 153: 5–26.
157. Schultze J, Nadler LM, Gribben JG: B7-mediated co-stimulation and the immune response. Blood Rev 1996; 10: 111–127.
158. Arulanandam AR, Moingeon P, Concino MF, et al: A soluble multimeric recombinant CD2 protein identifies CD48 as a low affinity ligand for human

158. ...CD2: Divergence of CD2 ligands during the evolution of humans and mice. J Exp Med 1993; 177: 1439–1450.
159. Hahn WC, Menu E, Bothwell ALM, et al: Overlapping but nonidentical binding sites on CD2 for CD58 and a second ligand CD59. Science 1993; 256: 1805–1807.
160. Menu E, Tsai BC, Bothwell ALM, et al: CD59 costimulation of T cell acrtivation. CD58 dependence and requirement for glycosylation. J Immunol 1994; 153: 2444–2456.
161. Hollander N, Shin ML, Rosse WF, et al: Distinct restriction of complement-and-cell-mediated lysis. J Immunol 1989; 142: 3913–3916.
162. Gregory CD, Dive C, Henderson S, et al: Activation of Epstein-Barr virus latent genes protects human B cells from death by apoptosis. Nature 1991; 349: 612–614.
163. Tudela M, Jarque I, Perez-Sirvent ML, et al: Clinical profile and course of paroxysmal nocturnal hemoglobinuria. Sangre (Barc) 1993; 38: 301–307.
164. Issaragrisil S, Piankijagum A, Tang-naitrisorana Y: Corticosteroids therapy in paroxysmal nocturnal hemoglobinuria. Am J Hematol 1987; 25: 77–83.
165. Rosse WF: Treatment of paroxysmal nocturnal hemoglobinuria. Blood 1982; 60: 20–23.
166. Hartmann RC, Jenkins DE, McKee C, et al: Paroxysmal nocturnal hemoglobinuria: Clinical and laboratory studies relating to iron metabolism and therapy with androgen and iron. Medicine (Baltimore) 1966; 45: 331–363.
167. Harrington WJ Sr, Kolodny L, Horstman LL, et al: Danazol for paroxysmal nocturnal hemoglobinuria. Am J. Hematol 1997; 54: 149–154.
168. Sholar PW, Bell WR: Thrombolytic therapy for inferior vena cava thrombosis in paroxysmal nocturnal hemoglobinuria. Ann Intern Med 1985; 103: 539–541.
169. Zimmerman D, Bell WR: Venous thrombosis and splenic rupture in paroxysmal nocturnal hemoglobinuria. Am J Med 1980; 68: 275–279.
170. Young NS, Barrett AJ: The treatment of severe acquired aplastic anemia. Blood 1995; 85: 3367–3377.
171. Paquette RL, Yoshimura R, Veiseh C, et al: Clinical characteristics predict response to antithymocyte globulin in paroxysmal nocturnal haemoglobinuria. Br J Haematol 1997; 96: 92–97.
172. Sanchez-Valle E, Morales-Polanco MR, Gomez-Morales E, et al: Treatment of paroxysmal nocturnal hemoglobinuria with antilymphocyte globulin. Rev Invest Clin 1993; 45: 457–461.
173. Schrezenmeier H, Hertenstein B, Wagner B, et al: A pathogenetic link between aplastic anemia and paroxysmal nocturnal hemoglobinuria is suggested by a high frequency of aplastic anemia patients with a deficiency of phosphatidylinositol glycan anchored proteins. Exp Hematol 1995; 23: 81–87.
174. Van Kamp H, van Imhoff GW, de Wolf JT, et al: The effect of cyclosporine on haematological parameters in patients with paroxysmal nocturnal haemoglobinuria. Br J Haematol 1995; 89: 79–82.
175. Stoppa AM, Vey N, Sainty D, et al: Correction of aplastic anaemia complicating paroxysmal nocturnal haemoglobinuria: Absence of eradication of the PNH clone and dependence of response on cyclosporin A administration. Br J Haematol 1996; 93: 42–44.
176. Nakao S, Yamaguchi M, Takamatsu H, et al: Expansion of a paroxysmal nocturnal hemoglobinuria (PNH) clone after cyclosporine therapy for aplastic anemia/PNH syndrome (letter). Blood 1992; 80: 2943–2944.
177. Antin JH, Ginsburg D, Smith BR, et al: Bone marrow transplantation for paroxysmal nocturnal hemoglobinuria: Eradication of the PNH clone and documentation of complete lymphohematopoietic engraftment. Blood 1985; 66: 1247–1250.
178. Graham ML, Rosse WF, Halperin F.C, et al: Resolution of Budd-Chiari syndrome following bone marrow transplantation for paroxysmal nocturnal haemoglobinuria. Br J Haematol 1996; 92: 707–710.
179. Medof ME, Nagarajan S, Tykocinski ML: Cell-surface engineering with GPI-anchored proteins. FASEB J 1996; 10:574–586.
180. Sloand EM, Maciejewski JP, Dunn D, et al: Correction of the PNH defect by GPI-anchored protein transfer. Blood 1998; 92: 4439–4445.
181. Kooyman DL, Byrne GW, McClellan S, et al: In vivo transfer of GPI-linked complement restriction factors from erythrocytes to the endothelium. Science 1995; 269: 89–92.
182. Field MC, Moran P, Li W, et al: Retention and degradation of proteins containing an uncleaved glycosylphosphatidylinositol signal. J Biol Chem 1994; 269:10830–10837.

5

Myelofibrosis (Agnogenic Myeloid Metaplasia)

Dimitrios Mavroudis, M.D.
John Barrett, M.D.

Many malignant and nonmalignant conditions are associated with an increased deposition of collagen in the bone marrow known as myelofibrosis. This chapter focuses on *idiopathic* or *primary myelofibrosis,* a term synonymous with myelosclerosis and agnogenic myeloid metaplasia (AMM). AMM is a chronic malignant hematologic stem cell disorder accompanied by reactive, nonclonal bone marrow fibrosis. AMM has certain typical features, including anemia, splenomegaly, a leukoerythroblastic blood picture, teardrop poikilocytosis, marrow fibrosis, and extramedullary hematopoiesis. The presence of these physical signs and laboratory findings help characterize the disease AMM. AMM was first described in 1879 by Heuck,[1] who reported two patients with severe bone marrow fibrosis combined with extramedullary hematopoiesis in the liver and spleen. Dameshek[2] was the first to recognize that AMM was a stem cell disorder, and he classified AMM with the chronic myeloproliferative disorders (MPDs) together with essential thrombocythemia (ET), polycythemia vera (PCV), and chronic myelogenous leukemia (CML). All chronic hematologic malignancies of stem cell origin, with varying degrees of marrow fibrosis, share the potential to evolve into acute leukemia. CML can be distinguished by a usually stereotypic clinical presentation and a unique chromosomal abnormality. The other MPDs overlap in their clinical characteristics and pathophysiology. ET and PCV have a tendency to evolve into AMM. All share common abnormalities of growth factor independence in erythroid, granulocytic, and megakaryocytic progenitors,[3] and similar chromosomal abnormalities, notably trisomy of chromosomes 5, 8, 13, and 20.[4] Table 5–1 lists the features which associate AMM with other MPDs.

Despite the recent progress in our understanding of the mechanisms underlying the fibrotic process, the prognosis and treatment of this condition have not significantly changed in the last 30 years. With the exception of allogeneic bone marrow transplantation (BMT), AMM remains an incurable disease, and current management remains palliative. Experimental therapies aimed at control of the malignant clone and the fibrotic component are currently being tested.

EPIDEMIOLOGY AND ETIOLOGY

AMM is the rarest of the MPDs, with an annual incidence estimated to be about 0.5/100,000.[5] It affects primarily elderly people with a median age at diagnosis of approximately 60 years. Rare cases of AMM have also been reported in children.[6] There is no evidence for a genetic predisposition to the disease. A slight predominance for males has been reported. Risk factors include prior radiation, chronic exposure to benzene, and administration of the radioactive contrast material thorium dioxide.[7–9] Thorium dioxide is a colloidal suspension containing ^{232}thorium, which is taken up by cells of the reticuloendothelial system and causes lifelong irradiation to the liver, spleen, lymph nodes, and bone marrow. Its use in radiographic studies before the early 1950s has been associated with the development of acute myeloid and lymphoid leukemias, myelofibrosis, and aplastic anemia.[9] Owing to the common induction of liver

TABLE 5–1 Comparison of Features of the Closely Associated Myeloproliferative Disorders

Features	Agnogenic Myeloid Metaplasia	Essential Thrombocytopenia	Polycythemia Vera
Stem cell disorder	Yes	Yes	Yes
Trisomy 8, 13, 20	Yes	Yes	Yes
Circulating committed progenitors	+++	+	+
Epo-independence	+	+	+++
G-CSF independence	++	++	++
Spontaneous megakaryocyte generation by PBMNCs	+++	++	+
Megakaryocyte abnormalities	+++	+++	+
Platelet function defects	+++	+++	++
Marrow fibrosis	+++	+ late	+ late
Marrow cellularity	↓↑	↑	↑
Anemia	+++	++	−
Thrombosis	±	+++	±
Platelet count	↓↑	↓↑	↓↑
Granulocyte count	↓↑	↓↑	↓↑

Epo, erythropoietin; G-CSF, granulocyte colony-stimulating factor; PBMNCs, peripheral blood mononuclear cells.
  +, occasional; ++, frequent; +++, always; ±, uncommon–never; ↑, increased; ↓, decreased; ↑↓, increased, normal, or decreased.

cirrhosis and splenic atrophy after exposure to thorium dioxide, patients who develop myelofibrosis may lack hepatosplenomegaly. The association of marrow fibrosis with avian leukemia virus in birds[10] raises the possibility that human AMM and its associated MPDs are of viral origin. However, apart from an intriguing but unconfirmed observation of the detection of possible retroviral RNA sequences and viral particles in the megakaryocytes of patients with AMM, PCV, and ET, no further evidence has been forthcoming.[11] Another interesting report is the case of a patient who developed myelofibrosis with extramedullary hematopoiesis in the skin, 20 years after the successful treatment of severe aplastic anemia.[12]

PATHOPHYSIOLOGY[13]

Stem Cell Origin

The clonal nature of hematopoiesis in AMM was first demonstrated by Jacobson et al.[14] with glucose-6-phosphate dehydrogenase (G6PD) isoenzyme analysis in a heterozygous female patient with AMM. Since then, other studies[15–17] have also confirmed that the primary defect is an abnormal clone at the stem cell level which gives rise to all blood cells in AMM patients, including T and B lymphocytes.[18] The marrow fibrosis in AMM is not of clonal origin and represents a secondary reaction of the stromal cells, an exaggeration of the normal marrow fibrous pattern.[14] Bone marrow fibroblasts from patients with AMM have physical characteristics similar to fibroblasts from normal marrows.[19] The reversibility of myelofibrosis with suppression or extinction of the malignant clone after prolonged chemotherapy or allogeneic BMT[20] provides further evidence that the fibrotic process is a consequence of the hematologic malignancy. In AMM there is a 10- to 20-fold increase in circulating progenitor cells as opposed to a threefold increase in other MPDs (Table 5–2) that are also associated with myelofibrosis.[21] These circulating progenitors give rise to erythroid and megakaryocytic colonies in the absence of exogenously added cytokines, a characteristic shared by all chronic MPDs.[22]

Abnormal Megakaryocytes and Marrow Fibrosis

The bone marrow stroma in AMM contains increased amounts of total collagen. In the early hypercellular phase of the disease, collagen is mostly soluble. With disease progression, the collagen becomes polymeric and insoluble due to extensive cross-linking.[23] With immunohistologic techniques, both interstitial and basement membrane collagens types I, III, IV, and V are significantly increased.[24] In advanced disease there is also an increased deposition of the glycoproteins fibronectin, tenascin, and vitronectin.[25–27] Ultimately, membranous or appositional new bone formation can occur, leading to osteosclerosis.

TABLE 5–2   Conditions Associated With Bone Marrow Fibrosis

Malignant diseases
    Myeloproliferative disorders
        Agnogenic myeloid metaplasia
        Essential thrombocythemia
        Polycythemia vera
        Chronic myelogenous leukemia
    Myeloid malignancies
        Acute myelogenous leukemia, AML M7
        Myelodysplasia with myelofibrosis
        Systemic mastocytosis
    Lymphoid malignancies
        Hairy cell leukemia
        Hodgkin's disease
        Non-Hodgkin's lymphoma
        Multiple myeloma
    Nonhematopoietic malignancies
        Metastatic adenocarcinoma (breast, prostate, stomach)

Nonmalignant Disorders
    Chronic infection
        Tuberculosis
        Histoplasmosis
    Autoimmune diseases
        Systemic lupus erythematosus
        Scleroderma
    Abnormalities of calcium metabolism
        Hyper- or hypoparathyroidism
        Renal osteodystrophy
        Vitamin D deficiency
    Other
        Gray platelet syndrome
        Gaucher's disease

The missing link between clonal hematopoiesis and reactive fibrosis was first suggested by Groopman,[28] who proposed that growth factors secreted by the hematopoietic malignant cells stimulated marrow fibroblasts to proliferate. The observation that collagen surrounds areas where abnormal megakaryocytes are clustered focused research on the identification of possible growth factors released from megakaryocytes and platelets. Platelet-derived growth factor (PDGF), transforming growth factor-β (TGF-β), and epidermal growth factor (EGF), all of which are contained in the alpha granules of platelets, stimulate bone marrow fibroblast proliferation.[29] Conflicting data exist for the concentration of PDGF in the platelets of AMM patients, with some studies reporting increased[30] and others decreased[31] levels. More convincing data exist for the role of TGF-β, because this glycoprotein is increased in concentration in platelets of AMM patients.[30] TGF-β promotes the formation and accumulation of extracellular matrix in the bone marrow, not only by enhancing gene expression for collagens type I, III, IV, and fibronectin but also by decreasing the synthesis of various collagenase-like enzymes that degrade collagen.[32] Furthermore, TGF-β controls other growth factors by stimulating PDGF production by bone marrow endothelial stromal cells[33] and by influencing the mitogenic activity of both PDGF and EGF.[29] In AMM there are changes in marrow vascularity, with dilation of the marrow sinusoids, endothelial hyperplasia, and neovascularization.[34] This effect may be also mediated by TGF-β, which stimulates angiogenesis.[35] The interaction of megakaryocytes with fibroblasts in the marrow stroma is illustrated in Figure 5–1.

Extramedullary Hematopoiesis

A unique and striking feature of AMM is the occurrence of extramedullary hematopoiesis in spleen, liver, and sometimes lymph tissues. The mechanism is unknown. However, the marrow fibrosis is associated with displacement of hematopoietic progenitor cells into the blood. Circulating stem cells likely then seed other tissues of the reticuloendothelial system and establish extramedullary sites of hematopoiesis. In turn, the process causing fibrosis in the marrow leads to fibrosis in the spleen; the spleen eventually can become massively and irreversibly enlarged. The mechanism of displacement of hematopoietic cells from the marrow mirrors that seen in the nonmalignant disorder of osteopetrosis, which is characterized by extramedullary hematopoiesis and large numbers of circulating stem cells (unpublished observation). In addition, the abnormal stem cells in AMM may have a greater capacity to proliferate outside the bone marrow microenvironment. The growth factor independence of committed progenitor cells has already been noted. Serum macrophage colony-stimulating factor (CSF-1) levels are increased in all chronic MPDs but the highest levels are detected in patients with extensive extramedullary hematopoiesis, suggesting that CSF-1 may also play a role in its pathogenesis.[36] The relative contribution of the bone marrow and the spleen in hematopoiesis in AMM has been extensively studied using radioisotopes. Although spleen and liver take up increased amounts of radiolabeled iron in AMM, very little is incorporated into circulating red blood cells. Thus, extramedullary hematopoiesis is largely ineffective.

Mechanisms of Anemia and Marrow Failure

Anemia in AMM is multifactorial (Fig. 5–2). Reduced red blood cell production is part of the MPD. This is complicated by dyserythropoiesis

Myelofibrosis (Agnogenic Myeloid Metaplasia)

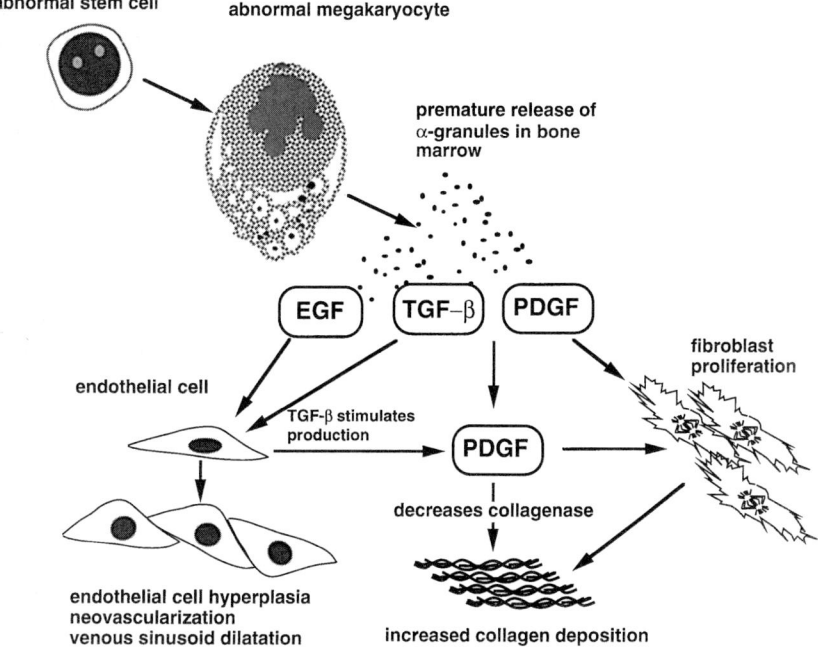

Figure 5–1 Pathophysiology of marrow fibrosis in agnogenic myeloid metaplasia. EGF, epidermal growth factor; TGF-β, transforming growth factor-β; PDGF, platelet-derived growth factor.

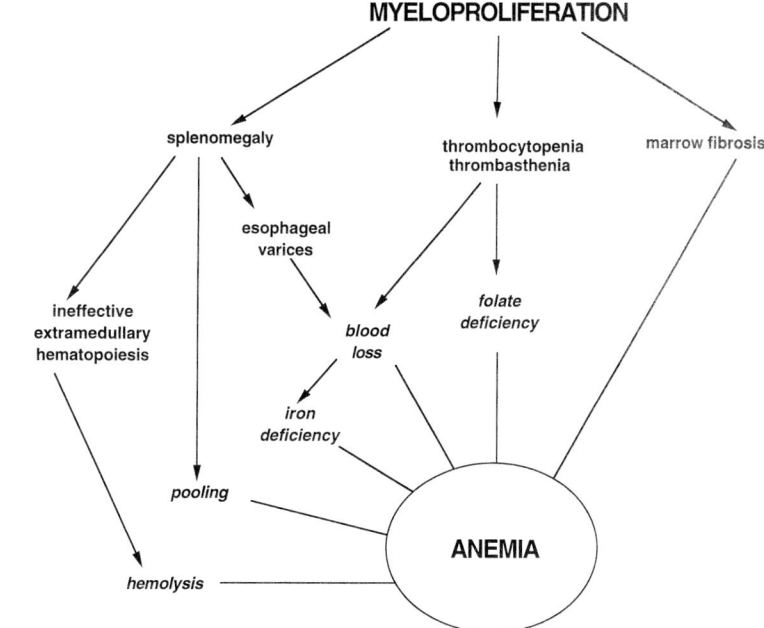

Figure 5–2 Multifactorial mechanisms in the anemia of agnogenic myeloid metaplasia.

and ineffective extramedullary erythropoiesis. There is also a hemolytic component to the anemia due to a reduced life span of the dyserythropoietic red blood cells. Rarely, a direct antiglobulin test–positive autoimmune hemolytic anemia occurs. Splenic pooling of blood aggravates the anemia and sequestration of platelets contributes to the thrombocytopenia. Patients have an increased tendency to bleed because of thrombasthenia and thrombocytopenia and from esophageal varices and peptic ulceration. In addition, they may become iron deficient from bleeding, and folic acid deficient from hypermetabolism. The pancytopenia which characterizes the "spent phase" of AMM may be due to a true reduction in functional marrow stroma caused by the severe fibrosis and osteosclerosis.

CLINICAL FEATURES

History

Typically, patients with AMM present with symptoms of anemia and splenomegaly. Early complaints are weakness, fatigue, palpitations, or exertional dyspnea. It is not unusual for symptoms of lassitude to be out of proportion to the degree of anemia, attributable to the hypermetabolic state associated with myeloproliferation. Patients with advanced AMM are frequently cachectic and may have fevers and night sweats. Gouty tophi can develop from increased urate production, although renal failure from hyperuricemia is rare. Pruritus exacerbated by increased temperature similar to that seen in PCV can be a presenting and disturbing symptom. Rarely, disease is preceded by the appearance of erythematous plaques of the skin, also known as Sweet's syndrome, as in many hematologic malignancies.[37]

Prominent enlargement of the spleen, which can extend from the left costal margin beyond the umbilicus to the right side of the pelvis, produces discomfort and a feeling of dull heaviness. Splenic compression of the stomach and intestine can cause dyspepsia, diarrhea, and especially early satiety, all of which contribute to weight loss. Splenic infarction can present as an acute abdominal emergency with severe pain.

Extramedullary hematopoiesis (ectopic myeloid metaplasia) has been described in almost any tissue, including the lungs, central nervous system, gastrointestinal or genitourinary tract, the peritoneum, and the pericardium.[38–40] The ectopic hematopoietic tissue can resemble tumors and cause pressure symptoms such as headaches, back pain, nerve paralysis, cough, or small bowel obstruction. Nevertheless, almost one fourth of patients are asymptomatic at diagnosis, and disease is discovered due to abnormalities on routine blood counts or the incidental finding of an enlarged spleen on a physical examination.

Physical Examination

The patient may have an anemic pallor, jaundice, peripheral edema, petechiae and ecchymoses due to thrombocytopenia or thrombasthenia, splenomegaly, hepatomegaly, and rarely lymphadenopathy. Portal hypertension may develop due to either increased blood flow from the spleen or thromboses of portal and hepatic veins.[41, 42] This may lead to ascites and esophageal varices, which can cause life-threatening bleeding episodes.

Laboratory Studies

Most patients are anemic and usually the red blood cells are normochromic and normocytic. Most commonly anemia is due to both ineffective erythropoiesis and shortened red blood cell survival. Splenic pooling can lead to dilutional anemia, secondary to an expanded plasma volume. Some patients may have hypochromic, microcytic anemia due to occult blood loss from peptic ulcer or esophageal varices. Not infrequently the anemia is macrocytic due to folate deficiency from the myeloproliferation and chronic hemolysis. Hemolysis is occasionally Coombs' test positive.[43] A "PNH [paroxysmal nocturnal hemoglobinuria]-like defect" on the red blood cells has also been described.[44] There is a single report of parvovirus B19–induced red blood cell aplasia in a patient with myelofibrosis.[45]

About one third of the patients may have leukocytosis or, less frequently, leukopenia. Thrombocytopenia occurs in one third of patients, but thrombocythemia is less common.[46] Thrombasthenia with abnormal platelet aggregation studies is a common finding in patients with AMM.[47] Bleeding times and prothrombin times are often prolonged.[46, 47] Frequently, patients have asymptomatic low-grade disseminated intravascular coagulation (DIC) with increased fibrin split products, and they are therefore at risk for catastrophic bleeding with surgical procedures if the coagulopathy is not corrected. Isolated deficiency of factor V and the presence of circulating anticoagulants have also been described.[46] Liver function tests are abnormal in half the patients[48] and the lipid profile is usually unfavorable despite a low total cholesterol.[49]

The leukoerythroblastic peripheral blood smear in established AMM is characteristic, showing red blood cells of different sizes and shapes with frequent teardrop forms (teardrop poikilocytosis), nucleated red blood cells, immature myeloid forms, and giant platelets, often accompanied by megakaryocyte fragments. The teardrop forms are reduced following splenectomy, underscoring the importance of the spleen in the generation of these cells.[50] The bone marrow cannot be aspirated ("dry tap") in most cases. However, even a hypocellular aspirate may reveal platelet clumps and a few abnormal megakaryocytes. A core biopsy is absolutely required to determine cellularity and the degree of bone marrow fibrosis. Marrow biopsies in AMM usually show patchy hypercellularity and increased numbers of dysplastic megakaryocytes, aggregated in clusters, surrounded by varying degrees of reticulin fibrosis. A histomorphometric evaluation of bone marrow biopsies at different stages of AMM showed that there was early hypercellularity with no or minimal reticulin fibrosis, which gradually progressed to a stage where fibrotic and osteosclerotic changes predominate.[51] During evolution of the disease there was a parallel increase in the number of dysplastic megakaryocytes.[51] In another report, bone marrow cellularity and fibrosis did not always correlate with other clinical signs of disease progression.[52] The diagnosis of AMM in its early stages can be more difficult. The aspirate is hypercellular and shows an increase in abnormal megakaryocytes. However, a reticulin stain of the biopsy should reveal a fine reticular pattern of fibrosis. Morphologic characteristics of blood and marrow in AMM are illustrated in Plate 5.

In cases where the bone marrow was aspirable at diagnosis, chromosomal abnormalities were detected in half of the patients with AMM.[53, 54] No specific abnormalities have been described, but the most commonly reported include trisomies 8, 9, and 21, partial trisomy 1q, and deletions in 13q and 20q.[55] Evolution to acute myelogenous leukemia is sometimes associated with acquisition of additional chromosomal aberrations.[56] The finding of a Philadelphia chromosome or bcr/abl rearrangement indicates a diagnosis of CML.

Magnetic resonance imaging (MRI) can easily distinguish cellular and fibrotic marrow, and in one report the patterns in the proximal femurs of patients with AMM correlated with the severity of the disease.[57] More studies are needed to evaluate the usefulness of MRI in the diagnosis, staging, evaluation of response to treatment, and follow-up of disease progression in patients with AMM.

Natural History

Since the onset of AMM is insidious, it is likely that the disorder has a lengthy preclinical phase with asymptomatic thrombocytosis, leukocytosis, and anemia (Fig. 5–3). In early AMM, splenomegaly is undetectable on clinical examination. Nevertheless, the marrow is hypercellular with increased reticulin. At this stage the disease is only distinguishable from ET by a lack of thrombotic complications. Patients are often diagnosed as having an atypical MPD or myelodysplastic syndrome (MDS) with marrow fibrosis. During this phase, which may last some years, patients remain active and require no transfusion support.

Since the initial stage of AMM is seldom symptomatic, most patients present with features of established AMM. In this phase of the disease, constitutional symptoms of weight loss and hypermetabolism are common. Gout may develop and splenomegaly becomes apparent. The blood picture shows leukoerythroblastic change with red blood cell abnormalities characteristic of myelofibrosis. The marrow may be difficult to aspirate and the biopsy shows marked increase in reticulin with patchy areas of hypercellularity. The anemia may respond to folate supplementation and myelosuppressive chemotherapy, which can also reduce the size of the spleen. However, transfusion support may ultimately be required.

The third phase is advanced myelofibrosis, characterized by massive fibrotic splenomegaly, transfusion-dependent anemia, and hemorrhagic complications from platelet dysfunction and thrombocytopenia. Patients develop complications from the enlarged spleen—infarcts and worsening cytopenias from sequestration of blood, esophageal varices, and marked constitutional symptoms. The blood picture changes to one of pancytopenia, the marrow is inaspirable, and the biopsy shows dense fibrosis and sometimes even osteosclerosis.

Most patients die from complications of pancytopenia and transfusion support. Transformation to acute leukemia occurs in 5% to 20% of patients in different series.[58] The leukemia is usually myeloid or myelomonocytic but other lineages have also been reported to be involved, producing megakaryocytic, erythroid, lymphocytic, or hybrid types of leukemia.[59] In contrast to the acute leukemia presenting as acute myelofibrosis (see below), the blastic phase of AMM is very resistant to induction chemotherapy and carries the same dismal prognosis as blast crisis of CML.

DIFFERENTIAL DIAGNOSIS

There is no difficulty in making a certain diagnosis of AMM in the typical elderly patient presenting

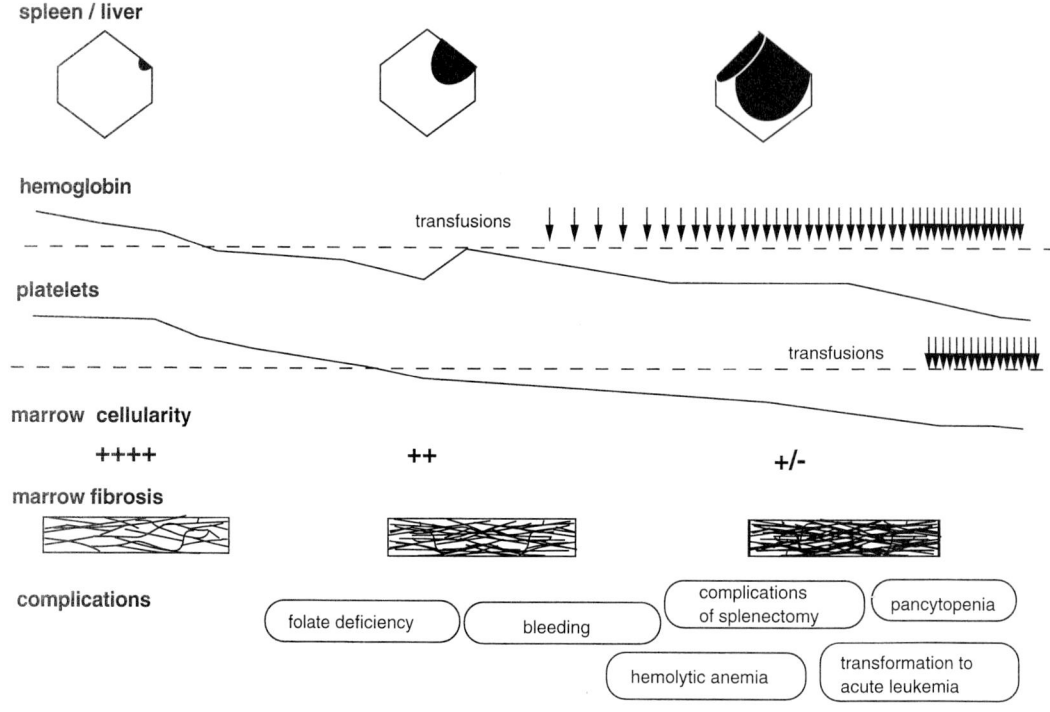

Figure 5–3 Natural history of agnogenic myeloid metaplasia.

with splenomegaly, leukoerythroblastic anemia, red blood cell poikilocytosis, and an inaspirable and fibrotic bone marrow on biopsy. However, in patients with less advanced disease, other hematologic disorders and causes of marrow fibrosis should be considered in the differential diagnosis (see Table 5–2).

Other Hematologic Disorders

A distinct presentation with pancytopenia, fever, and a fibrotic marrow containing immature myeloblasts with a megakaryocytic phenotype is sometimes called acute myelofibrosis (AMF).[60, 61] These patients do not have significant hepatosplenomegaly and teardrop cells are usually not present in the blood smear. AMF has a fulminant and fatal course with a median survival from diagnosis of only a few months.[60, 61] For practical purposes it is best to consider AMF as a form of acute megakaryocytic leukemia. Younger patients with AMF should be treated with acute leukemia induction therapy. In remission, which is often well-sustained, the fibrosis recedes. Allogeneic bone marrow transplantation can be curative.

Hairy cell leukemia should be considered in all patients presenting with cytopenia, splenomegaly, and marrow fibrosis. The diagnosis is based on the identification of hairy cells in the peripheral blood by morphology and cytochemistry. This B lymphocyte disorder is characterized by the presence of large circulating lymphocytes with characteristic cytoplasmic filamentous projections. The cells contain tartrate-resistant acid phosphatase. In some cases, when cells do not show characteristic morphology, flow cytometry for B cell markers and electron microscopy can be helpful in establishing the diagnosis.

Myelodysplastic syndromes (MDSs) are sometimes accompanied by significant marrow fibrosis and can be confused with AMM.[62] The clinical picture is similar, with cytopenias, teardrop forms, leukoerythroblastic blood smears, and megakaryocytic hyperplasia and dysplasia in the marrow with fibrosis. Unlike with AMM, splenomegaly is usually not prominent. The presence of myelofibrosis in patients with MDSs has been associated with a shorter survival.[63]

It is important to distinguish AMM from a subtype of CML, commonest in younger women, which presents with thrombocythemia and marrow fibrosis.[64] Marrow fibrosis can also be a manifestation of accelerated-phase CML. The diagnosis of CML is based on the detection of the Philadelphia chromosome by cytogenetics or the bcr/abl fusion gene product by gene amplification studies. Patients with CML and marrow fibrosis are at high risk for progression to blastic transformation and should be considered for early allogeneic BMT. Splenectomy before BMT reduces disease bulk and facilitates hematologic recovery.

ET is the disorder which most closely resembles AMM and, as discussed above, may indeed represent an earlier phase of the same disease. Thrombotic complications and platelet counts in the region of $10^6/\mu L$ distinguish ET from AMM. ET often progresses to myelofibrosis.[65] In general, splenomegaly is less pronounced and the marrow fibrosis is less dense in ET compared with AMM.

PCV evolves into postpolycythemic myeloid metaplasia in 5% to 15% of patients, 10 years or more after the initial diagnosis.[66] At that late stage the prognosis is poor and 25% to 50% of patients will develop acute leukemia. The clinical picture is identical to AMM and the distinction is based entirely on the previous history of polycythemia.

The gray platelet syndrome is a rare inherited disorder of megakaryocyte dysfunction characterized by a loss of PDGF and alpha granules from the mature megakaryocyte and platelet and a moderate degree of marrow fibrosis. The condition is distinguished from AMM by a family history of bleeding disorders and the absence of splenomegaly.

Nonhematopoietic Causes of Marrow Fibrosis

Marrow fibrosis sometimes accompanies metastatic spread of carcinoma (particularly breast and prostate) to the marrow or marrow involvement by lymphoma. The fibrosis is reversible with successful treatment of the neoplasm.[67, 68] Therefore, metastatic disease should be excluded before a diagnosis of AMM is established in a patient with a previous history of another malignancy: common carcinomas should be considered and the appropriate screening tests performed. Metastatic foci should be searched for in the bone marrow specimen, and radiographic evaluation of the bones may reveal lytic or blastic lesions suggestive of metastatic disease.

Myelofibrosis has also been reported in patients with autoimmune diseases, especially in association with systemic lupus erythematosus. For the majority of these patients, the cytopenias and perhaps the marrow fibrosis will improve following systemic steroid treatment.[69]

Systemic infections can sometimes cause diagnostic confusion. Disseminated tuberculosis and histoplasmosis can present with weight loss, fever, splenomegaly, moderate marrow fibrosis, and leukoerythroblastic anemia. Culture of the bone marrow for mycobacteria should be included in the diagnostic evaluation of these patients.

Finally, vitamin D deficiency from renal or dietary causes is associated with marrow fibrosis and osteosclerosis, but it is easily distinguished from AMM by the absence of splenomegaly and other hematologic abnormalities.

TREATMENT

Aim of Treatment

At present, AMM is curable only by allogeneic BMT. Unfortunately, transplant is not a realistic option for most patients because of their advanced age or the lack of a histocompatible sibling donor. Asymptomatic patients with AMM do not require treatment. However, therapy is eventually required for (a) symptomatic anemia, (b) severe thrombocytopenia, (c) symptomatic splenomegaly, (d) portal hypertension with gastrointestinal bleeding, and (e) symptomatic extramedullary hematopoiesis causing organ dysfunction such as spinal cord or nerve compression and pleural effusions. A schema for the treatment of AMM is shown in Figure 5–4.

Myelosuppressive Therapy

Single-agent chemotherapy, usually with hydroxyurea (20 to 30 mg/kg two to three times a week), is safe and effective treatment for symptomatic patients.[70] Hydroxyurea can alleviate the anemia and thrombocytosis, reduce the size of the spleen and liver, and to some extent improve marrow fibrosis.[70, 71] Since long-term treatment is often required for a persistent effect, hydroxyurea has the advantage of being well tolerated and associated with a low risk of leukemogenesis.[72]

Conflicting results have been reported recently for the use of interferon-α (IFN-α) in AMM (reviewed in Sacchi[73]). Treatment schedules have ranged from 0.5 to 3 million units daily or three

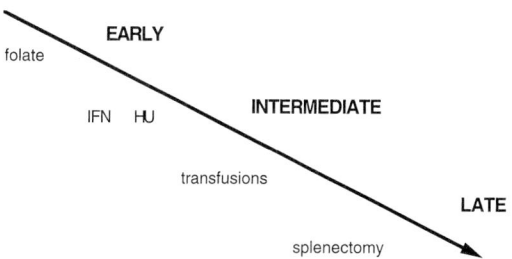

Figure 5–4 Treatment plan for agnogenic myeloid metaplasia. IFN, interferon; HU, hydroxyurea.

times a week. Reduction of thrombocytosis is achieved in most cases but anemia improved in only a few patients.[74, 75] Splenomegaly was reduced in fewer than half of the patients treated and marrow fibrosis was generally not reversed. Patients in the initial hyperproliferative stage of AMM were more likely to respond to IFN-α. Unfortunately, elderly patients did not tolerate the treatment very well because of frequent side effects, especially fever, anorexia, fatigue, depression, and insomnia, and often the interferon treatment must be discontinued due to cytopenias. More studies are needed to define the role of IFN-α in the management of AMM.

Supportive Care

In the treatment of anemia, potentially correctable causes such as iron deficiency from gastrointestinal blood loss or folate deficiency from increased hematopoiesis must be excluded. For direct antiglobulin test–positive hemolytic anemia, prednisone 1 mg/kg/day orally (PO) has been used successfully, but hemolysis often recurs with steroid withdrawal. Splenectomy also can be considered for these patients. Since ineffective hematopoiesis makes a major contribution to anemia in AMM, a trial of anabolic steroids (oxymetholone 50 mg twice to four times daily PO or danazol 400 mg twice a day PO for 3 to 6 months) is recommended.[5] About half the patients will respond to androgens but improvement is less common in patients with chromosomal abnormalities.[76] The patient should be informed of virilizing and other side effects, and hepatic function should be closely monitored. Both anabolic steroids and corticosteroids also can improve the thrombocytopenia.[5] Recombinant human erythropoietin (r-HuEpo) has recently been used in AMM patients with anemia with limited success.[77] In one report, seven AMM patients with pancytopenia and marrow fibrosis received a combination of r-HuEpo 200 units/kg three times per week and interferon 3 × 10⁶ units three times per week for 3 to 6 months and granulocyte-macrophage colony-stimulating factor (GM-CSF) 250 μg/m²/day for the first 3 weeks.[78] Anemia lessened in all patients, splenomegaly decreased significantly in four, and bone marrow fibrosis improved in two patients. These initial reports are promising, but prospective randomized studies are needed to determine the usefulness of growth factors in AMM. For the majority of patients with AMM who have failed, or are not candidates for, the above treatments, blood transfusions are used at regular intervals to correct severe anemia. Depending on the transfusion burden and prognosis of the individual patient, iron chelation with desferrioxamine should be considered to avoid organ damage from iron overload.

Splenectomy

Splenectomy is an option for selected patients with (a) refractory hemolytic anemia, (b) refractory severe thrombocytopenia, (c) painful splenomegaly refractory to other treatments, (d) portal hypertension associated with esophageal varices and gastrointestinal bleeding, and (e) pancytopenia in advanced AMM. When performed for these indications, the procedure improved anemia in 70% of patients, thrombocytopenia in 56%, splenomegaly in 97%, and portal hypertension in 83%.[79] Splenectomy is contraindicated in the setting of active DIC. Any coagulopathy should be corrected before surgery and the patient should otherwise be an acceptable surgical candidate. Operative mortality is high and even in the hands of experienced surgeons 10% to 15% may die secondary to the intervention.[79] Mortality risks are probably much lower when patients are carefully selected. The main complications of surgery are from hemorrhage and thrombosis due to the underlying platelet function defect, which can be exacerbated by massive thrombocytosis in the early postoperative period. Postsplenectomy compensatory increase in liver size usually occurs due to myeloid metaplasia of the liver.[80] The timing of splenectomy is critical. Splenectomy in the proliferative phase of the disease can cause a disastrous rise in the platelet count and lead to uncontrollable thromboses from massively increased circulating platelets and megakaryocytic fragments. At the other extreme, splenectomy in elderly patients with massive splenomegaly and pancytopenia can be dangerous. Nevertheless, splenectomy can be extremely beneficial and its accompanying risk therefore appropriate for patients whose quality of life has deteriorated because of severe pancytopenia.[81] For patients who are truly inoperable, splenic irradiation (200 to 300 cGy delivered in 10 to 15 daily fractions) can induce satisfactory responses lasting several months.[5, 82] Radiotherapy is effective treatment for extramedullary hematopoiesis causing neurologic or organ impairment or massive pleural or peritoneal effusions.[83]

Bone Marrow Transplantation

Allogeneic BMT can be a curative treatment for patients with AMM by establishing normal (donor) hematopoiesis and gradual resolution of marrow fibrosis.[84] Young patients (less than 50 years old) who have an HLA-matched sibling donor should be offered this option. Despite initial concerns about engraftment failure due to marrow fibrosis,[85] hematopoietic recovery occurs in most patients with only a few days added delay in the return of platelet counts.[86] In an analysis of the existing reports (reviewed in Singhal et al.[87]), post-transplant blood counts normalized earlier in splenectomized patients, and therefore elective splenectomy before transplant should be considered, especially if T cell depletion is used for graft-versus-host disease prophylaxis.

Experimental Approaches

New experimental treatments are aimed specifically at inhibiting pathogenetic processes responsible for fibrosis in AMM. Vitamin D_3 opposes the action of PDGF by reducing fibroblast proliferation and promoting collagenase activity[88]; vitamin D_3 deficiency is associated with marrow fibrosis. No responses were, however, observed in a study of vitamin D_3 in AMM.[89] In vivo, IFN-γ decreases intraplatelet levels of PDGF and TGF-β.[90] Anagrelide, a new platelet-lowering agent, which has been used successfully for the treatment of thrombocytosis in chronic myeloproliferative disorders, has also been observed to decrease the reticulin content of the marrow.[91] Since it is toxic to megakaryocytes, the main source of fibrinogenic cytokines in AMM, its clinical usefulness is currently under investigation.

PROGNOSIS

The median survival from diagnosis of AMM is approximately 5 years. Perhaps 20% of patients have prolonged survival, beyond a decade.[5] In a retrospective analysis of 133 patients, independent indicators of shorter survival included more than 10% circulating leukocyte precursors (blasts, promyelocytes, and myelocytes) and anemia with hemoglobin values of less than 10 g/dL.[92] In another report of 47 patients, survival was significantly worse in the presence of cytogenetic abnormalities (median 2.5 years) than without (median more than 6 years).[93] Transformed leukemias are usually refractory to treatment. Patients who do not succumb to leukemia die of cardiac causes, infection, bleeding, or thrombosis. In the future, new treatments directed at either the hematopoietic clonal disease or the fibrotic process may change the prognosis of patients with AMM.

REFERENCES

1. Heuck G: Zwei Fälle von Leukaemie mit eigenthümlichem Blut- resp. Knochenmarkbefund. Virchows Arch 1879; 78:475.
2. Dameshek W: Some speculations on the myeloproliferative syndromes. Blood 1951; 6:372.
3. Adams JA, Barrett AJ, Beard J, et al: Primary polycythaemia, essential thrombocythaemia and myelofibrosis—three facets of a single disease process? Acta Haematol 1988; 79:33–37.
4. Knuutila S: Lineage specificity in haematological neoplasms. Br J Haematol 1997; 96:2–11.
5. Tefferi A, Silverstein M, Noel P: Agnogenic myeloid metaplasia. Semin Oncol 1995; 22:327.
6. Sekhar M, Prentice H, Popat U, et al: Idiopathic myelofibrosis in children. Br J Haematol 1996; 93:394.
7. Anderson R, Hoshino T, Yamamoto T: Myelofibrosis with myeloid metaplasia in survivors of the atomic bomb in Hiroshima. Ann Intern Med 1964; 60:1.
8. Hu H: Benzene associated myelofibrosis. Ann Intern Med 1987; 106:171.
9. Johnson S, Bateman C, Beard M, et al: Long term hematological complications of Thorotrast. Q J Med 1977; 182:259.
10. Dodge WH: Avian monocytic leukaemia cells release fibroblast growth factor: Implications to associated myelofibrosis. Leuk Res 1985; 9:1559.
11. Boyd MT, Maclean N, Oscier DG: Detection of retrovirus in patients with myeloproliferative disease. Lancet 1989; 1:814.
12. Antonucci R, Walker R, Herion J: Myelofibrosis and aplastic anemia: First report of the two disorders occurring sequentially in the same person. Am J Med 1989; 86:352.
13. Reilly J: Pathogenesis of idiopathic myelofibrosis: Present status and future directions. Br J Haematol 1994; 88:1.
14. Jacobson R, Salo A, Fialkow P: Agnogenic myeloid metaplasia: A clonal proliferation of hematopoietic stem cells with a secondary myelofibrosis. Blood 1978; 51:189.
15. Lucas G, Padua R, Masters G, et al: The application of X chromosome gene probes to the diagnosis of myeloproliferative disease. Br J Haematol 1989; 72:530.
16. Anger B, Janssen J, Schrezenmeier H, et al: Clonal analysis of chronic myeloproliferative disorders using X-linked DNA polymorphisms. Leukemia 1990; 4:258.
17. Greenberg B, Woo L, Veomett I: Cytogenetics of bone marrow fibroblastic cells in idiopathic chronic myelofibrosis. Br J Haematol 1987; 66:487.
18. Buschle M, Janssen J, Drexler H, et al: Evidence for pluripotent stem cell origin of idiopathic myelofibrosis: Clonal analysis of a case characterized by a N-ras gene mutation. Leukemia 1988; 2:658.
19. Wang J: Myelopoietic effect of bone marrow fibroblasts cultured from patients with myelofibrosis. Am J Hematol 1988; 27:235.
20. Reversible myelofibrosis (editorial). Lancet 1985; 1:497.
21. Wang J, Cheung C, Fakhiuddin A, et al: Circulating granulocyte and macrophage progenitor cells in primary and secondary myelofibrosis. Br J Haematol 1983; 54:301.

22. Han Z, Briere J, Nedellec G, et al: Characteristics of circulating megakaryocyte progenitors (CFU-MK) in patients with primary myelofibrosis. Eur J Haematol 1988; 40:130.
23. Charron D, Robert L, Couty M, et al: Biochemical and histological analysis of bone marrow collagen in myelofibrosis. Br J Haematol 1979; 41:151.
24. Gay S, Gay R, Prchal J: Immunohistological studies of bone marrow collagen. In Berk P, Castro-Malaspina H, Wasserman L (eds): Myelofibrosis and the Biology of Connective Tissue. New York, Alan R Liss, 1982, pp 291–306.
25. Reilly J, Nash J, Mackie M, et al: Immunoenzymatic detection of fibronectin in normal and pathological haematopoietic tissue. Br J Haematol 1985; 59:497.
26. Soini Y, Kamel D, Apaja-Sarkkinen M, et al: Tenascin immunoreactivity in normal and pathological marrow. J Clin Pathol 1993; 46:218.
27. Reilly J, Nash J: Vitronectin (serum spreading factor): Its localization in normal and fibrotic tissue. J Clin Pathol 1988; 59:1269.
28. Groopman J: The pathogenesis of myelofibrosis in myeloproliferative disorders. Ann Intern Med 1980; 92:857.
29. Kimura A, Katoh O, Kuramoto A: Effect of platelet derived growth factor, epidermal growth factor and transforming growth factor B on the growth of human marrow fibroblasts. Br J Haematol 1988; 69:9.
30. Martyre M, Magdelenat H, Bryckaert M, et al: Increased intraplatelet levels of platelet-derived growth factor and transforming growth factor B in patients with myelofibrosis with myeloid metaplasia. Br J Haematol 1991; 77:80.
31. Katoh O, Kimura A, Kuramoto A: Platelet-derived growth factor is decreased in patients with myeloproliferative disorders. Am J Hematol 1988; 27:276.
32. Varga J, Rosenbloom J, Jimenez S: Transforming growth factor β (TGF-β) causes a persistent increase in steady-state amounts of type I and type III collagen and fibronectin mRNAs in normal human dermal fibroblasts. Biochem J 1987; 247:597.
33. Abboud S: A bone marrow stromal cell line is a source and target for platelet-derived growth factor. Blood 1993; 81:2547.
34. Charbord P: Increased vascularity of bone marrow in myelofibrosis. Br J Haematol 1986; 62:595.
35. Roberts A, Heine U, Flanders K, et al: Transforming growth factor β: Major role in regulation of extracellular matrix. Ann N Y Acad Sci 1990; 580:225.
36. Gilbert H, Prolaran V, Stanley E: Increased circulating CSF-1 (M-CSF) in myeloproliferative disease: Association with myeloid metaplasia and peripheral bone marrow expansion. Blood 1989; 74:1231.
37. Su W, Alegre V, White W: Myelofibrosis discovered after diagnosis of Sweet syndrome. Int J Dermatol 1990; 29:201.
38. Landolfi R, Colosimo C, De Candia E, et al: Meningeal hematopoiesis causing exophthalmus and hemiparesis in myelofibrosis: Effect of radiotherapy. Cancer 1988; 62:2346.
39. Lara J, Rosen P: Extramedullary hematopoiesis in a bronchial tumor. Arch Pathol Lab Med 1990; 114:1283.
40. Fedeli G, Certo M, Cannizzaro O, et al: Extramedullary hematopoiesis involving the esophagus in myelofibrosis. Am J Gastroenterol 1990; 85:1512.
41. Wanless I, Peterson P, Das A, et al: Hepatic vascular disease and portal hypertension in polycythemia vera and agnogenic myeloid metaplasia: A clinicopathological study of 145 patients examined at autopsy. Hepatology 1990; 12:1166.
42. Tsao M: Hepatic sinusoidal fibrosis in agnogenic myeloid metaplasia. Am J Clin Pathol 1989; 91:302.
43. Khumbanonda M, Horowitz H, Eyster M: Coombs' positive hemolytic anemia in myelofibrosis with myeloid metaplasia. Am J Med Sci 1969; 258:89.
44. Kuo C, van Voolen A, Morrison A: Primary and secondary myelofibrosis and its relationship to "PNH-like defect." Blood 1972; 40:875.
45. Soutar R, Birnie D, Bennett B: Parvovirus B19 induced red cell aplasia in myelofibrosis. Br J Haematol 1993; 85:623.
46. Silverstein M: Agnogenic Myeloid Metaplasia. Acton, Mass, Publishing Sciences Group, 1975.
47. Didsheim P, Bunting D: Abnormal platelet function in myelofibrosis. Am J Clin Pathol 1966; 45:566.
48. Varki A, Lottenberg R, Griffin R, et al: The syndrome of idiopathic myelofibrosis: Clinicopathological review with emphasis on the prognostic variables predicting survival. Medicine (Baltimore) 1983; 62:353.
49. Leglise D, Abgrall J, DesFontaine B, et al: Lipoprotein composition in agnogenic myeloid metaplasia. Biomed Pharmacother 1985; 39:135.
50. DiBella N, Silverstein M, Hoagland H: Effect of splenectomy on teardrop shaped erythrocytes in agnogenic myeloid metaplasia. Arch Intern Med 1977; 137:308.
51. Thiele J, Hoeppner B, Zankovich R, et al: Histomorphometry of bone marrow biopsies in primary osteomyelofibrosis/sclerosis (agnogenic myeloid metaplasia)—correlations between clinical and morphologic features. Virchows Arch 1989; 415:191.
52. Wolf B, Neiman R: Myelofibrosis with myeloid metaplasia: Pathophysiologic implications between bone marrow changes and progression of splenomegaly. Blood 1985; 65:803.
53. Miller J, Testa J, Lindgren V, et al: The pattern and clinical significance of karyotypic abnormalities in patients with idiopathic and post polycythemic myelofibrosis. Cancer 1985; 55:582.
54. Whang-Peng J, Lee E, Knutson T, et al: Cytogenetic studies in patients with myelofibrosis and myeloid metaplasia. Leuk Res 1978; 2:41.
55. Reilly J: Pathogenesis of idiopathic myelofibrosis: Present status and future directions. Br J Haematol 1994; 88:1.
56. Kerim S, Rege-Cambrin G, Scaravaglio P, et al: Trisomy 8 and an unbalanced t(5;17)(q11;p11)

characterize two karyotypically independent clones in a case of idiopathic myelofibrosis evolving to acute nonlymphoid leukemia. Cancer Genet Cytogenet 1991; 52:63.
57. Kaplan K, Mitchell D, Steiner R, et al: Polycythemia vera and myelofibrosis: Correlation of MR imaging, clinical and laboratory findings. Radiology 1992; 183:329.
58. Hernandez J, Miguel S, Gonzalez M, et al: Development of acute leukemia after idiopathic myelofibrosis. J Clin Pathol 1992; 45:427.
59. Kimura A, Kawaishi K, Nakata Y, et al: Leukemic transformation of primary myelofibrosis: Immunophenotype, genotype and growth characteristics of blast cells. Leuk Lymphoma 1995; 19:493.
60. Bearman R, Pangalis G, Rappaport H: Acute malignant myelosclerosis. Cancer 1979; 43:279.
61. Sultan C, Sigaux F, Imbert M, et al: Acute myelodysplasia with myelofibrosis: A report of eight cases. Br J Haematol 1981; 49:11.
62. Pagliuca A, Layton D, Manoharan A, et al: Myelofibrosis in primary myelodysplastic syndromes: A clinico-morphological study of 10 cases. Br J Haematol 1989; 71:499.
63. Maschek H, Georgi A, Kaloutsi V, et al: Myelofibrosis in primary myelodysplastic syndromes: A retrospective study of 352 patients. Eur J Haematol 1992; 48:208.
64. Clough V, Geary C, Hashimi K, et al: Myelofibrosis in chronic granulocytic leukemia. Br J Haematol 1979; 42:515.
65. Liberato N, Barosi G, Costa A, et al: Myelofibrosis with myeloid metaplasia following essential thrombocythemia. Acta Haematol 1989; 82:150.
66. Silverstein M: Postpolycythemic myeloid metaplasia. Arch Intern Med 1974; 134:113.
67. Kiely J, Silverstein M: Metastatic carcinoma simulating agnogenic myeloid metaplasia and myelofibrosis. Cancer 1969; 24:1041.
68. Kiang D, McKenna R, Keneddy B: Reversal of myelofibrosis in advanced breast cancer. Am J Med 1978; 64:173.
69. Paquette R, Meshkinpour A, Rosen P: Autoimmune myelofibrosis: A steroid-responsive cause of bone marrow fibrosis associated with systemic lupus erythematosus. Medicine (Baltimore) 1994; 73:145.
70. Manoharan A: Management of myelofibrosis with intermittent hydroxyurea. Br J Haematol 1991; 77:252.
71. Lofvenberg E, Wahlin A, Ross G, et al: Reversal of myelofibrosis by hydroxyurea. Eur J Haematol 1990; 44:33.
72. Nand S, Stock W, Godwin J, et al: Leukemogenic risk of hydroxyurea therapy in polycythemia vera, essential thrombocythemia and myeloid metaplasia with myelofibrosis. Am J Hematol 1996; 52:42.
73. Sacchi S: The role of α-interferon in essential thrombocythemia, polycythemia vera and myelofibrosis with myeloid metaplasia (MMM): A concise update. Leuk Lymphoma 1995; 19:13.
74. Barosi G, Liberato L, Costa A, et al: Induction and maintenance α-interferon therapy in myelofibrosis with myeloid metaplasia. Eur J Haematol 1990; 45 (suppl 52):12.
75. Furesi L, Laghi P, Forconi S: Interferon α-2b in the treatment of myelofibrosis. Haematologica 1990; 75:587.
76. Besa E, Nowell P, Geller N, et al: Analysis of the androgen response of 23 patients with agnogenic myeloid metaplasia. The value of chromosomal studies in predicting response and survival. Cancer 1982; 49:308.
77. Spiriti M, Latagliata R, Avvisati G, et al: Erythropoietin treatment of idiopathic myelofibrosis. Haematologica 1993; 76:371.
78. Bourantas K, Tsiara S, Christou L, et al: Combination therapy with recombinant human erythropoietin, interferon-α-2b and granulocyte-macrophage colony-stimulating factor in idiopathic myelofibrosis. Acta Haematologica 1996; 96:79.
79. Benbassat J, Gilon D, Penchas S: The choice between splenectomy and medical treatment in patients with advanced agnogenic myeloid metaplasia. Am J Hematol 1990; 33:128.
80. Towel B, Levine S: Massive hepatomegaly following splenectomy for myeloid metaplasia. Am J Med 1987; 82:371.
81. Barosi G, Ambrosetti A, Buratti A, et al: Splenectomy for patients with myelofibrosis and myeloid metaplasia: Pretreatment variables and outcome prediction. Leukemia 1993; 7:200.
82. Wagner H, McKeough P, Desforges J, et al: Splenic irradiation in the treatment of patients with chronic myelogenous leukemia or myelofibrosis with myeloid metaplasia. Effects of daily and intermittent fractionation with or without concomitant hydroxyurea. Cancer 1986; 58:1204.
83. Leinweber C, Order S, Calkins A: Whole-abdominal irradiation for the management of gastrointestinal and abdominal manifestations of agnogenic myeloid metaplasia. Cancer 1991; 68:1251.
84. Creemers G, Lowenberg B, Hagenbeek A: Allogeneic bone marrow transplantation for primary myelofibrosis. Br J Haematol 1992; 82:772.
85. Rajantie J, Sale G, Deeg H, et al: Adverse effect of severe marrow fibrosis on hematologic recovery after chemoradiotherapy and allogeneic bone marrow transplantation. Blood 1986; 67:1693.
86. Soll E, Massumoto C, Clift R, et al: Relevance of marrow fibrosis in bone marrow transplantation: A retrospective analysis of engraftment. Blood 1995; 86:4667.
87. Singhal S, Powles R, Treleaven J, et al: Allogeneic bone marrow transplantation for primary myelofibrosis. Bone Marrow Transplant 1995; 16:743.
88. McCarthy DM: Fibrosis of the bone marrow. Br J Haematol 1985; 59:1.
89. McCarthy DM, Hibbin JE, Goldman JM: A role for 1,25-dihydroxy vitamin D_3 in control of bone marrow collagen deposition? Lancet 1984; 1:78.
90. Martyre M, Magdelenat H, Calvo F: Interferon-gamma in vivo reverses the increased platelet levels of platelet-derived growth factor and transforming

growth factor-beta in patients with myelofibrosis with myeloid metaplasia. Br J Haematol 1991; 77:431.
91. Anagrelide Study Group: Anagrelide, a therapy for thrombocythemic states: Experience in 577 patients. Am J Med 1992; 92:69.
92. Visani G, Finelli C, Castelli U, et al: Myelofibrosis with myeloid metaplasia: Clinical and haematological parameters predicting survival in a series of 133 patients. Br J Haematol 1990; 75:4.
93. Demory J, Dupriez B, Fenaux P, et al: Cytogenetic studies and their prognostic significance in agnogenic myeloid metaplasia: A report on 47 cases. Blood 1988; 72:855.

6

Pure Red Cell Aplasia

Elizabeth M. Kang, M.D.
John F. Tisdale, M.D.

Pure red cell aplasia (PRCA) encompasses many disorders leading to the selective failure of erythropoiesis. In this chapter, we discuss acquired, congenital, acute, and chronic forms of the disease. We describe their clinical manifestations and associations, treatment strategies, and long-term prognoses, as well as elaborate on both the known and hypothesized causes for the different subsets of this heterogeneous disorder.

ACQUIRED PURE RED CELL APLASIA

Acquired PRCA is a rare disease. Only a few hundred cases have been reported (for reviews, see references 1 to 5). Although the exact cause is uncertain, PRCA is notably associated with clinical abnormalities of the immune system, and erythropoiesis appears to be suppressed by humoral or cellular immune effectors, or both. As with aplastic anemia, a variety of inciting causes may activate a similar immune response and result in an identical pathologic appearance of the bone marrow. Although viruses are suspected but unproven causative agents in general aplasia, a specific viral infection (parvovirus B19) can produce both transient and chronic PRCA. In children, acquired PRCA is often acute and self-limited such as seen in transient erythroblastopenia of childhood (TEC; see below); in contrast, acquired disease in the adult is almost always chronic.

Epidemiology, Case Definition, and Clinical Features

Immune-mediated disease more commonly affects women, with a male-female ratio of 1:2.1,[6] but males may predominate in series in which red cell aplasia is mainly associated with drugs or toxins[7] or with chronic lymphocytic leukemia (CLL).[8] The mean age of onset is about 60 years in immune-mediated disease.[6] There is no racial predisposition, and the disease is not apparently more common in Asia.

Anemia, reticulocytopenia, and absent marrow erythroid precursor cells define the syndrome.[9] The erythrocytes are usually normocytic or occasionally macrocytic. Neutrophil and platelet numbers are normal, but neutropenia, thrombocytopenia, or full pancytopenia can develop late in the course. A small proportion of patients may progress to leukemia: 2 of 58 patients developed acute myelogenous leukemia (AML) in one series.[2] Although normocellular, the bone marrow is remarkable for the complete lack, or at least a relative paucity, of recognizable erythroid precursor cells (Plate 6); there may rarely be an apparent "maturation arrest" with only early erythroblasts present.[10, 11] Diminished or ineffective marrow erythropoiesis can be measured with ^{59}Fe or ^{111}In scintigraphy.[12, 13] Cytogenetics is usually normal, but abnormal chromosomes can occur,[11] and their presence suggests the possibility of myelodysplasia,[14] including the 5q− syndrome.[15]

Only a few diseases have the distinctive marrow morphology of red cell aplasia (Table 6–1). The major practical distinction lies between the late presentation of Diamond-Blackfan anemia (DBA; see below) and acquired red cell aplasia; after a certain age, this distinction is arbitrary as there are usually no clinically distinguishing features or studies to differentiate the two.

Clinical Associations

Most cases are idiopathic, but there are a large number of associated illnesses (Table 6–2); the

TABLE 6–1 Differential Diagnosis of Pure Red Cell Aplasia

Self-limited
    Transient erythroblastopenia of childhood
    Transient aplastic crisis of hemolysis (parvovirus B19 infection)
Fetal red cell aplasia
    Nonimmune hydrops fetalis (in utero parvovirus B19 infection)
Hereditary pure red cell aplasia
    Diamond-Blackfan anemia
Acquired pure red cell aplasia

most interesting association is with thymoma. The often quoted 50% rate of associated thymoma has almost certainly been greatly exaggerated due to the propensity to report an unusual combination; the true proportion is probably closer to 10%.[1, 6, 15] Conversely, about 2% to 5% of thymomas have been estimated to be accompanied by red cell aplasia.[1] Nonetheless, the possibility of a mediastinal mass should be excluded by chest tomography.[16] Thymoma can precede the onset of PRCA by many years, and PRCA may appear or persist after removal of the tumor.[17, 18] The thymic mass is commonly composed of spindle cells, and while usually benign, can be malignant.[6, 15] Thymoma rarely occurs in children.

PRCA can occur in association with other "autoimmune" diseases, like myasthenia gravis,[19] collagen-vascular syndromes,[20] lichen planus,[21] and endocrine failure states,[22] either alone or associated with thymoma. PRCA also occurs in the context of other immunologic abnormalities, including hypoimmunoglobulinemia,[9, 21, 23, 24] monoclonal gammopathy,[25, 26] anergy, antinuclear antibodies, and autoimmune hemolysis.

PRCA complicates a wide variety of neoplasms (see Table 6–2), most frequently lymphoid,[8] as well as other hematologic malignancies and nonthymic solid tumors. The rate of red cell aplasia in CLL was estimated at 6% in one large series and anemia may be present at the time of diagnosis.[8] In 9 of 47 patients in a series from the Mayo Clinic, PRCA was associated with large granular lymphocytosis based on morphologic studies, T cell receptor rearrangements, and immunophenotyping[27] (see Chapter 10). T cell inhibition has been implicated in the pathophysiology of red cell aplasia in lymphoproliferative disease; however, many of these same illnesses, or their therapies, are immunosuppressive and would be permissive for persistent viral infection (see below). Many drugs have been associated with PRCA[1, 2] (see Table 6–2). One example is diphenylhydantoin: patients have developed marrow failure on drug rechallenge[28] and a drug-dependent antibody that inhibited in vitro erythropoiesis was demonstrated in one case.[29] However, most agents implicated as causative appear in single case reports without supporting in vitro studies.

Pathogenesis and Pathophysiology

PRCA appears to be immunologically mediated in idiopathic cases, and in patients with autoimmune diseases such as systemic lupus erythematosus (SLE), thymoma, and CLL. Red cell aplasia resulting from primary bone marrow failure occurs in myelodysplasia, myeloproliferative disease, and with isolated cytogenetic abnormalities. Parvovirus B19 infection may result in chronic red cell aplasia when defective immunity allows persistent infection (see below). Occasional cases of hereditary disease may not be discovered until adulthood.[30]

Antibodies to Erythroid Precursor Cells

A marrow-suppressing factor was first identified in a patient with PRCA, thymoma, and Hodgkin's disease.[31] An antibody-mediated pathophysiology was first proposed by Krantz and co-workers based on the presence in several patients of a plasma IgG that inhibited heme synthesis in suspension cultures of normal bone marrow cells[32] and, in the presence of complement, lysed erythroblasts.[33] Immunoglobulin preparations from some patients were later shown to inhibit colony-forming unit—erythroid (CFU-E)–derived erythroid colony formation but not myeloid colony formation, in the presence[35–37] or absence[38] of complement. An IgG inhibitor of blast-forming unit—erythroid (BFU-E) was also described during the course of a pregnancy complicated by red cell aplasia.[39] The prevalence of antibody to erythroid precursor cells in PRCA is difficult to assess due to limited patient numbers and reporting bias. In a cooperative European study, an antibody that inhibited erythropoiesis was found in 13 of 16 cases,[40] and a complement-dependent inhibitor was present in 7 of 19 cases in a Japanese series.[41] Antibody generally has not been detected in patients with red cell aplasia secondary to lymphoma and other malignancies.[8] A remarkable feature of the cytotoxic antibody in PRCA is its ability to inhibit erythropoiesis in rodent systems, including release of ^{59}Fe from murine cells in vitro, inhibition of red blood cell production after injection into mice, and depletion of CFU-E in treated animals. The target antigen on erythroid precursor cells has never been identified. In a total

TABLE 6–2 Clinical Classification of Acquired Pure Red Cell Aplasia

I. Thymoma and malignancy
    Thymoma
    Lymphoid malignancies: chronic lymphocytic leukemia (see text), malignant lymphoma, T cell immunoblastic lymphoma, malignant histiocytosis, Kaposi's sarcoma, acute lymphocytic leukemia, Hodgkin's disease, multiple myeloma
    Other hematologic diseases: myelodysplasia, chronic myelogenous leukemia, myelofibrosis
    Paraneoplastic to solid tumors, including carcinoma of the bronchus, breast, stomach, thyroid, bile duct, and skin

II. Collagen-vascular disease
    Systemic lupus erythematosus
    Juvenile rheumatoid arthritis
    Rheumatoid arthritis
    Sjögren's syndrome
    Multiple endocrine gland insufficiency

III. Virus
    Parvovirus B19
    Hepatitis
    Adult T cell leukemia virus
    Epstein-Barr virus

IV. Pregnancy

V. Drugs
    Probably causative:
        Antiepileptics (diphenylhydantoin, carbamazepine, sodium dipropylacetate, sodium valproate)
        Azathioprine
        Chloramphenicol (see Chapter 1) and thiamphenicol
        Sulfonamides (salicylazosulfapyridine, sulfasalazine, methazolamide [with hepatitis], chlorpropamide, sulfathiazole, metalozone, co-trimaxazole)
        Isoniazid
        Procainamide
    Occasional, possibly coincidental associations:
        Nonsteroidal anti-inflammatory drugs (aminopyrine, phenylbutazone, fenoprofen, sulindac)
        Allopurinol
        Halothane (and hepatitis)
        D-Penicillamine
        Maloprim (dapsone and pyrimethamine)
        Quinidine and quinacrine
        Gold
        Benzene and benzene-related compounds (pentachlorophenol, arsenicals, paraqua, insecticides such as lindane, and inhalation of air freshener aerosol (!)

V. Idiopathic

of four cases, erythropoiesis was inhibited by an antibody that bound directly to erythropoietin,[42–44] but in all others the antibody appears to bind to precursor cells and serum erythropoietin levels are high.[40] The strongest evidence of a pathophysiologic role for cytotoxic antibodies is their disappearance from the circulation when patients respond to therapy, including antilymphocyte sera, immunosuppressive drugs,[42] thymectomy,[45] and plasmapheresis.[46, 47] In contrast, an immunoglobulin that specifically stained erythroblast nuclei, which was also found in patient plasma, often persisted despite effective therapy and hematologic improvement,[48] and it may represent a secondary antibody directed to the contents of lysed erythroblasts. Alloimmunized patients can have other antibodies directed to antigens on mature erythrocyte surfaces which can be distinguished from the characteristic inhibitor of erythropoiesis.[35] In one case of PRCA and thymoma, a serum inhibitor of antigen-induced lymphocyte transformation was present[17]; such an activity might account for defective production of erythropoietic factors by lymphocytes in some patients.[36] IgG inhibitors of erythropoiesis have also been documented in children with TEC (see below).

Cytotoxic Lymphocytes

T cell inhibition of erythropoiesis may be a more common mechanism of depression of red blood cell production than is antibody formation.[49] Lymphocyte inhibition may be particularly common in PRCA associated with CLL.[8,50] T cell inhibition of either CFU-E– or BFU-E derived colony formation was present in eight of eight of such cases, while none showed a serum inhibitor of erythropoiesis,[8] and cells with the cytotoxic/suppressor lymphocyte phenotype and inhibitory function in erythropoietic colony culture were present in the early, nonanemic stages of disease in a high proportion of patients.[51] Similar to aplastic anemia, there may be increased numbers of lymphocytes with receptors for IgG (Tγ cells)[52,53] or with the cytotoxic T cell phenotype (CD8+),[53–55] which in some cases has been shown to inhibit erythroid colony formation by CFU-E and BFU-E progenitors. Genetic restriction of lymphocytic suppression of erythropoiesis by CD8+, HLA-DR+ lymphocytes was shown in one well-studied case.[56] T cell suppression specific for erythropoiesis in colony culture has been observed in patients with PRCA following Epstein-Barr virus infection[57] and in human T cell leukemia/lymphoma virus type 1 infection.[58] Clinical remission has correlated with the disappearance of the inhibitor cell population after immunosuppressive therapy– or chemotherapy-induced remission of CLL.[53,54,59] In some cases, the implicated population has contained true functional suppressor cells, capable of inhibiting in vitro immunoglobulin synthesis as well as erythropoiesis.[60,61]

Treatment

Basic to the management of patients with PRCA is red blood cell transfusion. The same principles as were described in Chapter 1 for the support of the patient with aplastic anemia should be applied to these patients, including chelation of iron when appropriate to avoid secondary hemochromatosis.

Transfusion-independence can be achieved in about two thirds of patients with PRCA following treatment with some form of immunosuppression, although sequential trials of different types of therapy may be necessary.[62–64] In one reported series, more than 80% of patients who responded ultimately achieved a normal hematocrit, but multiple courses of immunosuppression were often required.[49] There is little evidence that response rates are higher with combined modalities of more intensive regimens.[64] Prednisone alone can induce remission in about 45% of cases. Cytotoxic drug regimens have included azathioprine, cyclophosphamide, and 6-mercaptopurine, with dose titrated to leukopenia. A 3- to 4-month trial is generally adequate to assess responsiveness. Relapse occurs in about one half of treated patients and chronic cytotoxic chemotherapy may be required to maintain transfusion-independence.[65] Given the toxicities that are associated with chemotherapeutic agents, it is recommended to try more modest immunosuppressants first. In some cases, transfusion support may be preferable to chronic cytotoxic therapy.

Patients have responded to antithymocyte globulin (ATG),[10,42,66,67] cyclosporine (CsA),[68–71] and fludarabine,[72] including patients refractory to steroids. In one large series, 82% of patients responded to CsA, and CsA has been recommended by some as first-line treatment.[5] Plasmapheresis[46,47,73] and lymphocytopheresis[73] have been successful in inducing sustained remissions, and in some cases the clinical response has been correlated with removal of an antibody inhibitory to erythropoiesis in vitro.[46,47] Splenectomy may sometimes be helpful[62] but is rarely used now. Apparent responses have also been noted following treatment with androgens or high doses of intravenous immune globulin.[74–77] A spontaneous remission rate of around 15% complicates assessment of the overall response rates in small clinical trials.[7,62,64] Patients with PRCA that is secondary to malignant disease can also respond to immunosuppressive therapy or cytotoxic chemotherapy[8,62,78–80]; for example, CsA has been effective in the majority of patients in whom T cell suppression of erythropoiesis was secondary to large granular lymphocytosis[27,81,82] (Plate 7; see also Chapter 10).

The suspicion of thymoma based on the presence of an anterior mediastinal mass necessitates its removal for diagnosis and treatment of a possibly malignant chest mass, but the procedure itself probably benefits hematopoiesis in only a very small minority of patients. It is worth noting that PRCA can occur years after removal of a thymoma[6] and that spontaneous remission of red cell aplasia has occurred in a patient before thymectomy could be performed.[83]

PRCA is one of the few diseases in which hematopoietic colony cultures have clinical value in predicting response to treatment. In general, patients whose marrow contains CFU-E progenitors have a much higher likelihood of response to immunosuppression, compared with patients without detectable CFU-Es (Fig. 6–1).[49,84] These results confirmed the earlier observation that a proliferative response in suspension culture to added erythropoietin predicted clinical improvement with therapy.[32] Evidence of T cell suppression of BFU-E has correlated only with responsiveness to ATG treatment.[49] In contrast, the presence of an antibody to erythroid progenitors in coculture does not relate to outcome after immunosuppressive treatment, and antibodies are often undetectable in

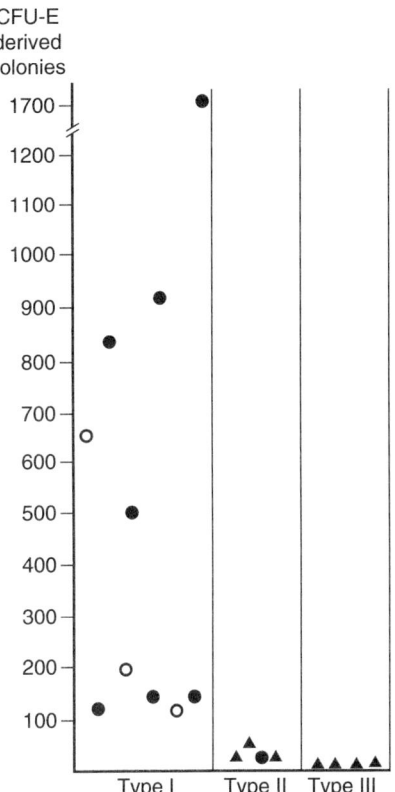

Figure 6–1 Graphic demonstration of correlation between CFU-E (colony-forming unit—erythroid) cultures and response to treatment.

patients who clinically appear to have an autoimmune process.[21]

Patients with PRCA have a relatively good long-term prognosis. Greater than 80% of patients either respond to treatment or have a spontaneous resolution. Fifty percent of patients who relapse will respond to subsequent therapy.[40, 62] Patients who remain transfusion-dependent require chelation with desferrioxamine administered subcutaneously, given a minimum of 5 days a week to avoid complications related to transfusional hemosiderosis and to maintain a normal life expectancy. There is a low risk of disease progression to either aplastic anemia or leukemia in nonresponders.[13]

PURE RED CELL APLASIA DUE TO PARVOVIRUS B19 INFECTION

Parvovirus B19 is the only virus in the parvovirus family known to be pathogenic to humans. It is a small spherical nonenveloped single-stranded DNA virus associated with different disease manifestations depending on the underlying condition of the infected patient; only the most common will be discussed here. The etiologic relationship of parvovirus B19 infection to both chronic and acute PRCA has been well documented and it has become routine to test for the presence of this virus in patients with PRCA.[85, 86] However, due to the prevalence of the virus in the general population and difficulties in interpreting the test results, many cases are incorrectly attributed to the parvovirus B19.

Epidemiology

The virus is endemic throughout the world. In North America, 50% of children by age 15 will have detectable anti-IgG levels and greater than 80% of the elderly will also become seropositive. Infection usually occurs in the late winter, spring, and early summer. The route of transmission appears to be respiratory, but the virus can be found in serum and transmitted by blood products. It is also heat resistant, and heat treatment of blood products is not generally effective in preventing transmission.

Clinical Features

In normal healthy patients, infection is often asymptomatic, but especially in children, parvovirus B19 causes erythema infectiosum (also known as slapped cheek or fifth disease). The illness is characterized by a nonspecific prodromal illness with symptoms such as fever, coryza, headache, nausea, and diarrhea. The prodrome is followed 2 to 5 days later by a typical erythematous facial rash from whence the disease derives its name "slapped cheek disease"; 1 to 4 days afterward, there is a second eruption of a maculopapular rash appearing on the trunks and limbs which, with resolution, takes on a lacy appearance. These cutaneous manifestations may be transient or recurrent, and they may be accompanied by pruritus, especially of the soles of the feet. Fifty percent of adults, and especially women, will develop a symmetrical small joint arthropathy with pain, swelling, and stiffness. These symptoms usually last for 1 to 3 weeks, although the arthropathy or even frank arthritis may develop and persist for years. There is no long-term damage to the joints.

Patients with underlying hemolytic disorders such as hereditary spherocytosis, thalassemia, sickle cell anemia, and red blood cell enzymopathies, or those under erythroid stress with iron deficiency anemia or hemorrhage, develop transient aplastic crisis (TAC) with parvovirus B19 infection. Even patients with normal hematologic values will have a decline in their red blood cell production but are well able to tolerate the short duration of failed erythropoiesis due to the long life span of erythrocytes already present in the circulation. Parvovirus B19 infection may be the presenting complaint of patients with otherwise well-compensated hemolytic disorders. Those patients who are dependent on rapid red blood cell turnover can experience a more precipitous and severe anemia, often requiring transfusion. Unlike those with erythema infectiosum, patients with TAC are usually viremic at presentation and therefore can be easily diagnosed by DNA studies. In immunocompetent patients, the infection is cleared, the anemia resolves, and the patients develop IgG antibodies with a subsequent lifetime immunity.

On the other hand, immunocompromised patients with or without other underlying hematologic problems may develop a chronic PRCA as a result of persistent parvovirus B19 infection. Fourteen percent of patients first diagnosed with PRCA, whose sera were examined retrospectively, were found to have active parvovirus infection.[87] In a large Japanese review, 11% of 150 cases (most with acute presentations) were blamed on the virus,[5] and parvovirus has appeared as an etiologic agent in other series.[41] Clinically, the anemia results in transfusion dependence and there may be associated neutropenia. The bone marrow contains giant pronormoblasts (Plate 8), the cytopathic signature of parvovirus infection, although these are usually infrequent. The diagnosis is established by detection of parvovirus B19 genome in the serum, blood, or bone marrow cells by dot blot hybridization; polymerase chain reaction (PCR) amplification of viral DNA may be necessary in rare cases but is prone to overinterpretation, as the virus may persist in bone marrow and visceral tissues in otherwise normal individuals.[88] Antibodies to parvovirus, as determined in capture immunoassays or enzyme-linked immunosorbent assay (ELISA), are not usually present, but a pattern of antibody response suggestive of early infection (IgM antibody and/or IgG antibody directed to the major capsid protein) may be found in patients with underlying congenital immunodeficiency.[89] A weak reaction on immunoblot testing is a consistent finding and correlates with poor neutralizing activity for the virus in erythroid colony assay.[89] Persistent parvovirus infection may be the dominant manifestation of some inherited immunodeficiency states.

Pathophysiology

The flulike symptoms seen initially in the course of erythema infectiosum are a result of the inflammatory cytokine responses to the viremia. The subsequent cutaneous eruptions arise from immune complex deposition during clearance of the virus. The joint symptoms also result from immune complexes: the virus itself can be found in both the synovium and the synovial fluid. Parvovirus B19 is directly cytotoxic to erythroid cells. This important property accounts for the reticulocytopenia seen even in hematologically normal patients. The virus infects and replicates in late erythroid progenitor cells using erythrocyte P antigen as a receptor. Persons who lack P antigen (p phenotype) are therefore not susceptible to infection by the virus. Viral propagation is dependent on the presence of erythropoietin: parvovirus does not readily propagate ex vivo in standard tissue culture systems, requiring other methods for detection and growth.

Persistence of the virus results from failure to mount a neutralizing antibody response; consequently, patients lack the typical immune complex–mediated symptoms (see above). Chronic PRCA that occurs in association with disorders in which defective antibody production is a feature or a result of its treatment may also represent occult viral infection.[90,91] Persistent parvovirus infection and PRCA have been documented in three patient populations: (1) congenital immunodeficiency (Nezeloff's syndrome),[92,93] (2) patients treated with immunosuppressive or cytotoxic drugs,[94–97] and (3) patients with the acquired immunodeficiency syndrome (AIDS).[98] Human immunodeficiency virus (HIV) infection predisposes patients to parvovirus B19 infection and in some patients it may be the first manifestation of AIDS.[99]

Treatment

Therapy consists of infusion of commercial immunoglobulin preparations. Parvovirus-specific immunoglobulin preparations are not necessary because most of the adult population has been exposed to the virus. One patient with congenital immunodeficiency was cured by a 10-day course followed by intermittent injections until virus had disappeared from his serum[93] (Fig. 6–2). Patients with AIDS have very high virus serum concentrations, and although immunoglobulin therapy is effective, relapse is common and demands retreatment.[98] The recommended course is 5 to 10 days of intravenous immune globulin at a dose of 0.4 g/kg. There are no differences among the commercial preparations and no consensus on the use of periodic immunoglobulin injection to prevent relapse.

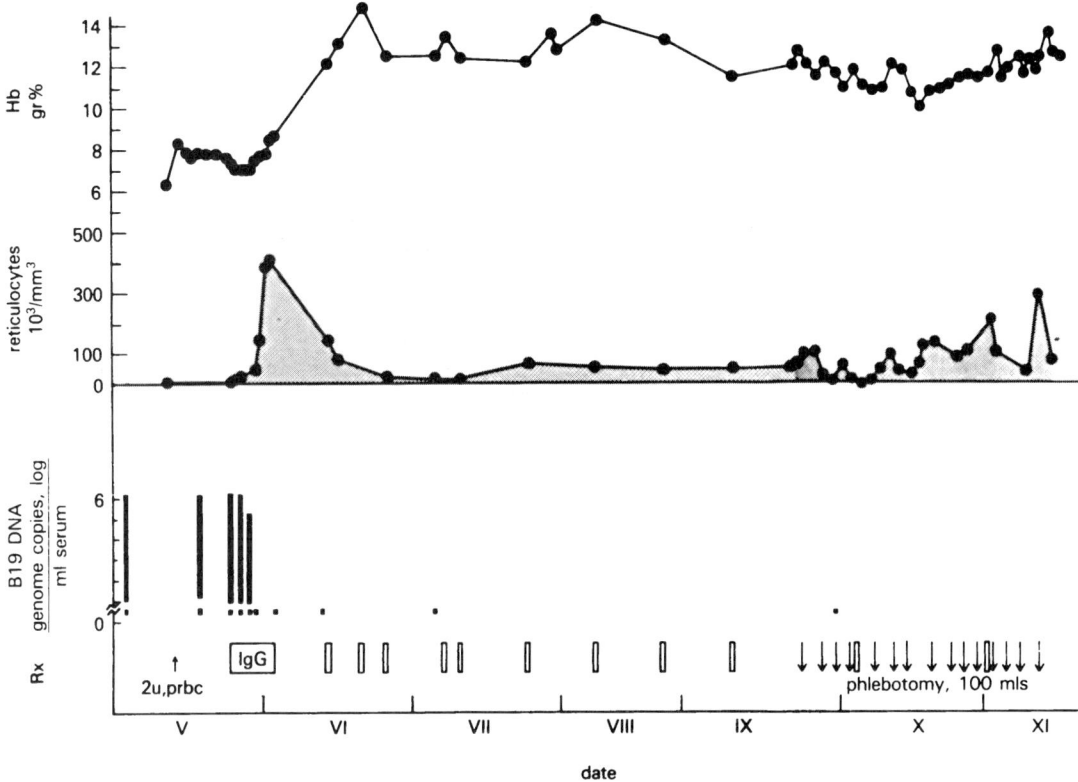

Figure 6–2 Response of chronic anemia due to persistent parvovirus infection to immunoglobulin therapy.[19] The patient initially was treated with immunoglobulin at 400 mg/kg/day for 10 days and then with periodic injections *(open rectangles)* until virus was no longer detected in the blood by the sensitive gene amplification method.

CONGENITAL PURE RED CELL APLASIA

In 1936, Josephs[100] described two cases of red cell aplasia occurring in infancy. Two years later, Diamond and Blackfan[101] reported four children with a "slowly progressive anemia beginning early in infancy, without any hemorrhagic tendency, with only moderate leukopenia and with the production of a small and inadequate number of reticulocytes from bone marrow which shows moderate hypoplasia." They used the term "congenital hypoplastic anemia" to indicate a partial pancellular marrow depression and to differentiate this syndrome from acquired aplastic anemia and Fanconi's anemia. The anemia was refractory to conventional treatments of the time, including intramuscular pentanucleotide; iron with cobalt or copper; bone marrow or spleen extract; vitamin C, both orally and intravenously; or supplemental vitamins. The original patients were easily managed by blood transfusions and the anemia in one of the four spontaneously remitted.[101] Since its first description, this entity of congenital hypoplastic anemia has had different appellations, including chronic congenital aregenerative anemia, chronic idiopathic erythroblastopenia with aplastic anemia, and probably most descriptively, erythrogenesis imperfecta; however, it is most commonly referred to as Diamond-Blackfan anemia, the name Josephs being lost from the eponym with time. A handful of patients were described over the next two decades, in whom the main therapy was blood transfusion support, and although supportive care permitted normal growth and development, iron overload inevitably led to severe liver disease and often liver failure.

In 1951, Gasser[102] reported a remission in a patient treated with corticosteroids and their use in the disorder soon became routine. By 1961, the first large series of corticosteroid-treated patients was reported by Allen and Diamond[103]: 12 of 22 treated patients experienced a remission manifested by a rapid reticulocytosis (within 2 weeks of the onset of therapy) and subsequent normalization of the hemoglobin. Those patients who were unresponsive never mounted an appreciable reticulocyte response, an observation useful in sparing nonresponders the side effects of long-term steroid treatment.[103] (However, an initial lack of a response to steroids does not preclude a subsequent trial.[104–106]) The treatment of DBA has changed very little since that time, with only a handful of case reports and very small series describing modest changes in transfusion requirements with alternative agents such as hematopoietic growth factors and immunosuppressive agents.

Epidemiology and Clinical Features

There is no significant sex difference, with male-female ratios of about 1:1. All races are affected, although the majority of reported patients are Caucasian.[107–110] More than 400 cases have been reported in the literature.[107, 111–113] The estimated disease incidence using data from a number of different European registries is from 4 to 10 per million live births,[114–116] and at a single American referral center, 78 patients were diagnosed over a 60-year period.[104] Some studies have suggested a seasonality to the incidence. Prevalence in the general population is perhaps not fully appreciated because of loss of follow-up in nonpediatric patients.

Clinically, DBA is defined as a constitutional congenital PRCA characterized by a hyporegenerative anemia. (The terms "congenital" and "constitutional" are often incorrectly interchanged, but congenital refers to manifesting at birth, whereas constitutional refers to the presence of a constellation of symptoms and signs such as physical abnormalities.)

Most patients present with pallor. Congenital anomalies may be present (in published data ranging from 24% to 45%) but are much less frequent and severe than those seen in Fanconi's anemia. For example, 50% of Fanconi's anemia patients have upper limb abnormalities, but the incidence is approximately 9% in DBA.[107] The most common of the abnormalities seen in DBA patients are craniofacial, but there are a multitude of anomalies described, including thumb abnormalities such as triphalangeal, bifid, accessory, absent, or hypoplastic digits, or subluxations, which may be unilateral or bilateral, and most often, a flattening of the thenar eminences or weakness of the radial pulse, singly or in combination, similar to that seen in patients with thrombocytopenia and absent radii syndrome (TAR). Other abnormalities described include short stature unrelated to steroid use (and in four of eight patients studied, growth hormone deficiency was found),[117] and even heart malformations (Table 6–3). The classic DBA facies was described by Cathie as having "tow col-

TABLE 6–3 Malformations in Diamond-Blackfan Anemia*

Malformations	Incidence
Craniofacial dysmorphism (glaucoma, hypertelorism, Cathie's facies, snub nose)†	19%
Upper limb abnormalities (triphalangeal thumbs; bifid, absent digits)	9%
Genitourinary (duplicate ureters, horseshoe kidney, hypoplastic genitalia, inguinal hernia)	7%
Growth disturbances	6%
Neck (web, Sprengel's deformity, Klippel-Feil syndrome)	4%
Skeletal (scoliosis, aseptic necrosis)	3%
Cardiac (aortic stenosis, atrial septal defect, patent ductus arteriosus)	2%
Other	3%

*Of 436 cases reviewed, 114 (26%) had at least one anomaly.
†Examples given are not inclusive but represent the most common findings.
Adapted from Young NS, Alter BP: Aplastic Anemia Acquired and Inherited. Philadelphia, WB Saunders, 1994, p 364.

oured hair, snub nose, wide set eyes, thick upper lip, and an intelligent expression."[118] DBA patients have been thought to resemble each other more than they do their own relatives. These anomalies, however, are rarely pronounced enough to be the presenting complaint.

There is a higher incidence of prematurity and low birth weight in affected neonates and an apparently increased rate of miscarriage in families with affected children, although these observations may be related to recall bias.[107] Unlike patients with TEC, DBA patients do not have a viral prodrome and they are also usually younger: 80% present within the first year of life.[106] Distinct from acquired PRCA in children, there are no associated underlying autoimmune or malignant disorders.

Reported inheritance patterns in affected families are both autosomal dominant and autosomal recessive, but most cases are sporadic. With apparent dominant inheritance, the numbers of males and females were equal, the incidence of physical abnormalities was similar to that in all other DBA patients, and the disease generally followed a milder clinical course.[107] In the reported cases of recessive inheritance, there were twice as many affected males as females, the abnormalities were similar in incidence and severity, and again the clinical course seemed to be milder than in sporadic disease.[107] A number of these families were consanguineous, making dominant inheritance with incomplete penetrance less likely as an explanation. The predominance of males suggests an X-linked inheritance in some cases but obviously not in all. There are also reports of sibling sets, fraternal and identical twins along with affected siblings, and male cousins being affected.[119–122] Sporadic DBA could be due to new mutations, acquired disease, variable penetrance, or any combination of these, within families.

Patients have a normocytic or macrocytic anemia, reticulocytopenia, normal to increased numbers of platelets, and occasionally a mild neutropenia.[123] Indirect and direct Coombs' testing is negative. Serum levels of iron, ferritin, folic acid, vitamin B_{12}, and erythropoietin are normal or elevated. In one study the hemoglobin at presentation ranged from 1.5 g/dL to 12.4 g/dL and the mean corpuscular volume (MCV), from 70 to 140 fL, with a mean of 93 fL.[104] There are suggestions that the macrocytosis may be less pronounced in those presenting with disease at younger ages (during the first 3 months of life).[104] DBA patients do not have pancytopenia, nor do they show increased chromosomal instability as found in Fanconi's anemia patients.[112] Aplastic crisis with acute parvovirus infection or aplasia secondary to chronic parvovirus infection can be excluded by serologic and DNA testing. There are reported cases of patients presenting with a congenital anemia secondary to a maternal infection of parvovirus B19 while in utero. These children had parvovirus evident in their bone marrows but not in their sera, and they did not appear to respond to immune globulin therapy (see also above).[124]

The diagnosis of DBA relies on examination of the bone marrow (Plate 9). The diagnostic criteria include significant erythroid hypoplasia, and almost always the erythroid aplasia is complete. Occasionally, there are normal numbers of erythroid precursors with an apparent maturation arrest, and fewer than 5% of patients have erythroid hyperplasia with maturation arrest.[125] It is unclear whether those patients with erythroid hyperplasia have a different disorder altogether or a variant of the same etiology. The other hematopoietic lineages should appear normal in the marrow, and the overall cellularity is usually normal or mildly hypocellular.[126] There are no giant pronormoblasts as would be seen with parvovirus infection.

Pathogenesis

The pathogenesis of DBA is as yet unknown, but given the heterogeneity of the clinical manifestations, disease course, and inheritance patterns, there are likely multiple causes. An intrinsic progenitor cell defect in DBA is presumed as bone marrow transplant is curative, but the single lineage defect is puzzling, suggesting selective disruption of erythroid differentiation.

Genetics

Unlike in Fanconi's anemia, there are no consistent chromosomal aberrations. Cytogenetic analysis is usually normal, although there have been cases with an abnormal chromosome 16, either due to enlargement, breaks, or endoreduplication, and an abnormal chromosome 1.[127–130] Sister chromatid exchange is also normal. Recently, the gene in some familial cases and a few sporadic cases has been localized to a region of chromosome 19.[131] The protein and its function have yet to be identified and, until more information is obtained, it is believed that this gene will account for only 30% of the cases.

Enzymes

In their initial discussion, Diamond and Blackfan proposed an inborn error of metabolism as a possible cause of the disease.[101] Enzyme abnormalities have since been discovered, but they are either not relevant to the etiology or of unclear significance. The elevations of fetal hemoglobin, red blood cell i antigen, and pyrimidine enzymes orotate phosphoribosyltransferase and oritidine-5'-monophosphate decarboxylase are a reflection of the stress erythropoiesis induced by the anemia.[132] Elevated adenosine deaminase (ADA) levels, which are not normally associated with fetal erythropoiesis, were seen by one group in 26 out of 29 patients,[133–135] and elevated ADA levels were present in 9 of 19 patients and 2 of 15 relatives in another study.[136] ADA is a critical enzyme in the purine salvage pathway and has also been found to be increased in some cases of childhood acute lymphocytic leukemia (ALL). Other than being used to help differentiate DBA from TEC (see below) and broadly consistent with disordered erythropoiesis, it is unclear whether this enzyme elevation is a primary event or a secondary phenomenon.

Cytokines

An erythropoietin insensitivity has been hypothesized due to the hormone levels that are excessively elevated for the level of anemia. Long-term culture–initiating cell (LTC-IC) studies showed decreased CFU-E or BFU-E in more than 50 patients, but normal numbers in approximately 12.[107] In some laboratories very high concentrations of erythropoietin were found to improve colony growth of DBA cultures.[137–141] Others have found increased erythroid colony growth and erythropoietin sensitivity in bone marrow culture studies when BPA (burst-promoting activity; probably the equivalent of interleukin-3 [IL-3] or stem cell factor [SCF]) was added. This effect was increased with the removal of monocytes and lymphocytes, suggesting that BPA acted directly on the progenitor cells.[139] In vitro studies using IL-3 showed improved BFU-E growth, and four of four DBA marrows reached normal numbers of BFU-E with SCF and five of a separate six patients had increased blood BFU-E with SCF (but not to normal levels).[142] Initial enthusiasm for colony growth assays, as in vitro models of this disease, has waned. Moreover, two promising animal models, both of which have discrete cytokine- or growth factor receptor–derived abnormalities due to genetic mutations, have also been found to be irrelevant. The mouse W locus has a *c-kit* mutation causing an anemia cured by bone marrow transplantation (BMT),[143, 144] and the Steel mouse has a c-kit receptor mutation resulting in anemia cured by spleen transplantation.[145] However, these animals do not respond to prednisone and, more importantly, there has been no evidence of c-kit or erythropoietin receptor mutations seen in DBA patients.[146, 147] The expression of the hematopoietically active SCF transcription factor is normal as well.[148] None of these in vitro or animal data have translated to any significant clinical benefit in trials using cytokine growth factors[119, 149-151] (see below).

Immunology

The response to steroids in the majority of patients implicates an immunologic mechanism, which has been further supported by occasional responses to other agents such as ATG, CsA, or cyclophosphamide.[152-154] The mechanism of action of corticosteroids in DBA is unknown. Prednisone could act as an immunosuppressant or hematopoietic stimulant, or both. Corticosteroids have been shown to increase colony growth in vitro. It is also unclear whether the other drugs used also have in vivo hematopoietic stimulatory effects.[155-162]

In vitro studies using colony growth measured directly or indirectly in the presence of either lymphocytes or sera from DBA patients have shown evidence of both serologic and cellular inhibition of erythroid growth.[163, 164] Other assays have shown altered lymphocyte CD4/CD8 ratios, decreased T cell numbers, and impaired proliferation of lymphocytes and suppressor cell function, as well as increased sensitivity of lymphocytes to radiation stress.[165, 166] Not all results have been consistently reproducible and the role of secondary alloimmunization has not been excluded in these often highly transfused patients.[167, 168]

Despite the heterogeneity of this disease, there is a common failure of erythroid development, most likely due to blocks in the differentiation pathway, perhaps involving signaling pathways dependent on cytokine stimulation as an intracellular signal transduction defect, a receptor-ligand defect, or even the presence of an inhibitory cytokine.[169] Determination of the function of the chromosome 19 DBA gene should help to elucidate not only the etiology of DBA but also fundamental aspects of erythropoiesis in general.

Course of Disease and Treatment

Without transfusions or other treatment the majority of patients would die from profound anemia and its complications, as was described in the initial case reports. Although remissions and even spontaneous cures can occur, most patients will need some form of long-term treatment. Currently, corticosteroids are the recommended first-line therapy (Table 6–4). Seventy percent of patients respond to prednisone, usually given at an initial dose of 2 mg/kg/day, and their hemoglobin levels can be maintained at lower doses once an initial response is established.[107] Transfusion-independence may be sustained on extremely low doses—1 to 2 mg/day—but most patients require chronic treatment.[114] Corticosteroids can sometimes be completely withdrawn but there is a significant relapse rate. A proportion of patients will respond to steroids on a second trial, even if there was no response on first exposure, and a

TABLE 6–4 Treatment Algorithm for Diamond-Blackfan Anemia

1. Prednisone 2 mg/kg/day—expect response (reticulocytosis) in approximately 2–4 wk
   If response, taper to as low a dose as possible; if patient develops resistance or side effects from steroids, go to 3
   If relapse after weaning, retry steroids at initial dose
   If no response, go to 2
2. High-dose corticosteroids 4–6 mg/kg/day intravenous or oral
   If response, taper; if unable to taper, go to 3
   If no response, go to 3
3. Begin transfusion therapy with desferrioxamine as appropriate; consider experimental protocols
4. If patient remains transfusion dependent and has HLA-matched sibling donor, consider for transplant
5. Retry steroids every few years

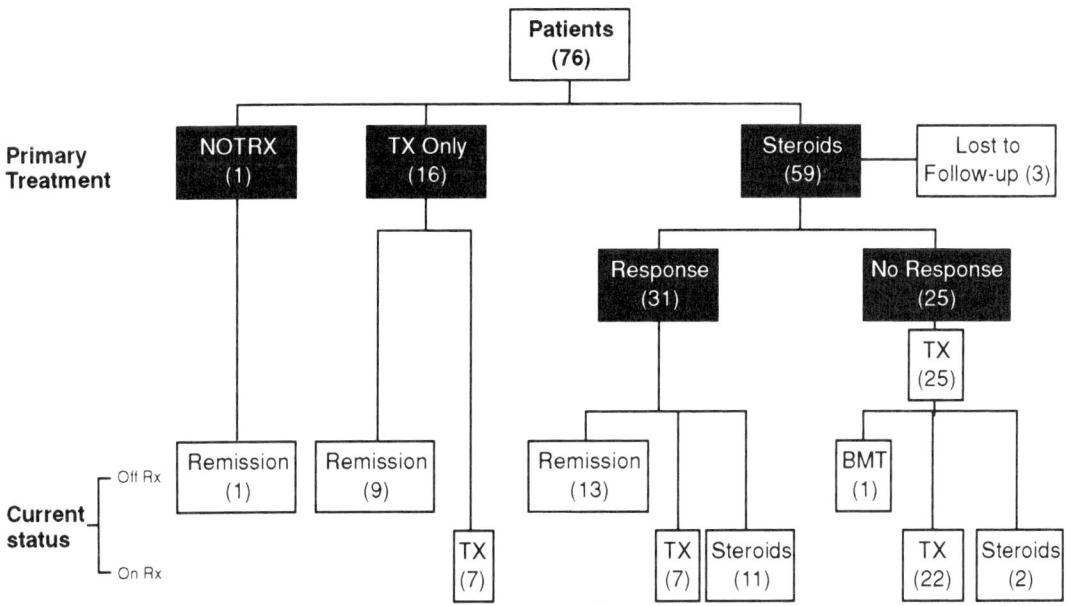

Figure 6–3 Corticosteroid responses in patients with Diamond-Blackfan anemia. (From Janov A, Leong T, Nathan D, Guinan E: Diamond-Blackfan anemia—Natural history and sequelae of treatment. Medicine [Baltimore] 1996; 75:80–86.) (Tx = transfusion.)

similar proportion will subsequently become refractory despite a good early response. In a Boston series of 76 patients, 59 were treated with steroids, 25 of whom did not respond initially, but two later did improve on subsequent retrial. Of the other 21, 11 required continued therapy, and 13 had a complete remission (Fig. 6–3). Of all the patients followed, both treated and not, there were 23 who became transfusion-independent, although the hemoglobin values did not necessarily return to normal.[104] To date, no study has been able to clearly identify prognostic factors, including malformations, age at presentation, or response to steroids, which relate to long-term outcome.

Chronic corticosteroid therapy is associated with many short- and long-term complications, including osteoporosis, cushingoid features, diabetes, hypertension, severe growth retardation, aseptic necrosis, glaucoma, and cataracts. Those who become refractory to, are resistant to, or are intolerant of corticosteroids require chronic red blood cell transfusions. Desferrioxamine is used to prevent iron overload after multiple transfusions.[169]

Occasional responses have been observed with androgens, very-high-dose methylprednisolone, IL-3, ATG, CsA, and cyclophosphamide.[119, 149, 152–154, 171] Of 19 patients with DBA anemia followed in the Hematology Branch of the National Heart, Lung, and Blood Institute (NHLBI) over the past two decades, eight patients have received CsA, with two responding. One of 19 patients had been treated with both ATG and CsA. This patient had both congenital PRCA and cyclic neutropenia: the neutrophil count improved but the anemia did not. One other patient had been treated with ATG alone but had no apparent benefit.

BMT is an option in patients with a histocompatible sibling and who have failed corticosteroids, but it has been infrequently employed. For patients and their families the long-term effects of chronic red blood cell transfusion seem to be preferable to the morbidity and mortality associated with transplant. BMT has usually been performed late in the course of the disease, when there are heavy transfusion burdens with hemosiderotic organ damage as well as alloimmunization, and as a result DBA patients tend to have a high treatment-related mortality and morbidity. The first DBA patient to be transplanted received the transplant in 1976 with the use of antilymphocyte globulin (ALG), ^{32}P, and total body irradiation (TBI) as the preparative regimen. The engraftment was successful, but the patient died on day 55 with pneumonia.[172] Since then 20 more patients have received transplants[173–179] (Table 6–5). Some experts do not recommend the use of transplant in patients with DBA, but given current results, and continuing improvements in relevant techniques,

TABLE 6–5 Bone Marrow Transplantation (BMT) in Diamond-Blackfan Anemia

Age (yr)	Recipient/Donor Sex*	Blood Transfusion History (units)	Steroid History	Type	Conditioning†	Prophylaxis	Acute/Chronic GvHD	Survival Post BMT
13	M	238	NA	sib	ALG-P-TBI	NA	NA	55 days—DIP
5	M	89	NA	sib	BU-CY-TBI	NA	NA	>21 mo
6	F	40	NA	sib	BU-CY	NA	NA	>21 mo
5.5	M/F	100	NR	sib	ATG-BU-PRO-CY	MTX	+ + / +	>1320 days
16	M/M	150	std—9,NR	sib	ATG-BU-PRO-CY	MTX	+ + / −	>520 days
5	M/F	100	NR	sib	ATG-BU-PRO-CY	MTX	+ + / + +	>540 days
5	F/M	100	NR	sib	ATG-BU-CY	MTX	+ + / −	>1180 days
31	M	14	NA	sib	BU-CY-TLI	NA	NA	>38 mo
5.5	F/F	84	NR	sib	BU-CY	NA	+ + /sli	>10.6 yr
5	F/F	80	NR	sib	BU-CY	NA	+ + /s	>7.4 yr
31	F/M	100	sti—22,NR	sib	BU-CY-ATG	NA	−	>3.0 yr
9	M/M	130	NR	sib	BU-CY	NA	+ + + /sl	35 days—DIP
6	F/F	40	NA	sib	BU-CY	MTX	−	>87 mo
1	M/F	12	NA	sib	BU-CY	MTX	−	>64 mo
1	M/M	5	NA	sib	TLI-BU-CY	MTX + CSA	−	>60 mo
5	M/F	51	NA	sib	TBI-CY	MTX	y/y	>43 mo
12	M/M	376	NA	sib	BU-CY-ATG	MTX-CSA-ATG	−	>37 mo
6	F/M	8	NA	sib	TLI-CY	MTX-CSA + Ster	−	>5 mo
3	M/M	18	NA	sib	BU-CY	CSA	−	5 mo—pneumonia
5	M/F	51	NA	sib	BU-CY	CSA + Ster	−	1.6 mo—graft failure
8	F/F	55	NA	Mother (HLAi)	TLI-BU-CY	MTX + CSA	ne	0.4 mo—sepsis
14	M/F	150	NA	Unrelated	TBI-CY	CSA	+ + + +	0.4 mo—acute GvHD

M, male; F, female; NA, not available; NR, no response; std—9, steroid dependent until age 9; sti—22, steroid independent until age 22; sib, matched sibling; HLAi, HLA identical; ALG, antilymphocyte globulin; P. ³²P; TBI, total body irradiation; BU, busulfan; CY, cyclophosphamide; ATG, antithymocyte globulin; PRO, procarbazine; TLI, total lymphoid irradiation; MTX, methotrexate; CSA, cyclosporine; Ster, steroids; GvHD, graft-versus-host disease; s, skin; l, liver; i, intestine; y/y, presence or absence; ne, not evaluable; DIP, diffuse interstitial pneumonitis. The number of plus signs equals the degree of GvHD.

*If only one given, it is the recipient.
†Doses varied per patient.

including molecular typing methods, nonmyeloablative regimens, better graft-versus-host disease prophylaxis and treatment, and even the use of cord blood as a stem cell source, most physicians agree that a steroid-resistant patient with a related HLA-matched donor should at least be referred to a transplant center for evaluation.[180] Studies are needed to determine the best timing and type of transplant for these patients.

A benefit for prolactin has been postulated based on anecdotal reports of cases improving after puberty. We are examining the use of combined immunosuppressive regimens in a National Institutes of Health (NIH) protocol. With determination of the chromosome 19 gene function, protein replacement and even gene therapy become possibilities.

Patients who are corticosteroid responsive have a better overall prognosis than those who are corticosteroid resistant. Many will go on to lead normal lives.[181] As stated previously, a percentage of patients may be maintained on minimal steroid doses and others will undergo spontaneous remission. Patients who are transfusion-dependent do not fare as well. Prior to the use of desferrioxamine, they had a shorter life expectancy as a result of complications from iron overload, especially due to cardiomyopathy and hepatic cirrhosis. Currently, the median life expectancy with the use of desferrioxamine is 30 to 40 years[104, 107, 181] (Fig. 6–4). DBA patients also appear to have an increased risk of myelodysplasia or leukemia (with a published relative risk of 200 later in life).[104] There may be evolution with time of decreased cellularity and the development of other clinically significant cytopenias.[182] In 29 patients seen at the NIH, 24 patients had a hypocellular marrow on biopsy and five patients have had a progressive decline in either their neutrophil counts only or also platelets (three patients) (N. Giri, personal communication, June 1999).

TRANSIENT ERYTHROBLASTOPENIA OF CHILDHOOD

TEC is an acquired, self-limited red cell aplasia affecting normal children. In 1949, Gasser[183] described acute erythroblastopenia occurring secondary to apparent toxic, allergic, or infectious insult in 12 children, in whom there was complete recovery with no evidence of permanent anemia. The term transient erythroblastopenia of childhood first appeared in a publication in 1970 by Wranne[184]; currently over 450 cases have been described in the literature.[107] The differential diagnosis includes parvovirus B19 infection, DBA, Fanconi's anemia, nutritional deficiencies, thymoma-associated PRCA, drug effects, and other reticulocytopenic anemias (Table 6–6). The final diagnosis is made retrospectively after spontaneous resolution of the anemia.

Clinical Features and Epidemiology

The epidemiology of this disease has not been well documented given the transient nature of the illness and the probability of omitting patients with only mild signs and symptoms. A Swedish population-based study approximated an annual incidence of 4.3 per 100,000 children who were less than 3 years of age and 2.5 per 100,000 children less than 4 years old,[185] and a retrospective study from England reported an estimated incidence of $5/10^6$.[186] In one study evaluating the bone marrows of 25 patients with childhood anemia, 15 were given the diagnosis of TEC; four,

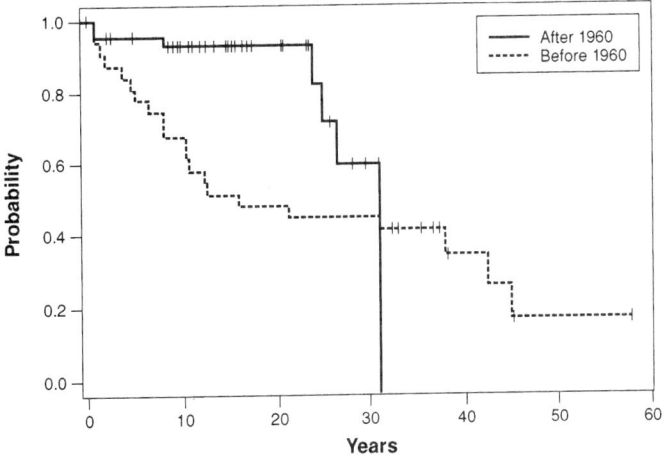

Figure 6–4 Kaplan-Meier survival curves of patients with Diamond-Blackfan anemia. (From Janov A, Leong T, Nathan D, Guinan E: Diamond-Blackfan anemia—Natural history and sequelae of treatment. Medicine [Baltimore] 1996; 75:80–86.)

TABLE 6–6   Differential Diagnosis of Pure Red Cell Aplasia in Children

Parvovirus B19—positive DNA or bone marrow PCR, suggestive history, usually immunocompromised patients
DBA—may have elevated adenosine deaminase levels, younger age
Fanconi's anemia—increased chromosomal breakage, characteristic phenotype
Acquired pure red cell aplasia—associated with other immune disorders; does not resolve spontaneously; otherwise a diagnosis of exclusion
Nutritional deficiencies—characteristic laboratory indices, i.e., macro- or microcytic; measurable serum levels
Drug-induced aplasia—concordant history, resolution with discontinuation of drug (otherwise very difficult to differentiate from idiopathic acquired pure red cell aplasia)

PCR, polymerase chain reaction; DBA, Diamond-Blackfan anemia.

nutritional anemia; and one each of congenital dyserythropoietic anemia, anemia of chronic disease, spherocytosis, and blood loss, and two were indeterminate.[187] In another study of 33 children evaluated for red cell aplasia, 22 were given the diagnosis of TEC; seven, parvovirus B19 aplasia; and four, DBA.[188] A single-institution prospective evaluation of 50 cases, 14 of which were already recovering at the time of diagnosis, showed a mean age of 22 months and an equal distribution of female-to-male cases.[188]

The mean age of presentation is about 2 years.[107] Ninety percent of patients are older than 1 year of age at diagnosis, and only 10% of patients are older than 3 years. Five percent of reported cases are less than 6 months of age; however, it is suggested that the incidence in infants is underestimated.[189]

Patients usually present with pallor; they may have a flow murmur and tachycardia on physical examination. There are no associated congenital anomalies. More than half will have had a preceding viral illness affecting either the upper respiratory or gastrointestinal systems. There have also been case reports of patients with neurologic manifestations such as seizures, transient ischemic attacks, and paralysis, coinciding with the anemia.[190–192] For the majority, the anemia lasts approximately 4 weeks; the longest documented period was 8 months.

Laboratory Studies

The usual presentation is of a normocytic, normochromic, reticulocytopenic anemia. Hemoglobin values range from 2 to 10 g/dL. Ninety percent of patients will have a reticulocyte percentage of less than 1%.[188] A few patients have had thrombocytopenia or leukopenia, as well as leukocytosis, but these are rare associations.[107, 188, 192–194] The bone marrow is consistent with erythroblastopenia; 90% have no erythroid precursors and 10% demonstrate maturation arrest to the erythroblast stage only. Occasionally lymphoid aggregates may mimic the appearance of lymphoid leukemia. There are no giant pronormoblasts. In the recovery phase, stress erythropoietic values are seen, with elevated levels of hemoglobin F, red blood cell I antigen, and reticulocytosis.[107, 188] ADA is normal in TEC. The mean nadir hemoglobin in those with reticulocytopenia at diagnosis was 6.8 g/dL with an MCV of 81 and white blood cell count of 8100/mm^3. The indices are similar in the recovery phase except for the reticulocytosis. Platelet counts may also be elevated.[188]

Pathophysiology

In bone marrow culture studies of over 50 patients by different laboratories, 50% of patients had decreased CFU-E growth and 30% decreased BFU-E growth.[107]

Serum or IgG inhibitors of normal progenitors were detected in four patients, with one having autologous inhibition.[195] In 30 other patients, 18 (60%) were positive for autologous or allogeneic serum inhibitors. Cellular inhibitors, again both autologous and allogeneic, have been seen in 30% of cases examined.[107] A T cell–mediated process has been proposed based on the evaluation of a 4-year-old child in whom CFU-E growth was initially 28% of the control but which increased fivefold after T cell depletion of the patient's marrow. T cell depletion had less effect on CFU-E when the samples were obtained at a later stage in the disease.[196] In contrast to adult PRCA, no patient has had evidence of both serum and cellular inhibitors.

Familial

Familial TEC has been described. Five sets of siblings, including identical and fraternal twins, have been reported with anemia occurring either simultaneously or, in two cases, separated by 2 to 3 years.[193, 197–199] In a Swedish study of 52 affected children, there were four pairs of siblings, with the probability of this occurring by chance alone estimated to be less than in 1 in 10^6. Of note, one sibling set was treated for 6 months with prednisone, with reticulocytosis evident at 3 weeks. In two of the other sibling sets, the fathers also had had a history of transient anemia during childhood, suggesting an autosomal inheritance pattern.[185]

Seasonality

Clustering of small cases within June to October or November to March have been reported,[193, 194, 197, 200, 201] but tabulation of all cases reported in the literature does not support a seasonal effect.

Viral

The clinical prodrome points to a virus as a causative agent. The presence of human herpesvirus 6 (HHV6) was found by PCR in two marrows of children affected with TEC; controls, which consisted of other children with anemia but distinct diagnoses from TEC, were negative.[202] HHV6 is a CD4+ lymphotropic virus causative of exanthem subitum in children, and other illnesses in immunocompromised patients. No other viruses to date have been consistently identified, and further analyses are needed before confirming HHV6 as an etiologic agent.

A unifying theory would suggest that the erythroid elements are an innocent bystander in the immune-mediated attack against a viral agent. A specific virus may not be needed and the variety of clinical manifestations of preceding illness ranging from none to seizure-like neurologic symptoms would depend on the etiology and host immune response. Increased familial incidence would also correlate with a viral cause, in terms of either a common exposure or susceptibility in the immune system response or erythroid cell sensitivity.

Evaluation and Treatment

Given that TEC is the most common diagnosis of immunocompetent patients presenting with anemia at a young age, evaluation, other than the routine history and physical examination, should initially consist of only routine laboratory studies.[106] Further investigations, including bone marrow aspiration and laboratory tests for parvovirus B19, should be undertaken and other diagnoses entertained only if the anemia persists for more than 2 months. Treatment is expectant. Corticosteroids have not shown any benefit in shortening the duration of the anemia.[106, 107] Depending on the extent and duration of the anemia, the patient's symptoms, and also the comfort level of the physician, an occasional red blood cell transfusion may be required. Children often tolerate very low hemoglobin levels with no sequelae, and unnecessary transfusions should be avoided. Recurrence has been documented in only two cases, and it is unclear whether these were truly TEC or some other diagnosis.[203]

REFERENCES

1. Dessypris EN: Pure Red Cell Aplasia. Baltimore, Johns Hopkins University Press, 1988.
2. Dessypris EN: The biology of pure red cell aplasia. Semin Hematol 1991; 28:275.
3. Freedman MH: Pure red cell aplasia in childhood and adolescence: Pathogenesis and approaches to diagnosis. Br J Haematol 1993; 85:246.
4. Erslev AJ, Soltan A: Pure red-cell aplasia: A review. Blood Rev 1997; 10:20.
5. Mamiya S, Itoh T, Miura AB: Acquired pure red cell aplasia in Japan. Eur J Haematol 1997; 59:199.
6. Hirst E, Robertson TI: The syndrome of thymoma and erythroblastopenic anemia. Medicine (Baltimore) 1967; 46:225.
7. Schmid JR, Kiely JM, Pease GL, et al: Acquired pure red cell agenesis. Acta Haematol 1963; 30:255.
8. Chikkappa G, Zarrabi MH, Tsan MF: Pure red-cell aplasia in patients with chronic lymphocytic leukemia. Medicine (Baltimore) 1986; 65:339.
9. Ammus SS, Yunis AA: Acquired pure red cell aplasia. Am J Hematol 1987; 24:311.
10. Jacobs AD, Champlin RE, Golde DW: Pure red cell aplasia characterized by erythropoietic maturation arrest. Am J Med 1985; 78:515.
11. Fitzgerald PH, Hamer JW: Primary acquired red cell hypoplasia associated with a clonal chromosomal abnormality and disturbed erythroid proliferation. Blood 1938; 71:325.
12. Bunn HF, McNeil BJ, Rosenthal DS, et al: Bone-marrow imaging in pure red blood cell aplasia. Arch Intern Med 1976; 136:1169.
13. Schmid JR, Kiely JM, Harrison EG Jr, et al: Thymoma associated with pure red-cell agenesis. Cancer 1965; 18:216.
14. Dessypris EN, Gogo A, Russell M, et al: Studies on pure red cell aplasia. X. Association with acute leukemia and significance of bone marrow karyotype abnormalities. Blood 1980; 56:421.
15. DiBenedetto J Jr, Padre-Mendoza T, Albala MM: Pure red cell hypoplasia associated with long-arm deletion of chromosome 5. Hum Genet 1979; 46:345.
16. Baron RL, Lee JKT, Sagel SS, et al: Computed tomography of the abnormal thymus. Radiology 1982; 142:127.
17. Geary CG, Byron PR, Taylor G, et al: Thymoma associated with pure red cell aplasia, immunoglobulin deficiency and an inhibitor of antigen-induced lymphocyte transformation. Br J Haematol 1975; 29:479.
18. Murase T: Bilineage hematopoietic inhibitor and T lymphocyte dysfunction in a patient with pure red cell aplasia, myasthenia gravis and thymoma. Exp Hematol 1993; 21:451.
19. Socinski MA, Ershler WB, Frankel J, et al: Pure

RBC aplasia and myasthenia gravis. Arch Intern Med 1983; 143:43.
20. Ustun C, Karavelioglu D, Ilhan O, et al: A case report of a patient who has pure red cell aplasia and rheumatoid arthritis. Int J Hematol 1997; 66:505.
21. McManus KG, Allen MS, Trastek VF, et al: Lipothymoma with red cell aplasia, hypogammaglobulinemia, and lichen planus. Ann Thorac Surg 1994; 58:1534.
22. Souadjian JV, Enriquez P, Silverstein MN, et al: The spectrum of diseases associated with thymoma. Arch Intern Med 1974; 134:374.
23. Linsk JA, Murray CK: Erythrocyte aplasia and hypogammaglobulinemia. Response to steroids in a young adult. Ann Intern Med 1961; 55:831.
24. Purtilo DT, Zelkowitz L, Harada S, et al: Delayed onset of infectious mononucleosis associated with acquired agammaglobulinemia and red cell aplasia. Ann Intern Med 1984; 101:180.
25. Resegotti L, Dolci C, Palestro G, et al: Paraproteinemic variety of pure red cell aplasia. Acta Haematol 1978; 60:227.
26. Prasad AS, Berman L, Tranchida L, et al: Red cell hypoplasia, cold hemoglobinuria and M-type gamma G serum paraprotein and Bence Jones proteinuria in a patient with lymphoproliferative disorder. Blood 1968; 31:151.
27. Lacy MQ, Kurtin PJ, Tefferi A: Pure red cell aplasia: Association with large granular lymphocyte leukemia and the prognostic value of cytogenetic abnormalities. Blood 1996; 87:3000.
28. Brittingham TE, Lutcher CL, Murphy DI: Reversible erythroid aplasia induced by diphenylhydantoin. Arch Intern Med 1964; 113:764.
29. Dessypris EN, Redline S, Harris JW, et al: Diphenylhydantoin-induced pure red cell aplasia. Blood 1985; 65:789.
30. Balaban EP, Buchanan GR, Graham M, et al: Diamond-Blackfan syndrome in adult patients. Am J Med 1985; 78:533.
31. Field EO, Caughi MN, Blackett NM, et al: Marrow-suppressing factors in the blood in pure red-cell aplasia, thymoma and Hodgkin's disease. Br J Haematol 1968; 15:101.
32. Krantz SB, Kao V: Studies on red cell aplasia. I. Demonstration of a plasma inhibitor to heme synthesis and an antibody to erythroblast nuclei. Proc Natl Acad Sci U S A 1967; 58:493.
33. Krantz SB, Moore WH, Zaentz SD: Studies on red cell aplasia. V. Presence of erythroblast cytotoxicity in gamma G-globulin fraction of plasma. J Clin Invest 1973; 52:324.
34. Lowenberg B, Ghio R: An assay for serum cytotoxicity against erythroid precursor cells in pure red cell aplasia. Biomedicine 1977; 27:285.
35. Mangan KF, Besa EC, Shadduck RK, et al: Demonstration of two distinct antibodies in autoimmune hemolytic anemia with reticulocytopenia and red cell aplasia. Exp Hematol 1984; 12:788.
36. Mangan KF, Chikkappa G, Scharfman WB, et al: Evidence for reduced erythroid burst (BFUE) promoting function of T lymphocytes in the pure red cell aplasia of chronic lymphocytic leukemia. Exp Hematol 1981; 9:489.
37. Meyer RJ, Hoffman R, Zanjani ED: Autoimmune hemolytic anemia and periodic pure red cell aplasia in systemic lupus erythematosus. Am J Med 1978; 65:342.
38. Browman GP, Freedman MH, Blajchman MA, et al: A complement independent erythropoietic inhibitor acting on the progenitor cell in refractory anemia. Am J Med 1976; 61:572.
39. Baker RI, Manoharan A, De Luca E, et al: Pure red cell aplasia of pregnancy: A distinct clinical entity. Br J Haematol 1993; 85:619.
40. Peschle C, Marmont A, Perugini S, et al: Physiopathology and therapy of adult pure red cell aplasia (PRCA): A cooperative study. In Hibino S, Takaku F, Shahidi NT (eds): Aplastic Anemia. Baltimore, University Park Press, 1978, p 285.
41. Takahashi M, Nikkuni K, Tanaka I, et al: Serum erythropoietic inhibitors in patients with pure red cell aplasia. Ann Hematol 1991; 63:9.
42. Marmont A, Peschle C, Sanguineti M, et al: Pure red cell aplasia (PRCA): Response of three patients to cyclophosphamide and/or anti-lymphocyte globulin (ALG) and demonstration of two types of serum IgG inhibitors to erythropoiesis. Blood 1975; 45:247.
43. Casadevall N, Dupuy E, Molho-Sabatier P, et al: Brief report: Autoantibodies against erythropoietin in a patient with pure red-cell aplasia. N Engl J Med 1996; 334:630.
44. Peces R, De La Torre M, Alcazar R, et al: Antibodies against recombinant human erythropoietin in a patient with erythropoietin-resistant anemia. N Engl J Med 1996; 335:523.
45. Al-Mondhiry H, Zanjani ED, Spivack M, et al: Pure red cell aplasia and thymoma: Loss of serum inhibitor of erythropoiesis following thymectomy. Blood 1971; 38:576.
46. Messner HA, Fauser AA, Curtis JE, et al: Control of antibody-mediated pure red-cell aplasia by plasmapheresis. N Engl J Med 1981; 304:1334.
47. Freund LG, Hippe E, Strandgaard S, et al: Complete remission in pure red cell aplasia after plasmapheresis. Scand J Haematol 1985; 35:315.
48. Barnes RD: Refractory anaemia with thymoma (letter). Lancet 1966; 2:1464.
49. Charles RJ, Sabo KM, Kidd PG, et al: The pathophysiology of pure red cell aplasia: Implications for therapy. Blood 1996; 87:4831.
50. Hoffman R, Kopel S, Hsu SD, et al: T cell chronic lymphocytic leukemia: Presence in bone marrow and peripheral blood of cells that suppress erythropoiesis in vitro. Blood 1978; 52:255.
51. Mangan KF, D'Alessandro L: Hypoplastic anemia in B cell chronic lymphocytic leukemia: Evolution of T cell-mediated suppression of erythropoiesis in early-stage and late-stage disease. Blood 1985; 66:533.
52. Linch DC, Cawley JC, MacDonald SM, et al: Acquired pure red-cell aplasia associated with an increase of T cells bearing receptors for the Fc of IgG. Acta Haematol 1981; 65:270.

53. Abkowitz JL, Kadin ME, Powell JS, et al: Pure red cell aplasia: Lymphocyte inhibition of erythropoiesis. Br J Haematol 1986; 63:59.
54. Akard LP, Brandt J, Lu L, et al: Chronic T cell lymphoproliferative disorder and pure red cell aplasia. Am J Med 1987; 83:1069.
55. Milnes JP, Goorney BP, Wallington TB: Pure red cell aplasia and thymoma associated with high levels of the suppressor/cytotoxic T lymphocyte subset. BMJ 1984; 289:1333.
56. Lipton JM, Nadler LM, Canellos GP, et al: Evidence for genetic restriction in the suppression of erythropoiesis by a unique subset of T lymphocytes in man. J Clin Invest 1983; 72:694.
57. Socinksi MA, Ershler WB, Tosato G, et al: Pure red blood cell aplasia associated with chronic Epstein-Barr virus infection: Evidence for T cell–mediated suppression of erythroid colony forming units. J Lab Clin Med 1984; 104:995.
58. Levitt LJ, Reyes GR, Moonka DK, et al: Human T cell leukemia virus-I–associated T-suppressor cell inhibition of erythropoiesis in a patient with pure red cell aplasia and chronic T-gamma-lymphoproliferative disease. J Clin Invest 1988; 81:538.
59. Hanada T, Abe T, Nakamura H, et al: Pure red cell aplasia: Relationship between inhibitory activity of T cells to CFU-E and erythropoiesis. Br J Haematol 1984; 58:107.
60. Nagasawa T, Abe T, Nakagawa T: Pure red cell aplasia and hypogammaglobulinemia associated with Tr-cell chronic lymphocytic leukemia. Blood 1981; 57:1025.
61. Shionoya S, Amano M, Imamura Y, et al: Suppressor T cell chronic lymphocytic leukaemia associated with red cell hypoplasia. Scand J Haematol 1984; 33:231.
62. Clark DA, Dessypris EN, Krantz SB: Studies on pure red cell aplasia. XI. Results of immunosuppressive treatment of 37 patients. Blood 1984; 63:277.
63. Firkin FC, Maher D: Cytotoxic immunosuppressive drug treatment strategy in pure red cell aplasia. Eur J Haematol 1988; 41:212.
64. Marmont AM: Therapy of pure red cell aplasia. Semin Hematol 1991; 28:285.
65. Zaentz SD, Krantz SB, Brown EB: Studies on pure red cell aplasia VIII. Maintenance therapy with immunosuppressive drugs. Br J Haematol 1976; 32:47.
66. Mangan KF, Shadduck RK: Successful treatment of chronic refractory pure red cell aplasia with antithymocyte globulin: Correlation with in vitro erythroid culture studies. Am J Hematol 1984; 17:417.
67. Harris SI, Weinberg JB: Treatment of red cell aplasia with antithymocyte globulin: Repeated inductions of complete remissions in two patients. Am J Hematol 1985; 20:183.
68. Leonard EM, Raefsky E, Griffith P, et al: Cyclosporine therapy of aplastic anaemia, congenital and acquired red cell aplasia. Br J Haematol 1989; 72:278.
69. Tötterman TH, Höglund M, Bengtsson M, et al: Treatment of pure red-cell aplasia and aplastic anaemia with cyclosporin: Long-term clinical effects. Eur J Haematol 1989; 42:126.
70. Chikkappa G, Pasquale D, Zarrabi MH, et al: Cyclosporine and prednisone therapy for pure red cell aplasia in patients with chronic lymphocytic leukemia. Am J Hematol 1992; 41:5.
71. Nakao S, Masaoka H, Shiobara S, et al: Dramatic improvement of pure red cell aplasia refractory to combined cyclosporine and prednisolone therapy induced by prednisolone dose escalation. Br J Haematol 1991; 79:520.
72. Lee TK: Fludarabine therapy of pure red cell aplasia. Blood 1997; 90(suppl 1):16b.
73. Berlin G, Liedén G: Long-term remission of pure red cell aplasia after plasma exchange and lymphocytapheresis. Scand J Haematol 1986; 36:121.
74. Lippman SM, Durie BGM, Garewal HS, et al: Efficacy of danazol in pure red cell aplasia. Am J Hematol 1986; 23:373.
75. Needleman SW: Durable remission of pure red cell aplasia after treatment with high-dose intravenous gammaglobulin and prednisone. Am J Hematol 1989; 32:150.
76. Katakkar SB: Pure red blood cell aplasia: Response to intravenous immunoglobulins, a blocking antibody (letter). Arch Intern Med 1986; 146:2288.
77. Clauvel JP, Vainchenker W, Herrera A, et al: Treatment of pure red cell aplasia by high dose intravenous immunoglobulins. Br J Haematol 1983; 55:380.
78. Battle JD Jr, Hewlett JS, Hoffman GC: Prolonged erythroid aplasia in chronic lymphocytic leukemia: Favorable response to adrenocortical steroids in four cases (letter). Ann Intern Med 1963; 58:731.
79. Slater LM, Schultz MJ, Armentrout SA: Remission of pure red cell aplasia associated with nonthymic malignancy. Cancer 1979; 44:1879.
80. Hunt FA, Lander CM: Successful use of combination chemotherapy in pure red cell aplasia associated with malignant lymphoma, histiocytic type. Aust N Z J Med 1975; 5:469.
81. Yamada O, Mizoguchi H, Oshimi K: Cyclophosphamide therapy for pure red cell aplasia associated with granular lymphocyte-proliferative disorders. Br J Haematol 1997; 97:392.
82. Molldrem JJ, Mavroudis D, Jiang YZ, et al: Hematological response in cya-treated T-cell large granular cell leukemia (T-LGL) correlates with an increase in killer inhibitory receptor (KIR) expression and loss of CFU-GM inhibition (abstract). Blood 1997; 90(suppl 1):503a.
83. Ito M, Imoto S, Nakagawa T, et al: Spontaneous remission in pure red cell aplasia associated with thymoma. Int J Hematol 1991; 54:209.
84. Lacombe C, Casadevall N, Muller O, et al: Erythroid progenitors in adult chronic pure red cell aplasia: Relationship of in vitro erythroid colonies to therapeutic response. Blood 1984; 64:71.

85. Anderson LJ, Young NS (eds): Human Parvovirus B19. Monogr Virol; 20. Basel, Karger, 1997.
86. Young NS: Parvovirus. In Fields BN, Howley MM (eds): Virology, ed 3. Philadelphia, Lippincott-Raven, 1996, pp 2199–2215.
87. Frickhofen N, Cohen B, Young NS, et al: Parvovirus B19 as a cause of acquired pure red cell aplasia (abstract). Blood 1991; 78(suppl 1):366a.
88. Frickhofen N, Young NS: Persistent parvovirus B19 infections in humans. Microb Pathog 1989; 7:319.
89. Kurtzman G, Cohen R, Field AM, et al: The immune response to B19 parvovirus infection and an antibody defect in persistent viral infection. J Clin Invest 1989; 84:1114.
90. Mintzer D, Reilly R: Pure red cell aplasia associated with human immunodeficiency virus infection: Response to intravenous gammaglobulin (abstract). Blood 1987; 70:124a.
91. Kho L-K: Erythroblastopenia with giant pro-erythroblasts in kwashiorkor. Blood 1957; 12:171.
92. Kurtzman G, Ozawa K, Hanson GR, et al: Chronic bone marrow failure due to persistent B19 parvovirus infection. N Engl J Med 1987; 317:287.
93. Kurtzman G, Frickhofen N, Kimball J, et al: Pure red-cell aplasia of 10 years' duration due to persistent parvovirus B19 infection and its cure with immunoglobulin therapy. N Engl J Med 1989; 321:519.
94. Kurtzman G, Cohen B, Myers P, et al: Persistent B19 parvovirus infection as a cause of severe anemia in children with acute lymphocytic leukemia in remission. Lancet 1988; 2:1159.
95. Coulombel L, Morinet F, Mielot F, et al: Parvovirus infection, leukaemia, and immunodeficiency. Lancet 1989; 1:101.
96. Corral D, Darras F, Jensen C, et al: Parvovirus B19 infection causing pure red cell aplasia in a recipient of pediatric donor kidneys. Transplant 1993; 55:427–430.
97. Nour B, Green M, Michaels M, et al: Parvovirus B19 in pediatric transplant patients. Transplant 1993; 56:835–838.
98. Frickhofen N, Abkowitz J, Safford M, et al: Persistent parvovirus infection in patients infected with human immunodeficiency virus type 1 (HIV-1): A treatable cause of anemia in AIDS. Ann Intern Med 1990; 113:926.
99. Gottlieb F, Deutsch J: Red cell aplasia responsive to immunoglobulin therapy as initial manifestation of human immunodeficiency virus infection. Am J Med 1992; 92:331–333.
100. Josephs HW: Anemia of infancy and early childhood. Medicine (Baltimore) 1936; 15:307.
101. Diamond LK, Blackfan KD: Hypoplastic anemia. Am J Dis Child 1939; 464–467.
102. Gasser C: Aplastische Anämie (chronische Erythroblastophthise) und Cortison. Schweiz Med Wochenschr 1951; 81:1241.
103. Allen D, Diamond LK: Congenital (erythroid) hypoplastic anemia. Am J Dis Child 1961; 102:416–423.
104. Janov A, Leong T, Nathan D, et al: Diamond Blackfan anemia—Natural history and sequelae of treatment. Medicine (Baltimore) 1996; 75:80–86.
105. Alter BP: The bone marrow failure syndromes. In Nathan DG, Oski FA (eds): Hematology of Infancy and Childhood, ed 3. Philadelphia, WB Saunders, 1987, pp 195–205.
106. Glader BE: Diagnosis and management of red cell aplasia in children. Hematol Oncol Clin North Am 1987; 1:431–447.
107. Young NS, Alter BP: Aplastic Anemia Acquired and Inherited. Philadelphia, WB Saunders, 1994.
108. Kinoti SN, Kasili EG, Bwibo NO: Congenital pure red cell aplasia (case reports from Kenya). East Afr Med J 1978; 55:530.
109. Ogasawa T, Kasahara H, Watanabe T, et al: A case report of constitutional erythroid hypoplasia (Josephs Diamond Blackfan type) with immunodeficiency. Jpn J Pedodontics 1987; 25:174.
110. Shada DC, Seif Eldin SA, Qattawi S: Congenital (erythroid) hypoplastic anemia (Diamond Blackfan syndrome). Indian Pediatr 1982; 19:803–805.
111. Diamond LK, Wang WC, Alter BP: Congenital hypoplastic anemia. Adv Pediatr 1976; 22:349.
112. Alter BP, Nathan DG: Red cell aplasia in children. Arch Dis Child 1979; 54:263.
113. Alter BP, Young NS: The bone marrow failure syndromes. In Nathan DG, Oski FA (eds): Hematology of Infancy and Childhood, ed 4. Philadelphia, WB Saunders, 1993, p 216.
114. Ball SE, McGuckin CP, Jenkins G, et al: DBA in the U.K.: Analysis of 80 cases from a 20 year birth cohort. Br J Haematol 1996; 94:W-653.
115. Kynaston JA, West NC, Reid MM: A regional experience of red cell aplasia. Eur J Pediatr 1993; 152:306–308.
116. Dianzani I, Garelly E, Ramenghi U: Diamond Blackfan anemia: Congenital defect in erythropoiesis. Haematologica 1996; 81:560–572.
117. Becker RE, Maurer H, Bowyer FP, et al: Growth hormone deficiency (GHD) in Diamond-Blackfan anemia (DBA) (abstract). Pediatr Res 1991; 29:74A.
118. Cathie IAB: Erythrogenesis imperfecta. Arch Dis Child 1950; 25:313.
119. Dunbar CE, Smith D, Kimball J, et al: Treatment of DBA with haematopoietic growth factors, granulocyte-macrophage colony stimulating factor and interleukin 3: Sustained remissions following IL-3. Br J Haematol 1991; 79:316–321.
120. Waterkotte GW, McElfresh AE: Congenital pure red cell hypoplasia in identical twins. Pediatrics 1974; 54:646.
121. Bello A, Dorantes S, Alvarez-Amaya C: La anemia hipoplastica en la edad pediatrica. Bol Med Hosp Infant Mex 1983; 40:718.
122. Madanat F, Arnaout M, Hasan M, et al: Red cell aplasia resembling Diamond-Blackfan anemia in seven children in a family. Am J Pediatr Haematol Oncol 1994; 16:260–265.
123. Schofield KP, Evans D: Diamond Blackfan syndrome and neutropenia. J Clin Pathol 1991; 44:742–744.
124. Brown K, Green S, de Mayolo JA, et al: Congeni-

125. Lipton JM: Congenital pure red cell aplasia. *In* Hoffman R, Benz E, Shattil SJ, et al. Hematology: Basic Principles and Practice. New York, Churchill Livingstone, 1995; pp 312–370.
124. tal anaemia after transplacental B19 parvovirus infection. Lancet 1994; 343:895–896.
126. Giri N, Tisdale JF, Kim S, et al: Diamond Blackfan anemia: In vitro and in vivo assessment of multi lineage hematopoiesis and natural history (abstract). Blood 1998; 92(suppl 1):16b.
127. Philippe N, Requin CH, Germain D: Etudes chromosomiques dans 6 cas d'anémie de Blackfan-Diamond. Pediatrie 1971; 26:47.
128. Brizzard CP, Fayard C, Fraisse J, et al: Anémie par anérythroblastoses (type Blackfan-Diamond) chez une enfant porteuse d'anomalies chromosomiques constitutionelles. Pediatrie 1971; 26:305.
129. Heyn R, Kurczynski E, Schmidel R: The association of Blackfan-Diamond syndrome, physical abnormalities and an abnormality of chromosome 1. J Pediatr 1974; 85:531.
130. Tartaglia AP, Propp S, Amarose AP, et al: Chromosome abnormality and hypocalcemia in congenital erythroid hypoplasia (Blackfan-Diamond syndrome). Am J Med 1996; 41:990.
131. Gustavsson P, Garelli E, Wraptchinskaia N, et al: Genetics of Diamond Blackfan anemia: Analysis of the chromosome 19q13.2 region in familial and sporadic cases. Nat Genet 1997; 16:368.
132. Zielke HR, Ozand PT, Luddy RE, et al: Elevation of pyrimidine enzyme activities in the RBC of patients with congenital hypoplastic anemia and their parents. Br J Haematol 1979; 42:381.
133. Glader BE, Backer K, Diamond LK: Elevated erythrocyte adenosine deaminase activity in congenital hypoplastic anemia. N Engl J Med 1983; 309:1486.
134. Glader BE, Backer K: Comparable activity of erythrocyte adenosine deaminase and orotidine decarboxylase in Diamond Blackfan anemia. Am J Hematol 1986; 23:35.
135. Glader BE, Backer K: Elevated red cell adenosine deaminase activity: A marker of disordered erythropoiesis in Diamond-Blackfan anaemia and other haematologic diseases. Br J Haematol 1988; 68:165.
136. Whitehouse DB, Hopkinson DA, Pilz AJ, et al: Adenosine deaminase activity in a series of 19 patients with Diamond Blackfan syndrome. Adv Exp Med Biol 1986; 195(pt A):85.
137. Hasegawa D, Kojima S, Tatsumi E, et al: Elevation of the serum Fas ligand in patients with hemophagocytic syndrome and Diamond-Blackfan anemia. Blood 1998; 91:2793–2799.
138. Perdahl E, Naprstek B, Wallace W, et al: Erythroid failure in Diamond-Blackfan anemia is characterized by apoptosis. Blood 1994; 83:645–650.
139. Halperin DS, Estrov Z, Freedman MH: Diamond Blackfan anemia: Promotion of marrow erythropoiesis in vitro by recombinant interleukin-3. Blood 1989; 73:1168.
140. Chan HSL, Saunders EF, Freedman MH: Diamond Blackfan anemia I. Erythropoiesis in prednisone responsive and resistant disease. Pediatr Res 1982; 16:474.
141. Lipton JM, Kudisch M, Gross R, et al: Defective erythroid progenitor differentiation system in congenital hypoplastic (Diamond Blackfan) anemia. Blood 1986; 67:962.
142. Tsai PH, Arkin S, Lipton JM: An intrinsic progenitor defect in Diamond-Blackfan anemia. Br J Haematol 1989; 73:112.
143. Freedman MH, D'Amato D, Saunders EF: Erythroid colony growth in congenital hypoplastic anemia. J Clin Invest 1976; 157:673–677.
144. Abkowitz JL, Sabo KM, Nakamoto B, et al: Diamond Blackfan anemia: In vitro response of erythroid progenitors to the ligand for *c-kit*. Blood 1991; 78:2198.
145. Chabot B, Stephenson DA, Chapman BM, et al: The proto-oncogene *c-kit* encoding a transmembrane tyrosine kinase receptor maps to the mouse W locus. Nature 1988; 335:88.
146. Geissler EN, Ryan MA, Housman DE: The dominant white spotting (W) locus of the mouse encodes the *c-kit* proto-oncogene. Cell 1988; 55:185.
147. Huang E, Nock K, Beier DR, et al: The hematopoietic growth factor KL is encoded by the Sl locus and is the ligand of the c-kit receptor, the gene product of the W locus. Cell 1990; 63:225.
148. Alter BP, Gaston T, Lipton JM: Lack of effect of corticosteroids in W/Wv and Sl/Sld mice: These strains are not a model for steroid-responsive Diamond-Blackfan anaemia. Eur J Haematol 1993; 50:275–278.
149. Dianzani I, Garelli E, Dompe C, et al: Mutations in the erythropoietin receptor gene are not a common cause of Diamond-Blackfan anemia. Blood 1996; 87:2568–2572.
150. Zhang MY, Clawson G, Olivieri N, et al: Expression of SCL is normal in transfusion dependent Diamond Blackfan anemia but other BHLH proteins are deficient. Blood 1997; 90:2068–2075.
151. Olivieri N, Felig S, Valentino L, et al: Failure of recombinant human interleukin-3 therapy to induce erythropoiesis in patients with refractory Diamond Blackfan anemia. Blood 1994; 83:2444–2450.
152. Neimeyer CM, Baumgarten E, Holidack J, et al: Treatment trial with recombinant human erythropoietin in children with congenital hypoplastic anemia. Contrib Nephrol 1991; 88:276.
153. Ball SE, Tchernia G, Wranne L, et al: Is there a role for interleukin-3 in Diamond-Blackfan anaemia? Results of a European multicentre study. Br J Haematol 1995; 91:313–318.
154. Splain J, Berman B: Cyclosporine A treatment for DBA. Am J Hematol 1992; 38:208–211.
155. Abkowitz J, Powell J, Nakamura J, et al: Pure red cell aplasia; Response to therapy with antithymocyte globulin. Am J Hematol 1986; 23:363–371.
156. Marmont AM: Congenital hypoplastic anaemia refractory to corticosteroids but responding to cyclophosphamide and anti lymphocyte globulin. Acta Haematol 1978; 60:90–99.

157. Bacigalupo A, Frassoni F, Podesta M, et al: Cyclosporine A- (CyA) does not enhance CFU-C growth in patients with severe aplastic anemia. Scand J Haematol 1985; 34:133.
158. Greco B, Bielory L, Stephany D, et al: Antithymocyte globulin reacts with many normal human cell types. Blood 1083; 62:1047–1054.
159. Lopez-Karpovitch X, Zarzosa ME, Cardenas MR, et al: Changes in peripheral blood mononuclear cell subpopulations during antithymocyte globulin therapy for severe aplastic anemia. Acta Haematol 1989; 81:176.
160. Nydegger E: Suppressive and substitutive immunotherapy: An essay with a review of recent literature. Immunol Lett 1985; 9:185.
161. Nusenblatt RB, Palestine AG: Therapeutic review. Cyclosporine: Immunology, pharmacology, and therapeutic uses. Surv Ophthalmol 1986; 31:159.
162. Kronke M, Leonard WJ, Depper JM, et al: Cyclosporine A inhibits T-cell growth factor gene expression at the level of mRNA transcription. Proc Natl Acad Sci U S A 1984; 81:5214.
163. Shevach EM: The effects of cyclosporine A on the immune system. Annu Rev Immunol 1985; 3:397.
164. Maraguche A, Butler JL, Kehrl JH, et al: Selective suppression of an early step in human B-cell activation by cyclosporine A. J Exp Med 1983; 158:690.
165. Hoffman R, Zanjani E, Zalusky R, et al: Diamond Blackfan syndrome: Lymphocyte mediated suppression of erythropoiesis. Science 1976; 193:899–900.
166. Ortega J, Shore NA, Dukes PP, et al: Congenital hypoplastic anemia inhibition of erythropoiesis by sera from patients with congenital hypoplastic anemia. Blood 1975; 45:83–89.
167. Finlay JL, Shahidi NT, Horowitz S, et al: Lymphocyte dysfunction in congenital hypoplastic anemia. J Clin Invest 1982; 70:619–626.
168. van Diemen PCM, Maasdam D, Darroudi F, et al: X-ray sensitivity of lymphocytes of aplastic- and Diamond-Blackfan–anemia patients as detected by conventional cytogenetic and chromosome painting techniques. Mutat Res 1997; 373:225–235.
169. Nathan DG, Hillman DG, Chess L, et al: Erythroid precursors in congenital hypoplastic (Diamond-Blackfan) anemia. J Clin Invest 1978; 61:489.
170. Freedman MH, Saunder EF: Diamond-Blackfan syndrome: Evidence against cell-mediated erythropoietic suppression. Blood 1978; 51:1125.
171. McGuckin C, Liu W, Ball SE, et al: Diamond Blackfan anaemia: Differential pattern of in vitro progenitor response to macrophage inflammatory protein 1-alpha. Br J Haematol 1996; 92:280–286.
172. Halperin DS, Freedman MH: Diamond-Blackfan anemia: Etiology, pathophysiology, and treatment. Am J Pediatr Hematol Oncol 1989; 11:380–394.
173. Bernini JC, Carillo J, Buchanan G: High dose intravenous methylprednisolone therapy for patients with DBA refractory to conventional doses of prednisone. J Pediatr 1995; 127:654–659.
174. August CS, King E, Githens JH, et al: Establishment of erythropoiesis following bone marrow transplantation in a patient with congenital hypoplastic anemia (Diamond-Blackfan syndrome). Blood 1976; 48:491–498.
175. Wiktor-Jedrzejczak W, Szczylik C, Pojda Z, et al: Success of bone marrow transplantation in congenital Diamond-Blackfan anaemia: A case report. Eur J Haematol 1987; 38:204–206.
176. Iriondo A, Garijo J, Baro J, et al: Complete recovery of hematopoiesis following bone marrow transplant in a patient with unresponsive congenital hypoplastic anemia (Blackfan-Diamond syndrome). Blood 1984; 64:348–351.
177. Lenarsky C, Weinberg K, Guinan E, et al: Bone marrow transplantation for constitutional pure red cell aplasia. Blood 1988; 71:262–229.
178. Zintl F, Hermann J, Fuchs D, et al: Correction of fatal genetic diseases using bone marrow transplantation. Kinderaerztliche Praxis 1991; 59:10–15.
179. Greinix H, Storb R, Sanders J, et al: Long-term survival and cure after marrow transplantation for congenital hypoplastic anaemia (Diamond Blackfan syndrome). Br J Haematol 1993; 84:515–20.
180. Mugishima H, Gale RP, Rowlings PA: Bone marrow transplantation for Diamond Blackfan anemia. Bone Marrow Transplant 1995; 15:55–58.
181. Alter BP: Childhood red cell aplasia. Am J Pediatr Hematol Oncol 1980; 2:121–139.
182. Casadavell N, Croisille, Isabelle A, et al: Age-related alterations in erythroid and granulopoietic progenitors in DBA. Br J Haematol 1994; 87:369–375.
183. Gasser C: Akute Erythroblastopenie. Schweiz Med Wochenschr 1949; 79:838.
184. Wranne L: Transient erythroblastopenia in infancy and childhood. Scand J Haematol 1970; 7:76.
185. Skeppner G, Forestier E, Henter JI, et al: Transient red cell aplasia in siblings: A common environmental or a common hereditary factor? Acta Paediatr 1998; 87:43–47.
186. Kynaston JA, West NC, Reid MM: A regional experience of red cell aplasia. Eur J Pediatr 1993; 152:306–308.
187. Farhi DC, Luebbers E, Rosenthal N: Bone marrow biopsy findings in childhood anemia—prevalence of transient erythroblastopenia of childhood. Arch Pathol Lab Med 1998; 122:638–641.
188. Cherrick I, Karayalcin G, Lanzkowsky P: Transient erythroblastopenia of childhood: Prospective study of fifty patients. Am J Pediatr Hematol Oncol 1994; 16:320–334.
189. Miller R, Berman B: Transient erythroblastopenia of childhood in infants < 6 months of age. Am J Pediatr Hematol Oncol 1994; 16:246–248.
190. Michelson AD, Marshall PC: Transient neurological disorder associated with transient erythroblastopenia of childhood. Am J Pediatr Hematol Oncol 1987; 9:161.
191. Young RSK, Rannels E, Hilmo A, et al: Severe anemia in childhood presenting as transient ischemic attacks. Stroke 1983; 14:622.
192. Labotka R, Maurer H, Honig G: Transient erythroblastopenia of childhood: Review of 17 cases,

including a pair of identical twins. Am J Dis Child 1981; 135:937–940.
193. Hays T, Lane PA, Shafer F: Transient erythroblastopenia of childhood. A review of 26 cases and reassessment of indications for bone marrow aspirate. Am J Dis Child 1989; 143:605.
194. Rogers ZR, Bergstrom SK, Amylon MD, et al: Reduced neutrophil counts in children with transient erythroblastopenia of childhood. J Pediatr 1989; 115:746.
195. Koenig HM, Lightsey AL, Nelson DP, et al: Immune suppression of erythropoiesis in transient erythroblastopenia of childhood. Blood 1979; 54:742.
196. Tamary H, Kaplinsky C, Shvartzmayer S, et al: Transient erythroblastopenia of childhood: Evidence for cell-mediated suppression of erythropoiesis. Am J Pediatr Hematol Oncol 1993; 15:386–391.
197. Rao SP, Miller ST, Brow AK: Transient erythroblastopenia of childhood in 2 pairs of siblings (abstract). Pediatr Res 1990; 27:148A.
198. Seip M: Transient erythroblastopenia of childhood in siblings. Acta Paediatr Scand 1982; 71:689.
199. Sorva R, Wegeluis R, Weber TH, et al: Transient erythroblastopenia of childhood. A retrospective study of 57 cases with a review of the literature. Eur Pediatr Haematol Oncol 1984; 1:189.
200. Kubic PT, Warkentin PI, Levitt CJ, et al: Transient erythroblastopenia of childhood (TEC) occurring in clusters. Pediatr Res 1979; 13:435.
201. Bhambhani K, Inoue S, Sarnaik S: Seasonal clustering of transient erythroblastopenia of childhood. Am J Dis Child 1988; 142:175–177.
202. Penchansky L, Jordan JA: Transient erythroblastopenia of childhood associated with human herpes virus type 6, variant B. Am J Clin Pathol 1997; 108:127–132.
203. Freedman MH: "Recurrent" erythroblastopenia of childhood. Am J Dis Child 1983; 137:458–460.

7

Agranulocytosis

Neal S. Young, M.D.

HISTORY

In 1922, Werner Schultz read a paper before the Society for Internal Medicine and Pediatrics in Berlin describing five women with fatal necrotic pharyngitis and absent polymorphonuclear cells, a disease which he termed agranulocytosis[1] (Fig. 7–1). The title of Schultz's talk, *Ueber eigenartige Halserkrankungen,* may be translated as "On Unusual Throat Diseases," and a popular name for the syndrome in the 1920s was agranulocytic angina. The dramatic findings in the throat dominated early case descriptions, and severe pharyngeal ulceration and extreme leukopenia, termed "putrid sore throat" and "primary gangrene of the throat," were described during the nineteenth century. In the early twentieth century, agranulocytosis seemed new: "The disease is one that is easily diagnosed, runs a dramatic and clear-cut course, and the fact that it was not observed before 1922 is practical assurance that it did not exist before that time. To state otherwise would be to reflect on the diagnostic acumen of our clinicians of the past. Blood counts have been taken for fifty years. We must consider, then, that granulopenia is a disease of modern times and one that has come among us during the past ten years."[2] In the late nineteenth century, leukopenia was considered rare and of mainly diagnostic interest, secondary to overwhelming or specific infections, especially typhoid fever, and depression of white blood cell production was seen during World War I after mustard gas poisoning. Türk had described absent myeloid cells in the autopsy marrow of a case of sepsis and absent granulocytes, which he termed "malignant neutropenia." Yet one Danish investigator's search of his hospital's records found no agranulocytosis cases before 1921 and a marked increase after 1930[3] (Fig. 7–2). The drama and novelty of agranulocytosis were conveyed in case histories, as in this extract from a report of Kracke and Parker: "For four days a strong man fifty-eight years of age feels sluggish and tired; the fifth day has a chill and fever; the sixth day a higher fever; the seventh day, a slight redness of the throat and a restless stupor; the eighth day, coma and death. There is a negative history of infection, a negative blood culture; only an absence of granulocytes from the blood stream and in the marrow an absence of granulocytes, myelocytes, and myeloblasts. What is it, and why is it?... These events develop and follow in an orderly sequence. We have had nothing like it before either in biology or in medicine."[4]

It was in America that the strong association of drug ingestion and agranulocytosis was recognized, and in the 1920s through the 1930s agranulocytosis was considered a new syndrome, specifically related to the introduction of drugs made from coal tar derivatives (Fig. 7–3). Agranulocytosis was first reported in the United States in 1924, and when the subject was reviewed a decade later almost 500 cases in the English literature could be collected. The analgesic aminopyrine was incriminated in the great majority of the early reports. An association with specific drug use—usually aminopyrine but also dinitrophenol, gold, and arsenic—was held responsible not only for the apparent increasing frequency of agranulocytosis in medical practice but also for the higher rate in the United States and Germany, in the middle and upper classes (especially among medical personnel), and among whites compared to blacks.

Aminopyrine had a central role in the elucidation of the mechanism of agranulocytosis. In 1933 Madison and Squier[5] at the University of Wisconsin reproduced agranulocytosis by readministration of a test dose of aminopyrine; in 1952 Moeschlin and Wagner[6] in Germany made a normal subject severely granulocytopenic by infusion

3 .November 1922 LITERATUR- UND VERHANDLUNGSBERICHTE 1495

Berlin, Medizinische Gesellschaft, 11. X. 1922.

Vor der Tagesordnung demonstriert V. Schilling einen Patienten aus Buchara mit einer **Filaria medinensis**, die in einem Furunkel am Unterschenkel steckt.

Tagesordnung. H. Lippmann: **Zur klinischen Diagnose des Morbus Gaucher.** Die Forschungen der letzten Jahre haben ergeben, daß die primäre Splenomegalie vom Typ Gaucher eine Erkrankung des gesamten hämatopoëtischen Systems ist. Die Krankheit tritt fast regelmäßig bei Geschwistern auf. Eine Vererbung ist nicht mit Sicherheit festgestellt, das weibliche Geschlecht ist stärker beteiligt, die Krankheit beginnt sehr frühzeitig, vielleicht kongenital. Das Hervorstechendste ist ein kolossaler Milztumor (bis 16 Pfund). Regelmäßig findet sich eine eigenartige Verfärbung der Haut, eine hämorrhagische Diathese und eine Verminderung der weißen Blutkörperchen. Der übrige Blutbefund sowie der Urinbefund sind normal. Bis zum letzten Stadium verläuft die Krankheit gutartig. Durchschnittsdauer der Morbidität 19,3 Jahre. Lippmann schildert ausführlich die Krankengeschichte eines von ihm beobachteten Falles. In der Familie sind weitere Kranke nicht gefunden worden. Die Haut ist bei der Aufnahme leicht ikterisch gewesen, jetzt aber kaum verändert. In der Hauptsache wurde ein großer Milztumor, Lebervergrößerung und Leukopenie festgestellt. Die Differentialdiagnose wird eingehend erörtert. Um den Verdacht auf Morbus Gaucher zu erhärten, wurde die Milz punktiert, und im Ausstrichpräparat fanden sich typische Gaucher-Zellen mit mehreren Kernen und Riffelung. Denselben Befund ergab ein ausgestanzter Milzzylinder. Es wurde in diesem Falle also zum ersten Male intra vitam geweblich die Diagnose gestellt. Von Milzexstirpation und Röntgenbestrahlung wurde wegen der damit verbundenen Gefahr abgesehen.

L. Pick: **Zur pathologischen Anatomie des Morbus Gaucher.** Pathologisch-anatomisch gleichen sich alle Fälle von Morbus Gaucher absolut. Pick verfügt über 3 Fälle, die noch nicht publiziert sind. Es handelt sich um eine Erkrankung des hämatopoëtischen Systems, die charakterisiert ist durch die typischen Gaucher-Zellen in Milz, Lymphdrüse, Knochenmark und Leber. Milz und Leber erreichen einen großen Umfang, während die Lymphdrüsen nicht vergrößert sind und auch am Knochenmark makroskopisch keine starken Veränderungen zu sehen sind. Ueberall findet man jedoch kleine, 60—80 μ große Herdchen aus Gaucher-Zellen. Weil die Zellen nestartig gelagert sind, faßte Gaucher die Krankheit als Karzinom auf. Man hat eifrig nach besonderen Stoffen in den Zellen gesucht. Es zeigt sich eine Xanthochromreaktion und regelmäßig Hämosiderose. Die einen glaubten, daß die Zellen von den Epithelien abstammen, es ist jedoch jetzt mit Sicherheit erwiesen, daß sie aus den Retikuloendothelien hervorgehen. Pick hat in der Milz Knochenmarksriesenzellen gefunden. Die hämorrhagische Diathese erklärt sich, wie auch die Hämochromatose, aus dem vermehrten Blutzerfall. — Von anderer Seite wurde die Beobachtung gemacht, daß sich beim Diabetes sowie bei tierexperimenteller Cholesterinfütterung ähnliche Zellen in der Milz finden. Ein Vergleich dieser Befunde mit dem Gaucher hält aber in keiner Weise stand. Histochemisch verhalten sich die Zellen völlig anders. Von Amerikanern wurde beim Gaucher eine Vermehrung der Blutlipoide festgestellt, und so ist es nicht ausgeschlossen, daß es sich um eine komplexe Störung des Eiweiß-, Lipoid- und Eisenstoffwechsels handelt. Demonstration zahlreicher makroskopischer und mikroskopischer Präparate, insbesondere von einem selbst beobachteten Falle, in dem sich die Einlagerung von Gaucher-Zellen in der Hauptsache im Knochenmark sämtlicher Knochen fand, mit einer teilweisen Zerstörung des Knochens, sodaß es zum Einbruch eines Wirbelkörpers gekommen war. Differentialdiagnostisch gegenüber der Tuberkulose ist das Erhaltensein der Zwischenwirbelscheibe von Wichtigkeit. In dem Knochenmark ließ sich eine Proliferation der Gaucher-Zellen nachweisen. Dresel.

Berlin, Verein für Innere Medizin und Kinderheilkunde (Pädiatrische Sektion), 9. X. 1922.

(Demonstrationsabend.)

Finkelstein: a) **Zur Nierenpathologie im Kindesalter.** Demonstration eines 12jährigen Knabens mit Granularatrophie der Nieren. Auffallend ist die beträchtliche Hypertonie und die Starre der peripherischen Arterien. Es besteht eine Hypertrophie des Herzens, Retinitis albuminurica und eine mäßige Störung der Wasser- und Kochsalzausscheidung. Ursache unbekannt. b) **Genuine Lipoidnephrose** bei einem 2jährigen Mädchen. Sehr starke Oedeme, die jeder Behandlung trotzen; aller Erfahrung nach ist der Tod innerhalb eines Jahres zu erwarten.

Besprechung. Hirschfeld (ad 1) hielt den Vergleich mit einer arteriosklerotischen Schrumpfniere nicht für berechtigt.

Davidsohn: **Drei Fälle von Fazialislähmung.** a) Traumatische Geburtslähmung nach Zangengeburt. b) Fazialis- und Gaumensegellähmung bei einem 4½ Monate alten Kinde im Anschluß an einen blutigen, diphtherischen Schnupfen, der mit 6000 I.E.Heilserum behandelt war. c) Fazialislähmung bei einem 4½ Monate alten kongenital-syphilitischen Säugling, bei dem die Lähmung wahrscheinlich durch eine interkurrente Varizellenerkrankung provoziert wurde. Lumbalpunktat nur Pleozytose als krankhafter Befund.

Karger: Heilung einer Miliartuberkulose. Demonstration eines Kindes, das klinisch und röntgenologisch den sicheren Befund einer **Miliartuberkulose** geboten hatte. **Heilung nach 7 Milzreizbestrahlungen.** Wahrscheinlich erklärt die Beschränkung der Aussaat auf ein Organ (Lungen) und das Verschontbleiben der Meningen den günstigen Ausgang.

Nathan: **Behandlung von Hautabszessen.** Bei einem zwei Wochen alten Säugling führten mächtige subkutane Abszesse am Oberschenkel und an der Brust zu einer Nekrose der Faszie und der Muskulatur. Nach zweimaliger Füllung der Wundhöhlen mit etwa 150 ccm Blut der Mutter und Naht aller vorher gesetzten Inzisionsöffnungen Besserung des Allgemeinbefindens und rasche Heilung mit völliger Bewegungsfreiheit des Beines.

Besprechung. Japha sah einen ähnlichen Fall nach 4 Caseosaninjektionen heilen und möchte die Heilung als Protoplasmaaktivierung deuten.

Karger zeigt an einem etwa 12jährigen Mädchen die Fähigkeiten der Eidetiker (Jensch), das sind Kinder, bei denen kurze Zeit gesehene Bilder außerordentlich lebhafte Anschauungsbilder hervorrufen, sodaß diese in allen Einzelheiten vom Kinde reproduziert werden können. Jenseits der Pubertät schwindet diese im Alter von 6 bis 12 Jahren häufige Fähigkeit. Die von Jensch behaupteten Beziehungen zur Tetanie und zum M. Basedow werden abgelehnt.

Nassau.

Berlin, Verein für Innere Medizin und Kinderheilkunde, 3. VII. 1922.

Offizielles Protokoll.

Vorsitzender: His. Schriftführer: Magnus-Levy.

Leschke: **Vergleichende Blutdruckmessungen in verschiedenen Gefäßgebieten und histologische Befunde bei Aortenklappeninsuffizienz.** (Als Orig.-Art. in Nr. 40 erschienen.)

Besprechung. Arnoldi: Bei dem Vergleich des Blutdrucks des rechten und des linken Armes kann man Unterschiede antreffen, auch ohne daß besondere Veränderungen an den Gefäßen anzunehmen sind.

Werner Schultz: **Ueber eigenartige Halserkrankungen. a) Monozytenangina.** Es handelt sich um eine Gruppe von diphtherieähnlichen, aber diphtherienegativen, oberflächlich nekrotisierenden oder pseudomembranösen Anginen, welche junge, syphilisfrei befundene Individuen zwischen 12 und 27 Jahren betrafen. Neben Halsbefund und regionärer Drüsenschwellung hatten von sieben beobachteten Fällen drei generalisierte Lymphdrüsenschwellung mit Beteiligung seltener befallener Drüsen, wie Thorakal- und Trapeziusdrüsen. Stets war die Milz vergrößert palpabel, und sechsmal bestand ebenfalls palpable Leberschwellung, nie Ikterus. Alle fieberten anfangs hoch (39,2 bis 40,8°), und die Fieberdauer war lang (zwischen 13 und 34 Tagen). Die palpablen Milzschwellungen waren in einigen Fällen 3 bis 4 Wochen verfolgbar, in anderen 2 bis 3 Monate, in einem Fall etwa 2 Jahre. Im Blute war die Gesamtleukozytenzahl entweder normal oder nur leicht erhöht (bis 16700), bei erheblicher Vermehrung der Monozyten (Höchstzahlen zwischen 27% und 78%), teilweise nahmen auch die Lymphozyten an der Vermehrung teil, wobei vielfach die Abgrenzung monozytoider lymphoider Formen von sicheren Monozyten schwierig war. Die Oxydasereaktion von Monozyten fanden wir nach der Technik von N. Rosenthal entweder negativ oder positiv, aber im letzteren Falle oft feiner und spärlich und immer deutlich unterscheidbar von der positiven Oxydasereaktion der polynukleären Neutro- und Eosinophilen. Für den oben beschriebenen Symptomenkomplex haben wir im praktisch klinischen Gebrauch die Bezeichnung „Monozytenangina" bei uns eingeführt. Die Fälle zeigen eine gewisse Verwandtschaft zu denen amerikanischer Beobachtungen. Auch Beobachtungen von Türk und Marchand gehören hierher. b) **Gangräneszierende Prozesse und Defekt des Granulozytensystems.** Sämtlich tödlich verlaufene Fälle betreffen normal ernährte Frauen von 38 bis 61 Jahren, ohne Syphilis, mit Ausnahme eines Falles (Aortitis). Krankheitsdauer drei bis vier Tage in 3 Fällen, in den beiden übrigen eine bzw. zwei Wochen. Die Erkrankungen verliefen hochfieberhaft, drei Fälle mit deutlichem, einer mit zweifelhaftem, einer ohne Ikterus. Alle hatten tiefgreifende nekrotisierende Prozesse, vier an einer oder beiden Mandeln, in einem der Fälle waren die Hauptprozesse im Bereiche von Zungengrund, Pharynx und Larynx, während nur eine Tonsille lakunär belegt war. Bemerkenswert ist das Auftreten von Gingivitis in zwei Fällen, von denen der eine anamnestisch bereits im Jahre vorher eine akute Gingivitis aufwies. Außer den Tonsillen waren von Gangrän befallen: die benachbarten Teile des weichen Gaumens, Uvula, Zunge, Pharynx und Larynx, je nach Ausbreitung des Prozesses. Einmal bestand gleich-

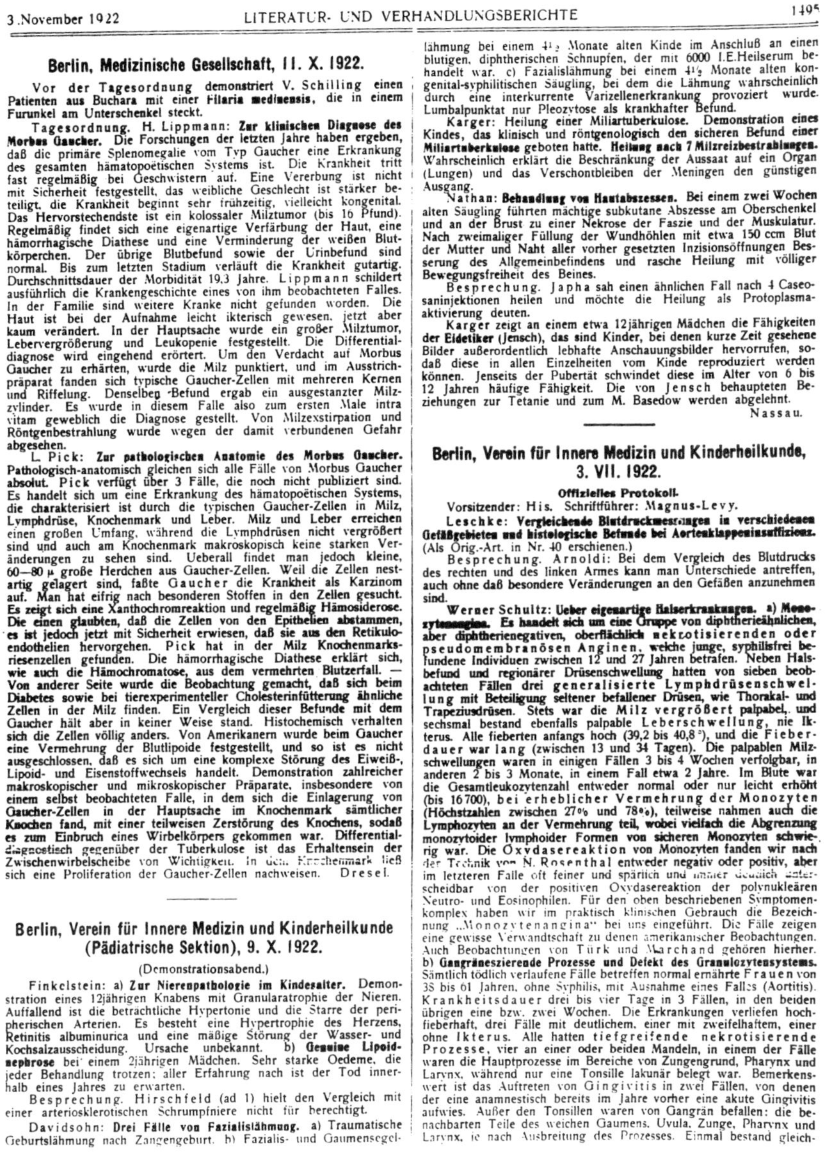

Figure 7–1 The first description of agranulocytosis: Schultz's report before the Society for Internal Medicine and Pediatrics, Berlin, July 3, 1922.[1]

of blood from an affected patient, and in finding drug-specific leukoagglutinins in the blood of neutropenic patients, established the immunologic mechanism of this form of agranulocytosis.[7] Agranulocytosis was considered a close relative of aplastic anemia (AA), especially because similar causative agents, like the antisyphilitic arsphenamine and benzene, were described for both types of marrow failure.

Careful observations of the clinical course of agranulocytosis led to the first recognition of the primary role of the depressed granulocyte number in the swift progress of trivial infection to sepsis, coma, and death. Study of bone marrow aspirates, obtained from patients at the onset of symptoms, as well as necropsy tissue, implicated failed myelopoiesis as the basis of agranulocytosis. The ability of drugs to elicit a damaging immune response was first recognized in the classic rechallenge and passive transfer experiments of the

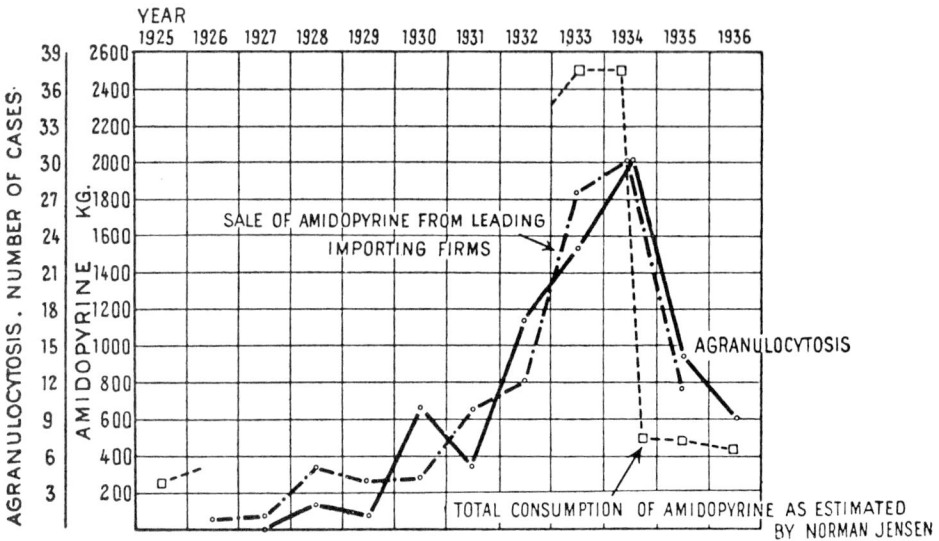

Figure 7-2 Close correlation between sales of amidopyrine and cases of agranulocytosis in Denmark in the 1930s.[3]

1930s. The history and clinical and laboratory aspects of agranulocytosis have been extensively reviewed.[8-12]

EPIDEMIOLOGY

The International Agranulocytosis and Aplastic Anemia Study (IAAAS) is the standard epidemiologic survey.[13] For this study, both community- and hospital-acquired cases were identified in eight European and Israeli metropolitan centers. Accurate incidence figures and case-control data for prior drug use were the main aims. About 116 million person-years were accumulated and 537 cases identified. The overall incidence of agranulocytosis was $3.4/10^6$ for a period that extended from 1980 to 1986. There was considerable variation in the incidence with geographic area, from high values of $7.0/10^6$ in Sweden and $6.5/10^6$ in Budapest to a low rate of $1.7/10^6$ in Milan. The rate of agranulocytosis rose with age: $1.1/10^6$ between 2 and 24 years, $2.7/10^6$ for 25 to 59 years, and $9.5/10^6$ for greater than 60 years. Only 10% of cases occurred in children and young adults, and more than half developed in older persons. Agranulocytosis was about twice as frequent among women as men. Both age and sex associations may only reflect more frequent medication use among women and the elderly. Some confirmatory results were obtained from an entirely different, faster, but also less comprehensive approach, the examination of computerized Medicaid billing data.[14] When computerized discharge diagnoses from the three American states for 1980 to 1985 were scanned for neutropenia, followed by chart review for substantiation, incidence rates of $2.3/10^6$ (Minnesota), $7.7/10^6$ (Michigan), and $15.4/10^6$ (Florida) were obtained, with an overall rate of $7.2/10^6$, figures quite similar to those of the IAAAS. As in the IAAAS, the rate of agranulocytosis increased with age. There also has been good agreement, for sulfonamide-associated agranulocytosis, in risk estimates derived from the Swedish Drug Monitoring System and a concurrent formal case-control study.[15]

Although incidence rates varied over time in the IAAAS, there were no consistent secular trends. Inexplicable differences in rates from one time period to another in this and other smaller studies have been blamed on underreporting due to ignorance of registries or loss of interest in protocols.[13] Rate differences are unlikely to be due to changes in drug use: the incidence of agranulocytosis in the Stockholm area has remained constant at about 0.01%, with new drugs supplanting older guilty agents removed from the market on the blacklists.

The rates of agranulocytosis and AA in the IAAAS appeared to be roughly inversely related,[13] and agranulocytosis is very rare in Thailand,[16] for example, where AA is relatively common. Note also that by comparison AA occurs mainly among young persons, and where sex ratios are not equal, they favor males rather than females. AA also is much less associated with drug use: in the IAAAS, about 65% of agranulocytosis cases were assigned

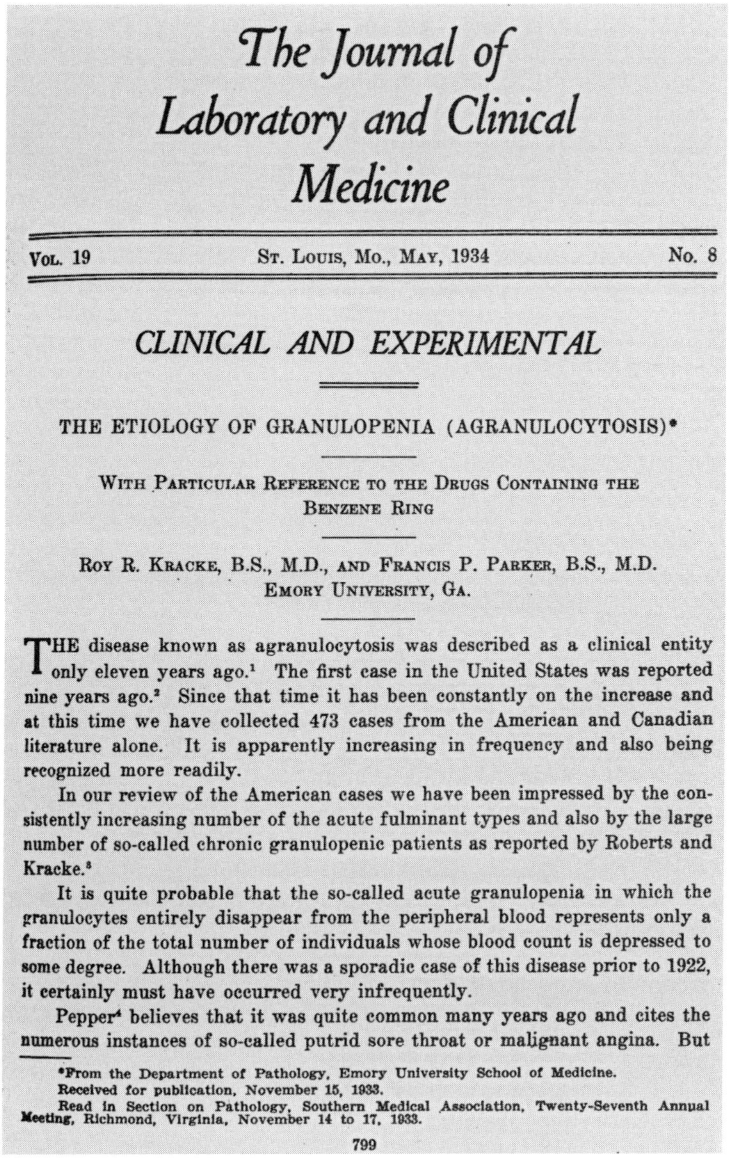

Figure 7–3 One of an important series of publications on the drug association of agranulocytosis was this by Kracke and Parker of Emory University.[2]

> # The Journal of Laboratory and Clinical Medicine
>
> VOL. 19   ST. LOUIS, MO., MAY, 1934   No. 8
>
> ## CLINICAL AND EXPERIMENTAL
>
> ### THE ETIOLOGY OF GRANULOPENIA (AGRANULOCYTOSIS)*
>
> WITH PARTICULAR REFERENCE TO THE DRUGS CONTAINING THE BENZENE RING
>
> ROY R. KRACKE, B.S., M.D., AND FRANCIS P. PARKER, B.S., M.D.
> EMORY UNIVERSITY, GA.
>
> THE disease known as agranulocytosis was described as a clinical entity only eleven years ago.[1] The first case in the United States was reported nine years ago.[2] Since that time it has been constantly on the increase and at this time we have collected 473 cases from the American and Canadian literature alone. It is apparently increasing in frequency and also being recognized more readily.
>
> In our review of the American cases we have been impressed by the consistently increasing number of the acute fulminant types and also by the large number of so-called chronic granulopenic patients as reported by Roberts and Kracke.[3]
>
> It is quite probable that the so-called acute granulopenia in which the granulocytes entirely disappear from the peripheral blood represents only a fraction of the total number of individuals whose blood count is depressed to some degree. Although there was a sporadic case of this disease prior to 1922, it certainly must have occurred very infrequently.
>
> Pepper[4] believes that it was quite common many years ago and cites the numerous instances of so-called putrid sore throat or malignant angina. But
>
> *From the Department of Pathology, Emory University School of Medicine.
> Received for publication, November 15, 1933.
> Read in Section on Pathology, Southern Medical Association, Twenty-Seventh Annual Meeting, Richmond, Virginia, November 14 to 17, 1933.
>
> 799

to a drug-attributable etiologic fraction by multiple logistic regression analysis, compared to 25% of aplasia cases.[13]

Relative risks for specific drugs are described in the discussions of individual agents below. Possibly ideal studies, in which the rate of a complication would be determined in a patient population receiving the drug by comparison with similar but untreated patients, are simply not available. A general trend is for early estimates of risk, usually gauged from small numbers of patients or collected series, to be much higher than when measured in formal epidemiologic studies. For example, in the case of aminopyrine and dipyrone, described at greater length below, the risk of agranulocytosis was early overstated as 1% to 4%, whereas the IAAAS upper estimate was about 1 in 50,000. Rate estimates of 1% to 2% agranulocytosis among treated cases probably represent the highest risk, for drugs like propylthiouracil, clozapine, and vesnarinone (see below). The probability of agranulocytosis is far lower for many other clearly associated agents: even arsenic compounds, given to more than 10% of naval personnel in 1932 as syphilis therapy, resulted in only a single case of agranulocytosis among 20,792 sailors treated![17] One understudied feature of drug induction of blood diseases is the role of host factors. For example, in a recent retrospective review of a large British database, agranulocytosis secondary to sulfasalazine and mesalazine occurred 10 times more frequently in patients receiving the drug for arthritis than in those with inflammatory bowel disease (Table 7–1), suggesting that patients with one form of an immunologically mediated disease might be particularly susceptible to a drug effect, also possibly immune-mediated.[18] HLA associations in agranulocytosis due to levamisole, clozapine, and methimazole (see below) may offer genetic markers for host susceptibility.

CLINICAL FEATURES

The classic presentation is fever and sore throat. Without treatment, agranulocytic pharyngitis is a severe syndrome: necrotic ulcerations with or without frank pus were commonly reported, with marked dysphagia or anginal pain and sometimes membrane formation. For example, in one early Canadian study of 30 patients, 60% had pharyngeal edema, 39% pharyngeal ulcerations, and 26% tonsillar ulcerations.[19] Systemic symptoms appeared out of proportion to the local throat findings, and tachycardia, lassitude, and prostration were present in advanced cases. Gangrenous stomatitis is recognized by spreading, dusky, purple or black lesions of the mucous membranes of the mouth or pharynx, and such frank tissue necrosis causes ulcerations (sloughed tissues appearing as pseudomembranes) and a fetid odor of the breath.[20] Tissue necrosis is probably the result of unopposed proliferation of the mixed endogenous mouth flora, anaerobic cocci, fusiform bacilli, vibrios, and spirochetes. In modern times, early application of antibiotics has much ameliorated neutropenic oral ulcerations. Now fever alone is probably the commonest symptom. Agranulocytosis may be entirely asymptomatic, especially when detected by weekly monitoring of blood counts in patients receiving drugs like clozapine.

The common complications of agranulocytosis reflect uncontrolled infection. Specific and localizing signs can be present on physical examination: abscesses of the head, neck, perineum and rectum; cellulitis; pneumonia; pseudomembranous enterocolitis; and bacteremic shock. Headache, fever, and prostration in patients and in volunteers who developed transient leukopenia after ingestion of small test doses of a suspected drug probably are mediated by massive release of cytokines from rapidly destroyed myelomonocytic cells. In comparison to patients who are leukopenic after cytoreductive chemotherapy, equivalent white blood cell levels in agranulocytosis are far more likely to be associated with symptoms.

Because of its drug relationship, agranulocytosis often occurs in patients with underlying illnesses requiring medication. However, unexpected signs like splenomegaly should point to an alternative diagnosis. Agranulocytosis can occur concomitantly with other drug toxicities like hepatitis and cutaneous eruptions.

Agranulocytosis has been divided into two clinical types corresponding to presumed pathophysiology: immune-mediated and direct drug toxicity. Immune agranulocytosis is described as typically having an acute course, and agranulocytosis related to toxic bone marrow depression as more insidious in onset and often asymptomatic. In my experience, the pattern of presentation is largely dependent on the degree of neutropenia and the likelihood of symptoms. In carefully monitored patients who developed agranulocytosis secondary to exposure to a single experimental cardiotonic

TABLE 7–1 Hematologic Complications of Sulfa Drugs in Two Diseases

Blood Disorder	Patients Treated for Arthritis (n = 3781)		Patients Treated for IBD (n = 6286)	
	Pts	Rate/1000 Users	Pts	Rate/1000 Users
Agranulocytosis	7	1.9	0	0.0
Neutropenia	7	1.9	2	0.3
Leukopenia	4	1.1	0	0.0
Pancytopenia	1	0.3	1	0.2
Thrombocytopenia	3	0.8	0	0.0
Hemolytic anemia	1	0.3	1	0.2
Totals	23	6.1	4	0.6

IBD, inflammatory bowel disease.
Adapted from Jick H, Myers MW, Deam AD: The risk of sulfasalazine- and mesalazine-associated blood disorders. Pharmacotherapy 1995; 15:176–181.

agent, some showed very rapid reduction in neutrophil number and soon developed symptoms, but in others the fall was more gradual and no symptoms developed despite days or a week or more of absolute neutropenia. Both patterns also have been described for clozapine. On rechallenge, neutropenia has recurred immediately with aminopyrine exposure, while severe neutropenia with phenothiazines has required longer exposure when the drug was reintroduced.

Laboratory Studies

Blood

All patients with agranulocytosis have a similar and characteristic blood picture. The blood smear shows absent neutrophilic granulocytes and usually no monocytes; bands and more immature myeloid forms are not seen, and toxic morphologic alterations in granulocytes are unusual in the absence of frank sepsis. Concomitant anemia in agranulocytosis is not uncommon, but thrombocytopenia is rare; reticulocytosis and thrombocytosis can occur during recovery. The degree of neutropenia in large clinical series is usually severe, perhaps the reflection of publication bias. Many drugs associated with agranulocytosis may also more commonly cause modest reductions in neutrophil number (examples include the phenothiazines, thiouracil derivatives, antiepileptics, and sulfa drugs), but such moderate leukopenia does not predict agranulocytosis, nor does continued treatment necessarily lead to worsened white blood cell counts.

Bone Marrow

The bone marrow morphology is more variable than the appearance of the peripheral blood smear (Plate 10). Absence of granulocytic precursor cells in the marrow defines agranulocytosis and distinguishes this syndrome from peripheral destruction of granulocytes, which also can be associated with drug administration. Marrow morphology spans the gamut from hypo- to hyperplasia of the myeloid series, even within series of patients with single drug exposures. In typical severe agranulocytosis, the marrow is empty of all granulocytic cells, but marrow aspirates from milder or convalescent cases may show early myeloid precursor cells from the promyelocyte to the myelocyte stage. Marrow hyperplasia may simply reflect late sampling during recovery; however, in some cases restriction of antibody binding or the drug effect to mature cells could lead to sparing of these precursors. "Maturation arrest," an unfortunate term that falsely implies a mechanism, almost certainly only reflects recovery of myelopoiesis.

In some serially sampled patients, myeloblasts, promyelocytes, and myelocytes appeared successively with marrow repopulation.[21] Total bone marrow cellularity has been directly correlated with the time to recovery, with samples containing myeloid cells most often observed within a week of appearance of granulocytes in the blood.[22, 23] Marrow lymphocytosis and plasmacytosis are inconsistent features. Some observers have suggested that lymphocytic infiltration early is a feature of immunologic agranulocytosis and delayed marrow lymphocytosis occurs with directly toxic effects of drugs.[8] Megakaryocytes are normal, but erythropoietic precursor cells have been decreased in some studies.

Other Laboratory Investigations

Antineutrophil antibodies have been measured by a variety of techniques, usually based on either physical binding or secondary effects on cell function.[24–26] Techniques include leukoagglutination; microagglutination; immunofluorescence; inhibition of granulocyte viability, metabolism, or of a specific neutrophil function such as phagocytosis-triggered release of $^{14}CO_2$; antibody-dependent lymphocyte-mediated granulocyte cytotoxicity; and protein A binding.

Leukoagglutinins were described in agranulocytosis due to aminopyrine and dipyrone and then phenylbutazone, the sulfonamides, mercurial diuretics, and chlorpromazine. Determination of antineutrophil antibodies in binding assays is more sensitive but less specific than the classic agglutination method. Demonstration of drug-dependent antibody binding is a reliable indicator of an underlying immunopathogenesis, but antibodies may be evanescent and their detection dependent upon the recent administration of the drug to the patient.[11]

Unfortunately, antineutrophil antibodies are not specific for either immune neutropenia or agranulocytosis. Tests may be positive in non-neutropenic patients with rheumatoid disease and high titers of rheumatoid factor or antinuclear antibodies. IgM autoantibodies are present in a significant proportion of normal persons, and antineutrophil antibodies appear after transfusion and pregnancy and in a wide variety of other conditions associated with neutropenia, including especially lupus erythematosus but also leukemia, lymphoma, paroxysmal nocturnal hemoglobinuria, liver disease, and in viral pneumonia. Antibodies directed to granulocyte cytoplasmic antigens may be present in vasculitis. In systemic lupus erythematosus, antinuclear antibodies that bind to DNA attached to cell surface receptors may be registered as antineutrophil antibodies. Antineutrophil antibodies can be found in other neutropenic states, including a large proportion of cases of chronic idiopathic neutropenia, Felty's syndrome and large granular lymphocytic leukemia. An assay for granulocyte-associated antibody rather than free antibody, analogous to the positive direct Coombs' test of autoimmune hemolytic anemia, has been suggested to be more sensitive and specific than measurement of free antibody to granulocytes; some patients with apparently immune-mediated neutropenia might have cell-associated antibody only.[27]

Pathogenic antibodies in agranulocytosis may be restricted to myeloid progenitor or precursor cells, while in immune neutropenia antibodies bind to peripheral blood granulocytes and not to precursor cells. For agranulocytosis, the presence of antibodies that inhibit myeloid colony formation in vitro[28] or that bind to immature myeloid cells[29] may correlate better with the clinical severity of the neutropenia than do antigranulocyte antibodies. In one case of acute agranulocytosis, the IgG appeared to recognize an Fc receptor,[30] and Fc receptors (NA1, NA2) are frequently the targets of antibodies in immune neutropenia. Specific experiments are required to demonstrate antibodies to myeloid precursor cells in individual patients; these are discussed below under Mechanisms.

Only occasionally have lymphocyte responses to drugs been measured, as for methimazole (see below), cimetidine (see below), sulfasalazine,[31] and indomethacin.[32]

While in vitro screening for drug effects on hematopoiesis is theoretically possible, the rarity of these syndromes cannot warrant the cost. In occasional cases, colony culture studies may point to one drug in a polypharmacy as an inhibitor.[10, 33]

DIFFERENTIAL DIAGNOSIS

Agranulocytosis should not be confused with other, more common, and usually more chronic forms of neutropenia (Table 7–2A–C). The diagnosis is immediate in the elderly woman with acute neutropenia and a history of ingestion of a suspicious drug. Although clearly age-related, agranulocytosis does occur in children, secondary, for example, to wide use of aminophenazone suppositories to suppress fever, and the distinction of a drug etiology from bacterial, viral, and idiopathic transient neutropenia may be difficult in young patients. In general, agranulocytosis is distinguished by the sudden fall in neutrophil number, the severity of the neutropenia, extreme local symptoms or frank sepsis, and the absence of anemia or thrombocytopenia. Although leukopenia of many causes is relatively common in internal medicine, the granulocyte level seen in genetic variations, secondary to infection, and as a feature of diseases like systemic lupus is relatively mildly depressed and rarely below 1000/µL. Secondary granulocytopenia also usually will be obvious from the clinical context. Importantly, such secondary neutropenia and neutropenia due to peripheral sequestration or destruction of granulocytes are almost always associated with a bone marrow aspirate showing abundant myeloid precursors. Severe neutropenia with myeloid *hypo*plasia is restricted to a very limited number of syndromes (Table 7–2C).

TABLE 7–2   Differential Diagnosis of Neutropenia*

Table 7–2A. Differential Diagnosis of Isolated Neutropenia
  Secondary to specific infectious agents
    Viruses, including viral hepatitis, Epstein-Barr virus, human immunodeficiency virus type 1
    Bacteria, especially in typhoid fever
    Rickettsiae
    Protozoa
  Secondary to overwhelming infection
    Sepsis
    Disseminated mycobacteria
  Collagen-vascular autoimmune diseases
    Systemic lupus erythematosus
    Felty's syndrome
  Starvation and kwashiorkor
  Alcoholism
  Ethnic and familial neutropenia ⎱ "Normal"
  Benign chronic neutropenia   ⎰ variation
  Myelodysplasia
  *Post chemotherapy, irradiation**
  Autoimmune neutropenia   ⎫
  Cyclical neutropenia   ⎪ Primary
  Pure white cell aplasia ⎬ hematologic
  Agranulocytosis   ⎪ diseases
  Large granular lymphocytic leukemia ⎭

Table 7–2B. Differential Diagnosis of Immune-mediated Neutropenia
  Agranulocytosis
  Pure while cell aplasia
  Autoimmune neutropenia
  Felty's syndrome
  Systemic lupus erythematosus
  Large granular lymphocytic leukemia

Table 7–2C. Differential Diagnosis of Isolated Neutropenia With Myeloid Hypoplasia
  Agranulocytosis
  Pure white cell aplasia
  Chronic idiopathic neutropenia
  Large granular lymphocytic leukemia
  Felty's syndrome (rarely)
  Myelodysplasia (rarely)

*Shown in italics are conditions in which the absolute neutrophil count is likely to be less than 500/µL.

Modest neutropenia, less than 1500/μL but rarely below 1000/μL, occurs normally among individual members and in families of some ethnic groups: American, West Indian, and African blacks; Arabs; and Yemenite and Ethiopian Jews. Hematopoiesis and bone marrow reserve are normal and there are no associated adverse clinical consequences. Although assumed to be familial and detectable in black American and African infants, leukopenia, at least among Africans, may be related to diet.[34] Familial neutropenia may be severe in the congenital neutropenias, lazy leukocyte syndrome, and myelocathexis. These syndromes are easily distinguished from agranulocytosis by their occurrence in families and the absence of a drug relationship. With mild neutropenia, symptoms will be absent; in patients with chronic moderate or severe neutropenia, infections of the skin, furunculosis or wound infection, and gingivitis are much more frequent than pharyngitis or sepsis.

Neutropenia accompanies a variety of specific infections, although the absence of leukocytosis or a low total white blood cell count is usually more striking and the absolute neutrophil numbers usually remain well above 500/μL. *Moderate* degrees of neutropenia are associated with specific bacterial infections (typhoid and paratyphoid fevers, brucellosis, tularemia, salmonellosis), rickettsial diseases (rickettsialpox, typhus, Rocky Mountain spotted fever, ehrlichiosis), viruses (flaviviruses and arenaviruses, hepatitis viruses), and protozoa (*Leishmania, Plasmodium*). The granulocyte number can be very low in bacterial sepsis and with advanced tuberculosis and other disseminated mycobacterial infections. Agranulocytosis can occur in severe kala-azar, in which the leishmaniasis is associated with splenomegaly. Severe neutropenia may persist for weeks in children recovering from respiratory tract infections, but their marrows show differentiating myeloid cells. Occasionally, absolute neutropenia and a marrow devoid of myeloid precursor cells—agranulocytosis—have occurred secondary to infection, as has been reported in cases of Epstein-Barr virus, typhoid fever, and viral hepatitis.

Modest neutropenia occurs in alcoholics, probably due to a combination of vitamin deficiency, splenomegaly, and a direct suppressive effect of ethanol on marrow function; alcoholics may be particularly slow to mobilize leukocyte reserves in the face of acute bacterial infection. Severe neutropenia (with anemia) can occur in copper deficiency; the marrow shows a deficiency of mature granulocytic cells.

In chronic idiopathic neutropenia, persistent neutropenia occurs in otherwise normal persons (usually young women), often in a familial pattern. Chronic neutropenia also occurs in children. Chronic neutropenia is more a syndrome than a disease. Despite the severe depression, even absence of neutrophils from the blood, severe infections are rare. Affected patients have cellular marrows with adequate myeloid CFU_{GM} progenitor numbers, and they mobilize granulocytes normally.

The most confusing aspects of the differential diagnosis are between agranulocytosis and other neutropenias with associated antineutrophil antibodies or associated myeloid hypocellularity (see Table 7–2B and C). Almost always the marrow in syndromes with antineutrophil antibodies shows the expected myeloid hypercellularity, but there are exceptional cases with myeloid hypoplasia. Diseases in which severe neutropenia is prominent often will be obvious from the characteristic clinical features or associated laboratory studies: isolated neutropenia with myeloid hyperplasia and joint symptoms implies Felty's syndrome; a physical examination will show splenomegaly in cases of splenic sequestration or primary splenic neutropenia. Other hematologic disorders will be defined by special bone marrow morphology, like the lymphocytic infiltration in large granular lymphocytosis.

MECHANISMS

That granulocyte production is affected far more frequently than red blood cell or platelet production by drugs and chemicals is likely due to the complex metabolic machinery of these cells and the development of degradative biochemical pathways at an early stage of myeloid maturation. The enzymes that process microbial pathogens also serve to alter drugs and chemicals into immunologically active or biochemically reactive compounds. Activated neutrophils may be especially efficient in oxidizing drugs, using enzymes like myeloperoxidase, to reactive metabolites that are able to form haptens with cell proteins and to induce antibody formation to cell membranes.[35] This type of mechanism has been implicated in agranulocytosis secondary to arylamines such as procainamide and dapsone; sulfhydryl-containing drugs such as propylthiouracil, captopril, and penicillamine; chloramphenicol (which can be reduced to an arylamine by gut bacteria); pyrazolones such as phenylbutazone; and anticonvulsants.

Two distinct mechanisms of drug-induced neutropenia have been advanced[8, 9, 36] (Table 7–3). This division is of heuristic value and widely accepted as the paradigm for drug mechanisms in agranulocytosis; however, for a particular case of

TABLE 7-3   Immune vs. Toxic Agranulocytosis

	Immune	Toxic
Paradigm drug	Aminopyrine	Phenothiazine
Time to onset	Days to weeks	Weeks to months
Clinical features	Acute, often explosive symptoms	Often asymptomatic or insidious onset
Rechallenge	Prompt recurrence with small test dose	Latent period, high doses required
Laboratory study	Leukoagglutinins; other antibody tests positive	Evidence of direct or metabolite-mediated toxicity to cells

agranulocytosis or new drug adverse reaction, inference of mechanism from clinical features is of dubious value; reports favoring both mechanisms have appeared for the same drug, and most cases of agranulocytosis will not be studied in the research laboratory.

Experiments in Humans

Not surprisingly, given its highly idiosyncratic nature, there is no animal model of agranulocytosis. Drugs have been readministered to patients after recovery from agranulocytosis. Madison and Squier reproduced neutropenia by readministration of amidopyrine to two recovered cases, in one man inducing absolute neutropenia within 12 hours (Fig. 7–4A).[5] Similar experiments with "test doses" (none of which could possibly be condoned by institutional review boards in our era) have been performed in susceptible patients and normal volunteers using aminopyrine[3, 37] and other drugs, including production of cutaneous wheal and flare reactions with local injection of drug or drug plus serum; even small amounts of aminopyrine injected intradermally can precipitate agranulocytosis.[38] Recurrent agranulocytosis has been well documented in many (but not all) patients ingesting aminopyrine derivatives. In contrast, prolonged administration of even high doses of amidopyrine does not lower granulocyte counts in nonsensitive patients.

Hematopoietic Colony Formation

Hematopoietic colony formation is not as consistently depressed in marrow samples from agranulocytosis cases as in AA. In many cases, colony formation by myeloid progenitor cells in the bone marrow is low, with 25%[39, 40] to 50%[22] of patients showing significantly decreased numbers of CFU_{GM}; compared to other types of neutropenia, a larger proportion of colony-forming cells are in active mitotic cycle.[40] Reduced myeloid colony formation during the acute phase of agranulocytosis with later recovery of colony numbers with convalescence has been reported for gold[41] and other agents. On the other hand, low colony formation by marrow sometimes has been observed weeks or months after recovery from neutropenia.[42] The normal colony formation that is frequently observed may reflect assay of a recovery marrow 1 to 2 weeks before return of granulocytes to the blood, or preservation of cells at the progenitor stage because of an insult to more differentiated precursor cells. Normal colony formation by marrow has been recorded even in the presence of a well-documented immunoglobulin inhibitor of myelopoiesis, suggesting that in some cases an antibody effect occurs during maturation after the CFU_{GM} stage.[43]

Serum Inhibitors

Moeschlin and Wagner[6] transfused blood from a patient with agranulocytosis due to aminopyrine into normal recipients and produced neutropenia within hours (Fig. 7–4B). The patient's plasma, after drug treatment or with the addition of the drug in vitro, but not the drug alone, agglutinated leukocytes in the test tube as well.[6] This early experiment established the causal relationship so strongly suggested by the clinical association of drug use and agranulocytosis. Later, leukocyte antibody activity was shown to be dependent on the presence of drug. Antibody plus drug also inhibited myeloid colony formation.[44]

In retrospect, the rapid decline in white blood cell number, often within minutes of the infusion, implicates a direct effect of a transferable factor on circulating cells as much as on marrow precursors. Opsonization of normal neutrophils can be demonstrated equally well with sera from patients whose neutropenia is associated with marrow depression as from those with peripheral leukocyte destruction. Reactivity with both myeloid progenitors and mature granulocytes was shown in one well-studied case of propylthiouracil agranulocytosis: a complement-dependent serum antibody bound myeloid progenitors and inhibited CFU_{GM}-derived colony formation, especially in the pres-

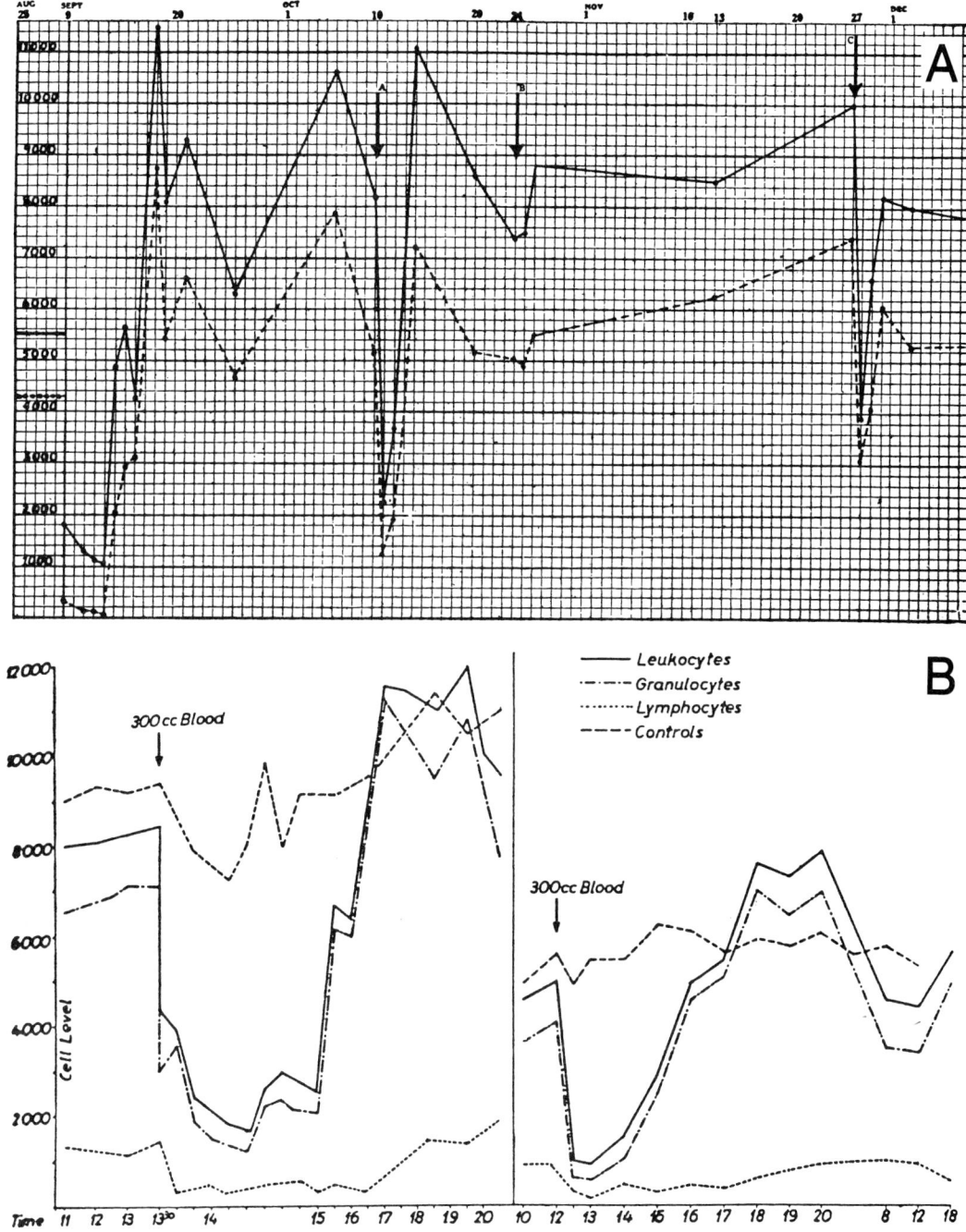

Figure 7–4 Blood count records after experimental reexposure of a sensitive patient to amidopyrine[5] **(A)**, and on infusion of serum from a patient with amidopyrine-induced agranulocytosis into a normal volunteer[6] **(B)**.

ence of added drug, and antibody also bound circulating granulocytes and monocytes.[45] Serum antibody inhibited erythroid as well as myeloid colony formation in this case, despite normal erythropoiesis in the patient's bone marrow, but consistent with depression of erythroid precursor cells in some instances of agranulocytosis. Plasma inhibitors of myelopoiesis, sometimes identified as antibodies, have been demonstrated in coculture with marrow cells either alone or in the presence of the drug, for many agents, including amidopyrine, thyrostatics, diphenylhydantoin, quinidine, chlorpropamide, ibuprofen, and clozapine. Inhibition in colony culture has been used to incriminate a single drug in a patient receiving dual antimalarial prophylaxis.[33] The relative specificity of a putative serum antibody for immature progenitors compared to granulocytes was nicely demonstrated for chlorpropamide agranulocytosis, in which the patient's serum inhibited CFU_{GM}-derived colony formation in a drug dose–dependent manner, but it did not inhibit erythroid progenitor–derived or mixed colonies, nor did the serum bind to either neutrophils or recognizable granulocytic precursor cells.[46]

Experiments to detect a plasma inhibitor of granulocytopoeisis cannot be routinely used to characterize an antibody in an individual case of agranulocytosis. The tests require adequate controls for the conditions of tissue culture, for inhibition by normal serum and its components, and to elicit antibody effects that may be dependent on the presence of the drug or on complement. Often the drug is insoluble in media. Tissue culture experiments, if performed, are seldom adequately controlled or rigorously designed. In some systematic studies, serum inhibitors were elusive and only could be demonstrated in a small minority (10%) of plasma samples using progenitor assays.[39]

The ability to detect an antibody in agranulocytosis can be much improved by employing multiple assays, some of which use granulocyte binding as a surrogate for colony culture testing of a progenitor effect. These tests are easier to perform, but they will miss cases in which antibodies are truly specific for a progenitor cell.[46] (In addition, as with other autoantibodies, it often is not possible to distinguish antibody formation that is secondary to cell destruction, with release of normally hidden cell antigens, from truly pathogenic cytotoxic antibodies.) IgG or IgM antibodies were detected in 13 of 13 cases of drug-associated agranulocytosis (with hypoplastic bone marrows) using enzyme-linked binding assays for antibodies to autologous or normal granulocytes.[47] Antibodies from agranulocytic patients also inhibit in assays of granulocyte metabolism.[48] Binding of antibodies to HL60 leukemic cells may be a substitute for marrow progenitor recognition; sera from patients with procainamide agranulocytosis showed equal reactivity to leukemic cells as to normal granulocytes (a pattern also seen with neutropenia in other conditions such as rheumatoid arthritis and large granular lymphocytosis).[49]

Intermediate metabolites of drugs might be expected to serve as better antigens than the parent compounds in these assays, as they are highly reactive and can covalently bind to macromolecules, including cell surface proteins, to create neoantigens. Serum reactivity to metabolite-cell mixtures has been enhanced after addition of a purified amodiaquine metabolite to target neutrophils[50] or only became apparent if metabolites, in the urine of treated patients, were added to the target cells.[47] Drugs may be selectively metabolized by activated neutrophils[51] or they may diffuse from one cell type and affect white blood cells secondarily.[52]

Cellular Immunity

Strong HLA class II associations in agranulocytosis among Ashkenazi Jewish patients receiving clozapine[53] and Japanese patients treated with methimazole[54] support a role for T cells in this form of marrow failure (Table 7–4). Lymphocyte inhibition of in vitro myelopoiesis has not been much studied and only described in a few cases of agranulocytosis,[55-57] including neutropenia secondary to chronic infection and Felty's syndrome. Patients with agranulocytosis secondary to clozapine had a high frequency of specific tumor necrosis factor (TNF) polymorphisms[58] (genetic differ-

TABLE 7–4 HLA Associations in Agranulocytosis

Disease	Population	Drug	HLA Antigen
Rheumatoid arthritis		Levamisole	B27
Schizophrenia	Ashkenazi Jewish	Clozapine	B38; DRB1*0402, DRB4*0101, DQB1*0302, DQA1*301
Graves' disease	Japanese	Methimazole	DRB1*08032

Data from references 53, 54, 136.

ences in the TNF-α affect gene transcription and the cytokine response to infections).

Direct Cytotoxicity

Direct toxicity by a drug or its metabolites was proposed early by analogy with benzene.[2] Evidence for a direct effect was provided by Pisciotta[59] for phenothiazine derivatives in the late 1960s. The antipsychotics chlorpromazine, promazine, and mepazine were most frequently reported. These phenothiazines were so often implicated in agranulocytosis that psychiatric patients routinely were monitored by weekly blood counts. Blood count monitoring also showed that about one tenth to one third of patients developed a transient and modest decrease in leukocytes early in treatment, unrelated to the rarer idiosyncratic reaction and perhaps dose-related.

Phenothiazine agranulocytosis had a pattern of leukocyte count depression sufficiently distinct from aminopyrine agranulocytosis to suggest a different mechanism. The phenothiazines' adverse effect required many weeks of treatment, usually to substantial cumulative doses, yet seldom occurred after 3 months of therapy. In contrast to aminopyrine, readministration did not produce a prompt decline in neutrophil number; large doses over time again were required to reinduce agranulocytosis, and some patients could be successfully re-treated with lower doses of drug.

Pisciotta studied the effect of chlorpromazine on human bone marrow in which DNA and RNA synthesis was measured by incorporation of radioactively labeled nucleotides.[59] The labeling index varied widely among hematologically normal persons and was less than 50% in about half, but a low labeling index in a hematologically normal marrow donor did not predict the occurrence of agranulocytosis with treatment. In contrast, in patients who had recovered from agranulocytosis due to chlorpromazine (but not for other types of agranulocytosis), cell proliferation was consistently lower, and thymidine incorporation could be further and completely suppressed by low concentrations of chlorpromazine. Bone marrow cells obtained during chlorpromazine treatment had a lower index but were no longer suppressed by chlorpromazine, suggesting the development of "resistance" under normal circumstances to the drug's effect on DNA synthesis. Chlorpromazine binds to proteins and can inhibit some DNA and RNA polymerases. These experiments support a nonimmune basis for agranulocytosis accompanying phenothiazine therapy. The variable degrees of inhibition of marrow cell proliferation by chlorpromazine in vitro would account for the common occurrence of modest leukopenia during treatment. Rarer and as yet undefined genetic defects in phenothiazine accumulation, metabolism, or detoxification would be responsible for idiosyncratic agranulocytosis.

Dose-dependent inhibition of in vitro colony formation has been demonstrated for other drugs implicated in agranulocytosis. Gold in the form of sodium aurothiomalate inhibited normal colony formation, at concentrations achieved in the bone marrows of treated patients, implicating altered metabolism of gold in the idiosyncratic reaction.[41] Several classes of antibiotics, including penicillins, β-lactams, and trimethoprim-sulfamethoxazole, also directly suppress myelopoiesis in vitro (see below). A metabolite of the antimalarial dapsone inhibited granulocyte colony formation in vitro, perhaps by generation of hydrogen peroxide and oxidant-mediated cytotoxicity.[60] In one systematic study of agranulocytosis, implicated drugs at plasma concentrations observed in patients inhibited hematopoietic colony formation in 10 of 14 cases.[61]

DRUGS

Agranulocytosis is the most common adverse hematologic reaction to drugs, and the great majority of cases of agranulocytosis are related to prior medical drug use (Tables 7–5 and 7–6). In collections of patients, a significant drug history can be obtained in 80% to 100% of cases. By the criteria of the IAAAS, the majority of cases of agranulocytosis were considered drug-related.[13] In most published series, aminopyrine or dipyrone has been most frequently linked to agranulocytosis, followed by sulfonamides, chlorpromazine, and other sulfa drugs.[19, 62] These associations were confirmed in the IAAAS, although the absolute number of cases of drug-associated agranulocytosis relative to the size of the population at risk was quite low (see Table 7–6).

Analgesics and Nonsteroidal Anti-inflammatory Drugs (NSAIDs)

The role played by analgesics and NSAIDs in the recognition of the drug component in the etiology of agranulocytosis has been described above. Pyrazolone was discovered in 1886; aminopyrine, dipyrone, antipyrine, and 4-aminoantipyrine are nearly identical molecules (see Fig. 7–5). Aminopyrine was introduced as an analgesic and antipyretic in 1897, and as an effective rival to the salicylates it gained worldwide popularity in the 1920s and 1930s. Almost 50 different proprietary preparations of aminopyrine were marketed in the

TABLE 7–5 Drugs Associated With Agranulocytosis*

Heavy metals
  Gold
  Arsenical compounds
  Mercurial diuretics
Analgesics and nonsteroidal anti-inflammatory drugs
  Aminopyrine, dipyrone, and related compounds (see text)
  Phenylbutazone and oxyphenbutazone, para-aminosalicylic acid, ibuprofen, indomethacin, diflunisal, benoxapren, sulindac, fenoprofen, tolmetin, etodolac
  Acetaminophen
  Cinchophen
Antipsychotics, sedatives, antidepressants
  Phenothiazines (e.g., chlorpromazine, mepazine, diethazine)
  Imipramine, desipramine, metapramine, clomipramine
  Chlordiazepoxide
  Amoxapine
  Meprobamate
  Pyrithyldione
  Barbiturates
  Minaprine
  Serotonin reuptake inhibitors
Anticonvulsants
  Phenytoin, diphenylhydantoin, methoin, trimethadione
  Ethosuximide
  Carbamazepine
Antithyroid drugs
  Propylthiouracil, methylthiouracil
  Methimazole
  Potassium perchlorate
  Thiocyanate
Cardiovascular drugs
  Procainamide, including sustained release form; tocainide
  Captopril
  Aprindine
  Propafenone
  Nifedipine
  Quinidine
  Ethacrynic acid (and other sulfa-based diuretics; see below)
  Propranolol
  Methyldopa
  Ajmalin (an antiarrhythmic)
Sulfa drugs
  Sulfonamides, including thiazide diuretics, spironolactone, methazolamide, and acetazolamide
  Oral hypoglycemics, including chlorpropamide and tolbutamide
  Sulfasalazine
  Dapsone
  Sulfa antibiotics (sulfathiazole, sulfadimethoxine, sulfadiazine, sulfamethoxypyridazine, sulfaguanidine, sulfapyridine, sulfanilamide, sulfamethoxazole-trimethoprim, sulfadiazine silver)
Pyritinol (antidepressant)
Antibiotics
  Sulfa antibiotics (see above)
  Penicillins (benzylpenicillin, penicillin G, oxacillin and cloxacillin, methicillin and nafcillin, carbenicillin, ticarcillin, ampicillin)
  Vancomycin
  Cephalosporins (cephalothin and derivatives, amoxicillin–clavulinic acid)
  Macrolides (erythromycin, roxithromycin)
  Streptomycin
  Gentamicin
  Clindamycin
  Nitrofurantoin
  Novobiocin
  Antituberculosis agents (isoniazid, rifampin, thiacetazone)
  Antifungals, including flucytosine, fluconazole
  Pyrimethamine (antitoxoplasmosis antifolinic)
  Mebendazole
  Levamisole (antihelmintic, also used in rheumatoid arthritis; see text)
  Antimalarials, including quinine, amodiaquine, chloroquine, hydroxychloroquine, quinacrine and dapsone (see above under Sulfa drugs)
  Zidovudine
Antihistamines
  Metiamide, cimetidine and ranitidine, omeprazole
  Tripelenamine, thenalidine, chlorpheniramine, brompheniramine, methaphenilene
  Mianserin
Miscellaneous drugs
  Isoretinoin
  Phenindione (anticoagulant)
  Colchicine
  Allopurinol
  Aminoglutethimide (an anticonvulsant, now used in Cushing's syndrome)
  Metoclopramide (antiemetic)
  Ticlopidine (antiplatelet agent)
  Tamoxifen
  Penicillamine
  1,2-Dimethyl-3-hydroxypyrid-40-one (L_1 oral iron chelator)
Miscellaneous chemicals
  Dinitrophenol
  Insecticides (DDT)
  Mustard gas
  Chinese herbal medicines, including yohimbine
  Hair dye

*Based on primary references and on published lists; sources and citations are available in Young and Alter.[12] Cases in which bone marrow examinations were not reported have been excluded to avoid confusion with peripheral granulocyte destruction.

TABLE 7-6 Drugs Associated With Agranulocytosis—International Aplastic Anemia and Agranulocytosis Study

Drug	RR	Excess Risk*
Cinepazide	∞	†
Sulfasalazine	∞	†
Antithyroid drugs	97	5.3
Macrolides	54	6.7
Procainamide	~50	3.1
Aprindine	~49	2.7
Dipyrone	16	0.6
Co-trimoxazole	16	1.7
Thenalidine	~16	2.4
Carbamazepine	11	0.6
Digitalis glycosides	2.5–9.9	0.1–0.3
Indomethacin	6.6	0.4
Troxerutin	6.0	0.3
Sulfonylureas	4.5	0.2
Corticosteroids	4.1	†
Butazones	3.9	0.2
Dipyridamole	3.8	0.2
β-Lactams	2.8	0.2
Propranolol	2.5	0.1
Salicylates	2.0	0.06

RR, multivariate relative risk estimate.
*Excess risk expressed as number of cases per 10^6 users in 1 week.
†Excess risk not calculated due to absence of exposed controls or, in the case of corticosteroids, confounding of causal relationship by the diagnosis of rheumatoid arthritis.
Data from Kaufman DW, Kelly JP, Levy M, et al: The Drug Etiology of Agranulocytosis and Aplastic Anemia. New York, Oxford University Press, 1991.

United States in the early part of the century, the multiplicity of names under which aminopyrine was marketed often confusing the investigation of individual cases of agranulocytosis. A prescription for aminopyrine was not required until 1938, around which time approximately 30 million were written in the United States annually. Dipyrone, a sulfonated chemical cousin of aminopyrine, remains a widely used analgesic and antipyretic in Europe, where it can be bought over-the-counter under a variety of labels; in Asia, where it (and phenylbutazone) are added to Chinese herbal remedies; and as an ingredient in alternative medicines in the United States ("Mexican aspirin").

Dipyrone and its derivatives dominate the agranulocytosis drug lists in modern European series.[62] Exposure has been cited in occasional cases of AA and leukemia as well. Skin contact with phenazone cream, chemically similar to aminopyrine, apparently has produced agranulocytosis, as has intravenous dipyrone used in trauma victims. Even with the recognition of agranulocytosis as a serious complication, aminopyrine still had advocates who argued its superiority to salicylates and corticosteroids for treatment of some chronic febrile states. However excellent an antipyretic and analgesic this class of chemicals, the available alternatives, aspirin and acetaminophen, have not been associated with agranulocytosis (although these drugs have other morbid effects).

From collections of reported series, the rate of aminopyrine-induced agranulocytosis was early estimated at almost 1%, with a mortality rate of about 0.5% for all patients who had received the drug[63]; more conservative estimates have been based on the number of prescriptions written (1 case per 10,000 drug courses)[38] or tablets sold (1 per 40,000[62]). The risks of pyrazolone induction of agranulocytosis have ranged over more than three orders of magnitude, from 1 in 116 to 1 in 466,000 exposures. High estimates usually have been based on reviews of published cases, but publication is often prompted by the occurrence of agranulocytosis (while negative series are not presented).[9] The 1% risk of agranulocytosis due to pyrazolone appears to be a gross overestimate and has been discredited by formal epidemiologic studies.[13, 64] Even assuming that every case of agranulocytosis identified in the IAAAS were indeed due to dipyrone, the absolute risk was estimated at only 3 to $19/10^6$ exposures.[65]

As described above, there is considerable evidence from in vivo and in vitro experiments that agranulocytosis secondary to aminopyrine is antibody-mediated. Drug-dependent leukoagglutinins and leukocytotoxins have been described in some, if not all, patients;[66] these leukoagglutinins can sometimes show extraordinary specificity for chemical structure.[67] Antibody-mediated inhibition of myelopoiesis is also drug dependent.[43, 44] Antibody and leukoagglutinin, as well as colony-inhibiting activity, can persist for months or more into convalescence, with clinical recovery presumably due to declining plasma drug levels.[43, 68] As Madison and Squier showed experimentally,[5] and has been observed in some recalcitrant patients, agranulocytosis occurs acutely on administration of aminopyrine. A latent reaction has been described to the closely related chemical antipyrine, with leukopenia developing 8 weeks after a single test dose with associated leukoagglutinins.[69] In vitro, aminopyrine can be metabolized by neutrophil hypochlorous acid to a highly reactive cation radical,[70] which could serve as a hapten or to alter a normal protein's conformation in the myeloid cell.

Phenylbutazone and aminopyrine are chemically similar, both sharing a phenyl-substituted pyrazolone core structure (Fig. 7–5). NSAIDs have been associated with agranulocytosis by both case reports[71, 72] and in epidemiologic surveys. In

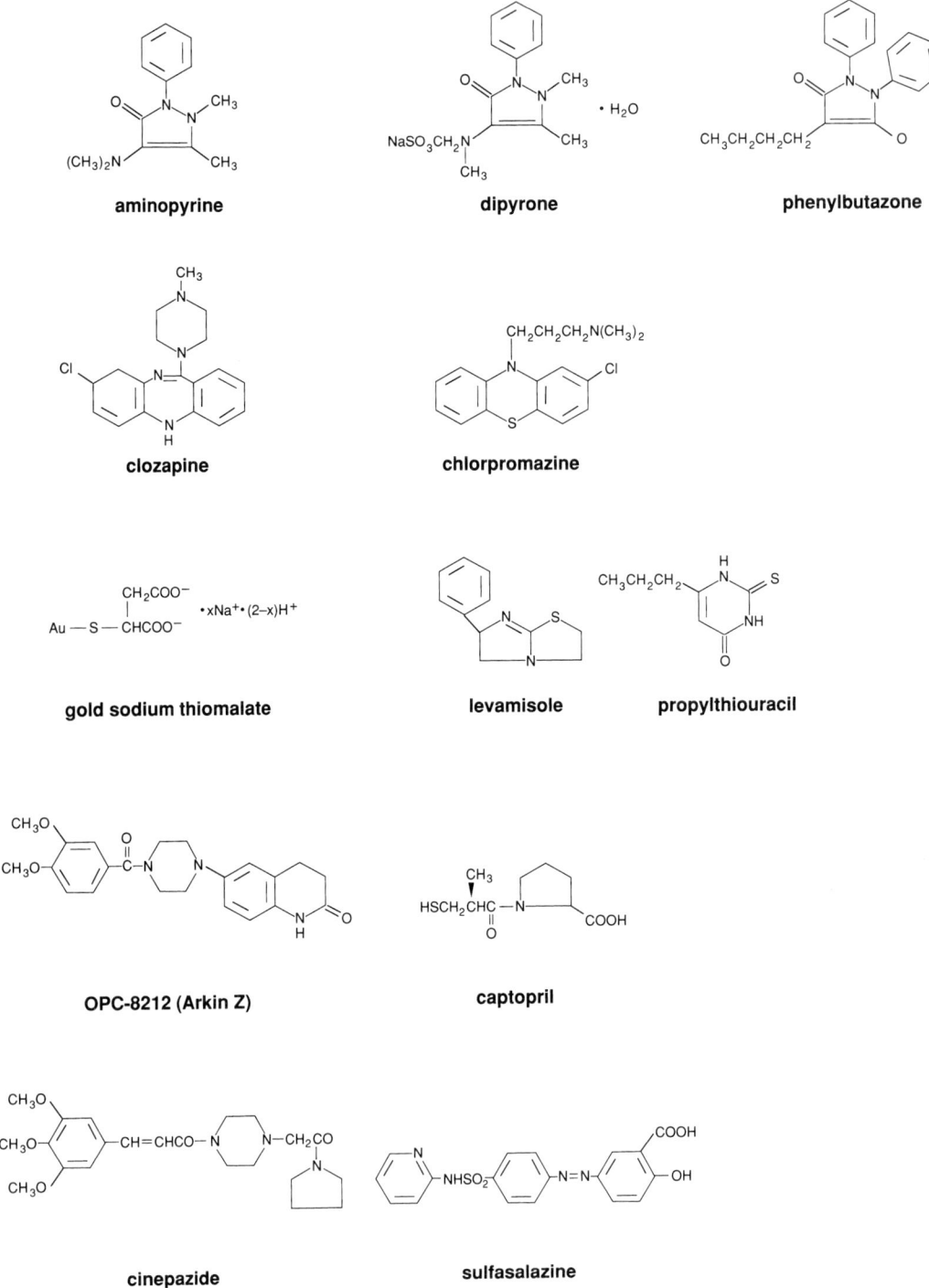

Figure 7–5 Structures of some chemicals and drugs associated with agranulocytosis.

the formal IAAAS, the relative risk of agranulocytosis with prior indomethacin exposure was 6.6, for butazones 3.9, and (nonsignificantly) elevated even for aspirin at 2.0[13] (see Table 7–6). Mild leukopenia can accompany phenylbutazone therapy and is probably unrelated to, if sometimes confused with, true agranulocytosis.[72, 73] Agranulocytosis is significantly associated but is still a rare complication of nonsteroidal drug use in collected series of patients and in populations. (Nonsteroidal drug use also has been associated with AA and, much less frequently, with pure red cell aplasia.) Susceptibility has been blamed on abnormal clearance of the drug,[74] increased sensitivity of the affected individual's marrow cells,[75] and immune mechanisms, both humoral[43] and cellular.[57]

Antithyroid Agents

Most estimates of risk have been based on extrapolations from cases of agranulocytosis identified in thyroid disease clinics. In early series, thiouracil was reported to cause agranulocytosis in about 2% of treated patients, and later estimates for propylthiouracil and methimazole ranged from 0% to about 10%.[76, 77] In a recent Japanese series of over 19,000 cases, only 70 patients developed agranulocytosis detectable by frequent blood count monitoring.[78] Agranulocytosis was significantly associated with antithyroid drugs in the IAAAS, where the relative risk for agranulocytosis with a history of recent use was over 100.[13] Nonetheless, this translated to only 6.3 excess cases of agranulocytosis per million users per week, a lower figure than suggested by the earlier clinic-based estimates.

Agranulocytosis has been associated with a variety of antithyroid drugs, including even thiocyanate and potassium perchlorate but chiefly with thioamides: methimazole and carbimazole, and thiouracil, propylthiouracil, and methylthiouracil. Patients who develop agranulocytosis are significantly older than other hyperthyroid patients, and they have received higher doses of antithyroid medication than the control population.[79] In a German review of a large clinic population, patients with agranulocytosis had been treated with significantly higher doses of methimazole, and most cases occurred within the first 2 months of therapy.[76] Recurrent agranulocytosis has occurred on exposure to a second, chemically different agent (methimazole after propylthiouracil)[80]; in vitro tests of immune recognition of drugs can also show apparent cross-reactivity in an occasional patient.[81] All these phenomena may be favored by the underlying immunopathology of Graves' disease.[81] Although agranulocytosis has been preceded by transient neutropenia,[82] moderate neutropenia is relatively common with propylthiouracil therapy and is not an indication for discontinuation of the drug. While agranulocytosis usually occurs within the first few months of therapy, it can appear after years of treatment or on reexposure after an uneventful first course of therapy.

Sera from patients with methimazole agranulocytosis have been shown to inhibit myeloid colony formation.[83, 84] More general tests of drug-induced lymphocyte transformation and drug-dependent antibody binding also are frequently positive.[81, 85, 86] A strong association between a histocompatibility class II antigen in Japanese patients with agranulocytosis secondary to methimazole has implicated a cellular immune mechanism.[54] Propylthiouracil accumulates in the bone marrow (more than in the thyroid) and is concentrated in neutrophils,[87] and granulocytes and thyroid cells share peroxidase enzyme systems that similarly metabolize antithyroid drugs to reactive intermediates.

Antibiotics

As a class, antibiotics may be the commonest agents associated with hospital-acquired neutropenia. In one review of 50 patients treated with a variety of antibiotics for chronic osteomyelitis after trauma, 30% experienced leukopenia and 6% developed agranulocytosis.[88] Virtually every antibiotic has been associated through case reports and small series of patients (see Table 7–5). The IAAAS took pains to exclude confounding of antibiotic use that was causal with antibiotic treatment of the first symptoms of leukopenia.[89] In this study, exposure during the 2 weeks prior to onset of agranulocytosis for the combination of trimethoprim and sulfamethoxazole carried a relative risk of 12 (confidence interval = 3.9 to 40) and macrolides were also associated with a high risk. Sulfonamides, β-lactams, tetracyclines, and other antibiotics, however, did not achieve statistical significance (no antibiotic was associated with the development of AA).

Trimethoprim and sulfamethoxazole are implicated in a variety of hematologic toxicities; of cases reported in Sweden over a decade, leukopenia was most common followed by bicytopenia, tricytopenia, thrombocytopenia, agranulocytosis, and anemia, and the overall probability of a hematologic complication of this treatment was estimated to be $5.3/10^6$ defined daily doses[90]; relative risks of agranulocytosis between 12 and 17 have been estimated from the Swedish drug monitoring system and a formal case control study, respectively.[15, 90] The risk for the sulfonamide sulfasalazine, used for treatment of inflammatory bowel disease and rheumatoid arthritis, was 1.2/10⁶ defined daily doses, with relative risks of 107 and 123. Mild neutropenia is common, occurring in 34% of children during the first week of therapy in one study.[91] The metabolic basis for trimethoprim-sulfamethoxazole inhibition of normal hematopoiesis appears to be inhibition on cellular dihydrofolate reductase.[92]

Historically both penicillin G and the semisynthetic penicillins have been associated with agranulocytosis.[93] Leukopenia has usually occurred in patients receiving large doses of penicillin after 2 weeks of therapy.[93, 94] The neutropenia appears in isolation, without other immune complex–mediated depression of peripheral blood counts, like penicillin-associated hemolytic anemia. The high dose-dependence, usually gradual decline in neutrophil number, absence of a correlation with antipenicillin antibody tests, and the frequent failure to detect antineutrophil antibodies have suggested direct toxicity as a mechanism, rather than hapten formation. Consistent with a direct mechanism was the long latent period to neutropenia on repeated (medically indicated) reexposure of one patient to carbenicillin.[95] On rechallenge in other patients, agranulocytosis reappeared within a few days,[96] more typical of an immune mechanism, and in some patients, drug-dependent antibody to granulocytes has been present in acute phase sera.[47, 94, 97] Neutropenia associated with the β-lactams also is related to dose and may occur in 5% to 15% of patients treated for more than 10 days with large amounts.[98] Patients rechallenged with a lower dose of cephalosporins did not develop recurrent neutropenia.[99]

Both penicillins and β-lactams have been reported to suppress myeloid colony formation in vitro in a dose-dependent manner.[98, 100] However, penicillin degradation products, which accumulate on storage in aqueous solution, were potent inhibitors of CFU_{GM} colony formation, while fresh penicillin was not suppressive in vitro.[101] Delivery of penicillin as a freshly prepared bolus reduced the rate of neutropenia in patients from 12 of 193 historical cases to 0 of 116 in a subsequent cohort.[102]

Psychotropic Drugs

Phenothiazine leukopenia, discussed above, is the paradigm. More recently, aplastic anemia in about 32 patients treated with the new antiepileptic felbamate led to discontinuation of marketing efforts, a marked reduction in numbers of treated patients, and severe impact on the research efforts and stock market share price of the manufacturer.[103] The most extensive literature concerns the antipsychotic clozapine; the survival of this drug, despite agranulocytosis as its most serious complication, is illustrative of broad scientific, medical, and social issues.

Clozapine is a piperazine-substituted dibenzodiazepine with remarkable efficacy in refractory schizophrenia. In early clinical trials, the rate of agranulocytosis was low, probably because the duration of treatment was quite short. However, not long after its introduction into clinical practice in the mid-1970s, a virtual epidemic of agranulocytosis occurred in Finnish hospitals; many of these patients died, and the estimated 0.5% risk of developing agranulocytosis led to severe curtailment of clozapine use in Europe and its withdrawal from clinical research trials.[104] The hazard of agranulocytosis was even higher in other European surveys, about a 2% cumulative risk after a year of therapy,[105] and much greater than for other neuroleptics. The U.S. experience has been similar, with an estimated risk of bone marrow failure usually cited as 1% to 3%.[106] Analysis of the data in the obligatory surveillance system, including 11,555 patients for 1990 to 1991, suggested cumulative incidence rates of 0.80% after 1 year and 0.92% after 1½ years of treatment.[107–109] Clozapine was reintroduced into use only with stringent selection of patients and a rigorous hematology monitoring system. Nonetheless, as of October 1992, of 40,000 monitored patients, 171 had developed agranulocytosis and there were seven fatalities, mainly due to gram-negative sepsis.[110]

Clozapine agranulocytosis resembles phenothiazine agranulocytosis in its latent period, with onset after months of treatment (usually between 3 and 12 weeks) not a high cumulative dose, and reversibility with drug discontinuation.[104, 111] Similar to agranulocytosis in general, older patients and women appear to be at greater risk.[107, 112] Almost all cases have occurred during the first 6 months and 75% to 90% in the first 18 weeks[107, 113] of therapy. Agranulocytosis has been observed in only an occasional patient after the first year of treatment. Both precipitous and gradual onsets have been described. Examination of monitored white blood cell counts has suggested that the neutrophil count may fall for a month before the patient develops the clinical syndrome,[107] but others have concluded that a sharp rise in the neutrophil count may herald agranulocytosis weeks later.[108] Patients usually recover within 2 to 3 weeks of discontinuing treatment.[112] On rechallenge, agranulocytosis occurs with a shorter latency period.

The mechanism of clozapine agranulocytosis is unknown. In contrast to phenothiazine, sera from patients with acute clozapine agranulocytosis are cytotoxic to granulocytes and inhibit myelopoiesis in vitro.[114] In vitro, clozapine is oxidized by leukocyte myeloperoxidase to reactive free radical forms, which can couple to protein.[115] Possibly conjugated drug could serve to target immune system cells. The major metabolite of clozapine, N-desmethylclozapine, inhibited human marrow progenitor cells in vitro, but at much higher concentrations than achieved in the plasma of treated patients.[116] The IgM fraction of sera from patients in the acute phase of agranulocytosis was toxic to granulocytes in the absence of drug, supporting an immune mechanism rather than direct cytotoxicity.[117]

A genetic basis for the high frequency of agranulocytosis among the Finnish patients was suspected but none could be established by pedigree analysis.[118] Among American Jewish patients with schizophrenia, the haplotype HLA-B38 (a variant of B16), DR4, DQw3 was implicated in the development of agranulocytosis[53, 119]: B38 was found in 83% of the affected cases and only 20% of the treated controls.[53] In a further refinement of the analysis, the haplotype DRB1*0402, DRB4*0101, DQB1*0302, DQA1*301 (which is linked to B38) was present in 9 of 10 Jewish patients; a different hapolytpe, HLA DR2, DQ1, was present in 13 of 21 non-Jewish cases.[120] Agranulocytosis secondary to clozapine has been reported in a Native American with a similar haplotype except that the B16 variant was B39,[121] but this gene has not been associated with clozapine agranulocytosis in Europe.[113] There is no evidence of cross-reactivity between clozapine and other drugs used in schizophrenia.[122]

The marketing of clozapine in the United States has been unique: clozapine was distributed as part of an obligatory and proprietary "patient management system," that included registration in a national database, weekly phlebotomy and blood count determination at a central laboratory, and reporting of that result to the physician. Early withdrawal of drug due to frequent, compulsory monitoring of the white blood cell count has been credited with the very low mortality rate of clozapine agranulocytosis[106]: among the first 12,000 American patients treated for 15 months under a monitoring protocol, there was only one reported death from agranulocytosis.[113] However, early termination of the drug may not prevent the development of agranulocytosis,[123] or low white blood cell counts may go unheeded.[124] Unfortunately, abrupt withdrawal can also precipitate severe and prolonged psychotic relapse. The "bundling" of clozapine, the arrangement by which weekly doses were dispensed only after a blood specimen for neutrophil counting was obtained, has been the source of bitter controversy, particularly as the manufacturer dictated the terms of drug use and, initially, the central laboratory to be used for blood counting.[125] Clozapine was precedent-setting in that its purchase price included not only production and profit but the ancillary laboratory services as well. As a result, the annual cost of clozapine per patient is about $10,000, and the projected cost nationally, even if the drug were used only for the strict indication of refractory schizophrenia, would be in excess of $1 billion.[106] A major motivation behind the monitoring system is clearly fear of litigation. Unfortunately, the patient population which benefits from clozapine is often poorly compliant and also often unable to afford such extraordinary costs, making it "a rich man's drug for a poor man's disease." Because the costs are so often passed on to public providers, clozapine has become a focus as well for arguments over drug pricing and cost-effectiveness, industry responsibility and liability, patient eligibility, and access to medical care. Monitoring of blood counts is now accomplished less expensively at private laboratories, and in the United Kingdom clozapine therapy is considered cost-effective by comparison with the resource use of hospitalization. The expected death rate from agranulocytosis due to clozapine, even without monitoring, is only one to three persons annually worldwide![126] In one thoughtful analysis, a price tag of about $62,000 was placed on each "quality-adjusted life-year" (a measure of both years of life saved and the quality of life gained or lost by drug use); cost effectiveness declined dramatically, more than 10-fold, during the second and subsequent years, due to the lower rates of agranulocytosis in patients after the first 6 months of therapy (and was particularly sensitive to the laboratory fee for blood count monitoring).[127]

Cardiac Drugs

In the IAAAS, a variety of drugs used to treat cardiovascular disease were associated with increased risk of agranulocytosis, including digoxin and its derivatives, dipyridamole, and propanolol; some associations, such as that with procainamide, were not surprising given earlier case reports, while the implication of digoxin was unexpected[13] (see Table 7–5). Except for cinepazide, the excess deaths were not numerous.

Captopril is especially interesting because of the relatively high risk of agranulocytosis associated with its use. While neutropenia was observed early in clinical trials, resulting in imposition on its use by the Food and Drug Administration (FDA), the rate after its introduction into wide clinical use appeared much higher, mainly due to the apparent susceptibility of some treated subpopulations: the frequency of neutropenia in all cases was estimated at 0.02% to 0.03% initially, but rose to 0.40% in patients with azotemia and to 7.2% in patients with collagen-vascular diseases such as systemic lupus erythematosus or scleroderma.[128] Both renal failure and probenicid increase blood levels of captopril and its metabolites. Severity of infections and mortality were also higher in these patients.[128] Agranulocytosis secondary to captopril has been confirmed by rechallenge.[129] Like procainamide (discussed below) captopril has diverse effects on the immune system: captopril readily conjugates proteins that then induce antibody formation in animals[130] and it can induce suppressor lymphocyte activity in culture of human cells.[131]

Agranulocytosis occurs with procainamide treatment at an apparently high rate, estimated at about 0.6% in one hospital series[132]; agranulocytosis secondary to tocainide has been estimated at 0.18%[133]; and at a Los Angeles hospital, 4.4% of patients recovering from open heart surgery developed severe neutropenia on the sustained release form of procainamide.[134] Similar to other drug-associated agranulocytosis, onset usually has occurred within 3 months of initiating treatment. Most patients have recovered upon discontinuation of the agent, but mortality has been estimated to be as high as 25%. Agranulocytosis has recurred on reexposure. Procainamide agranulocytosis may be accompanied by thrombocytopenia, marrow granuloma, and a lupus-like syndrome, the last a common independent toxicity of this family of drugs (but true agranulocytosis, as opposed to moderate neutropenia, is very unusual in idiopathic lupus). Procainamide-induced agranulocytosis also differs in serologic findings and time of onset from lupus secondary to the drug (yet antineutrophil antibodies are found in both groups!). The slow acetylation phenotype, associated with lupus-like laboratory abnormalities and the clinical syndrome, has not been linked to agranulocytosis. One possible mechanism for immune self-reactivity has been inferred from the ability of procainamide to inhibit DNA methylation and induce autoreactivity in cloned T cell lines.[135]

Levamisole

When levamisole was employed as a single-dose antihelmintic, it was virtually free of toxicity. Levamisole's immunostimulatory properties led to wider application as an adjuvant in cancer chemotherapy and in chronic rheumatic syndromes, and in these conditions it has been associated with agranulocytosis with a high frequency. In a retrospective survey of several thousand patients, leukopenia occurred in about 2% of cancer patients and 5% of rheumatic disease cases, severe enough almost always to lead to discontinuation of levamisole treatment[136]; in other series of levamisole-treated cases, of 60 patients with rheumatoid arthritis receiving the drug, 35% showed persistent leukopenia and 10% developed agranulocytosis,[137] and severe neutropenia was found in 8% of 192 breast cancer patients.[53] Bone marrow specimens obtained soon after the onset of agranulocytosis show hypocellularity with absence of cells more mature than promyelocytes.[136, 137] Agranulocytosis secondary to levamisole in rheumatoid arthritis was associated significantly with HLA B27 (present in 50% of cases, compared to 8% of the normal population; B27 is not associated with rheumatoid arthritis), but patients with ankylosing spondylitis, most of whom have the B27 antigen, were not unusually susceptible.[136, 138, 139] Rechallenge with levamisole can precipitate agranulocytosis within hours.[136] Granulocytotoxins, sometimes characterized as IgM antibodies, can be consistently detected in levamisole agranulocytosis sera, but these antibodies may also precede the episode by months, persist beyond its resolution, and they do not correlate with colony inhibition in vitro.[139–142]

Antihistamines

Both leukopenia and agranulocytosis have been linked to treatment with cimetidine and ranitidine (see Table 7–5), and histamine H_2 antagonists have been associated with other adverse hematologic effects, including thrombocytopenia, anemia, and bi- and tricytopenias.[143] Recurrent agranulocytosis with cimetidine rechallenge[144] or cimetidine exposure after recovery from ranitidine neutropenia[145] implicates these drugs as causal agents. The first H_2 antagonist used in man, metiamide, was never marketed because of fatal agranulocytosis and granulocytopenia in early clinical trials. Substitution of metiamide's thiouracil side chain for cimetidine's cyanoguanidine appeared to have eliminated agranulocytosis as a complication until case reports began to appear after its formal approval and with its widespread use.[146]

Cimetidine[147, 148] and ranitidine[149, 150] produce concentration-dependent inhibition of CFU_{GM}-derived colony formation. While the doses required to suppress myelopoiesis in vitro exceed the usual therapeutic plasma levels, these drugs may accumulate in some patients, especially if renal excretion is diminished.[149] Estrogens have blocked this direct effect of cimetidine on in vitro CFU_{GM} colonies,[151] and one study showed a greater susceptibility of marrow cells from males compared to females[152]; more men are reported with hematologic complications secondary to antihistamines.[143] A possible mechanism of cimetidine's action was suggested by the effect of H_2-receptor blockade on murine hematopoietic cells' entry into mitosis and DNA synthesis.[153] An immune basis for cimetidine's effect on blood cell production was inferred from the ability of cimetidine to induce lymphocyte blastogenesis and increase suppressor/cytotoxic lymphocytes in one patient.[56]

TREATMENT

Supportive Treatment

Once drug exposure ceases, recovery should follow. Dameshek in 1942 recognized that death in agranulocytosis was secondary to sepsis, not to the reduced white blood cell count itself. Rapid recovery in severely neutropenic cases treated with sulfathiazole and penicillin was described shortly thereafter. Relatively simple measures like handwashing, use of gowns, single-patient rooms or strict isolation, and antibiotics have appeared to reduce mortality in agranulocytosis. However, of paramount importance is the early introduction of broad-spectrum, parenterally administered antibacterials to the febrile neutropenic patient (see Chapter 1).

Hematopoietic Growth Factors

Very rapid improvement in granulocyte numbers in agranulocytosis has been reported in large numbers of case reports in patients who were treated with granulocyte-macrophage colony-stimulating factor (GM-CSF) or granulocyte colony-stimulating factor (G-CSF) for agranulocytosis secondary to a wide variety of drugs (for references, see Young and Alter[12]). The experience with 22 patients with drug-induced agranulocytosis treated with G-CSF at 4 to 10 µg/kg was summarized by Amgen, Inc.: recovery to a neutrophil count above 1000/µL occurred at a median of 4 days (range 1 to 15 days).[154] Prolonged neutropenia despite growth factor therapy has been reported only occasionally[155]; fatalities, despite their use, rarely.[156] However, the "natural history" of agranulocytosis, in which infections are treated without application of marrow-stimulating factors, is highly variable, and in particular the time to granulocyte recovery after discontinuation of an offending agent has a wide range. In my experience with a single experimental drug in a relatively uniform and closely monitored patient population, recovery from absolute neutropenia occurred as soon as 2 days to as late as 3 weeks after stopping drug; in comparing about a dozen patients who recovered spontaneously with a similar number who received G-CSF, the mean duration of neutropenia was shortened by about 3 days (from 9.5 to 6.5 days). Sixteen Japanese patients with Graves' disease and neutropenia or agranulocytosis secondary to antithyroid drug therapy were treated with a standard dose of G-CSF[157]; granulocyte counts increased promptly with G-CSF administration in the moderate cases, but in three patients with true agranulocytosis, recovery times were 6, 7, and 14 days, similar to the time course without treatment in historical controls.[157] In a small series of cases of clozapine-induced agranulocytosis, prompt administration of G-CSF appeared to shorten recovery time to about 8 days compared with historical recovery periods that averaged almost 16 days,[158, 159] but in another comparison of G-CSF-treated patients with historical controls, the average duration of agranulocytosis was no different (about 6.5 days).[160] Despite the lack of convincing evidence of efficacy, especially a controlled trial, growth factors are frequently recommended based on the accumulation of single case reports. Although G-CSF has few side effects, toxicity secondary to growth factors, including adult respiratory distress syndrome, has been reported in agranulocytosis patients.[161]

A rationale for the use of colony-stimulating factors in agranulocytosis is uncertain, other than their obvious ability to elevate neutrophil numbers in normal persons, after cytotoxic chemotherapy, and in some patients with bone marrow failure syndromes. Levels of serum G-CSF were surprisingly low in Japanese patients with methimazole-associated neutropenia[162] but increased at the onset of agranulocytosis in another.[157] In one patient with agranulocytosis followed serially, serum G-CSF levels rose to very high concentrations with onset of neutropenia and returned to undetectable levels with recovery.[163]

COURSE AND PROGNOSIS

Untreated, agranulocytosis is almost always fatal. In 1932, Doan[164] estimated mortality at greater than 90% in untreated "malignant neutropenia"; 40 of 43 (93%) patients reviewed in 1926[165] and 95 of 130 (73%) collected in 1939 died.[166] In the early antibiotic era, survival improved, and mortality was estimated at 20% to 50%: 19 (37%) of 51 dipyrone cases reported to 1964[167] and 12 of 30 (40%) in a Montreal series, observed from 1946 to 1964 and treated mainly with penicillin,[19] died. In the current era, the great majority of patients survive an episode of agranulocytosis: mortality was 9% in cases identified through the IAAAS of the 1980s.[13] Mortality from agranulocytosis, even with the development of superior antibiotics, has remained high in some series: 28 (30%) of 94 patients reported to the Swedish registry from 1966 to 1970[168]; 6 (15%) of 40 cases in Finland from 1960 to 1968[169]; 15 (25%) of 61 patients in Ulm, Germany, from 1968 to 1980[22]; and 27 (17%) of 158 patients from Barcelona, Spain from 1970 to 1989.[170] In my personal experience with an experimental cardiotonic drug alluded to above, the mortality rate was about 10%, despite an elaborate monitoring system to detect leukopenia early (once-weekly blood counts reported to a centralized data analysis center), a strict protocol for in-hospital observation, and a low threshold for initiation of treatment with broad-spectrum antibiotics. While these particular patients suffered from advanced cardiac disease, many who receive drugs and subsequently develop agranulocytosis will be similarly handicapped by an underlying illness and may suffer the worst consequences of neutropenia.

Old age, septicemia, shock, and metabolic complications of infection like renal failure are poor prognostic variables.[170] Although not deducible from published series, it is likely that the severity of neutropenia and especially its duration relate negatively to outcome. As described above, in patients with agranulocytosis who survive, the time to recovery of granulocytes in the blood is highly variable, 3 to 56 days in one series,[22] with a mean of about 12 days (to half-maximal granulocyte numbers[22] or reappearance of granulocytes in the blood[21]). In 44 Swedish patients with agranulocytosis secondary to sulfasalazine, the median recovery time was 12 days and all patients had granulocytes in their blood by 3 weeks.[171] Historically, monocytosis was cited as a signal of a good prognosis or a harbinger of recovery from agranulocytosis.[172]

The results of controlled readministration of a single dose of suspected drug vary from recurrent agranulocytosis, to modest depression of granulocyte number, to no effect at all[21]—but continued drug administration may be associated with a fatal outcome.[169] Recurrent agranulocytosis is well documented and occurred in 8 of 17 patients who were reexposed, including nine episodes in one woman treated with aminopyrine metabolite over a 6-year period![173] The therapeutic need must be compelling before intentional reexposure of a recovered agranulocytosis patient to the incriminated drug.

Patients with idiosyncratic drug-associated agranulocytosis are, not unexpectedly, susceptible to the same range of microorganisms as myelosuppressed cancer patients, and similar to other neutropenic patients, a microbiologic diagnosis can be established in only about 50% of cases.[174] A shift from infection with gram-negative to gram-positive organisms over the last decade has been observed in both populations, and empirical antibiotic therapy for agranulocytosis can be determined based on the experience with more common chemotherapy-induced neutropenia.[174] The old adage that patients with agranulocytosis often die as their white blood cell counts show signs of recovery has not been disproved: there is little satisfaction in observing a regenerating bone marrow at autopsy.[19] Neither vigilance nor antibiotic therapy should be relaxed prematurely.

PURE WHITE CELL APLASIA

Chronic hypoplastic neutropenia was described by Spaet and Dameshek[175] in 1952 in a report of four patients who suffered repeated infectious episodes; their bone marrows were hypoplastic in the myeloid series, in contrast to the myeloid hyperplasia typical of the neutropenia of hypersplenism. A few years later, Butler[176] reported a 21-year-old woman with chronic severe neutropenia and recurrent stomatitis, whose marrow showed no maturation beyond the metamyelocyte, and whose plasma contained a broadly reactive leukoagglutinin.[176] Those authors who have emphasized an immune etiology have termed this syndrome "immune panleukopenia"; other writers, who featured the marrow morphology, called it "chronic agranulocytosis" or "pure white cell aplasia" (the marrow also may show myeloid cells to the myelocyte stage of differentiation). In a case termed "autoimmune panleukopenia," episodic leukopenia was associated with an immunoglobulin that bound lymphocytes and granulocytes, and inhibited myeloid colony formation in vitro (both human and mouse, similar to pure red cell aplasia); the patient responded to cyclophosphamide.[177] In another patient, the inhibitor was defined as a complement-dependent IgG that was specific for CFU_{GM} but did not affect more primitive or erythroid progenitors or bind to mature granulocytes.[178] T cells, as well as a plasma inhibitor, were implicated in a woman with neutropenia and an assortment of autoimmune or allergic syndromes (hypothyroidism, eczema, alopecia)[179] and in another patient without a serum inhibitor.[180] In general, the syndrome is extremely rare, and only a few recent cases have been published.[180–182] There is little to distinguish pure white cell aplasia in the setting of drug exposure[43] from agranulocytosis, and the term is best used for chronic severe leukopenia without any suspicious drug history.

Pure white cell aplasia, like pure red cell aplasia, has been associated with thymoma, but the combination is rare—eight cases had been published by 1990.[183] The tumor is usually a malignant spindle cell carcinoma, and there may be clinically important hypogammaglobulinemia. A serum inhibitor of in vitro myelopoiesis has been shown in CFU_{GM} assays in two cases,[184, 185] and a T cell inhibitor in another.[180] As with pure red cell aplasia, the thymoma should be removed, but for the purpose of excising a malignancy rather than in expectation of a cure of the marrow deficiency. Some patients with pure white cell aplasia have responded to thymectomy,[186] and also to splenectomy,[181] plasmapheresis,[180] intravenous immune globulin,[182] cyclophosphamide,[177] azathioprine,[187] and cyclosporine.[179, 180]

REFERENCES

1. Schultz W: Ueber eigenartige Halserkrankungen. Dtsch Med Wochenschr 1922; 48:1495–1496.
2. Kracke RR, Parker FP: The etiology of granulopenia (agranulocytosis) with particular reference to the drugs containing the benzene ring. J Lab Clin Med 1934; 19:799–818.
3. Plum P: Clinical and Experimental Investigations in Agranulocytosis. Copenhagen, NYT Nordisk Forlag, HK Lewis, 1937.
4. Roberts SR, Kracke RR: Agranulocytosis: Its classification. Cases and comments illustrating the granulopenic trend from 8,000 blood counts in the South. Ann Intern Med 1931; 5:40–51.
5. Madison FW, Squier TL: The etiology of primary granulocytopenia (agranulocytic angina). JAMA 1934; 102:755–759.
6. Moeschlin S, Wagner K: Agranulocytosis due to the occurrence of leukocyte agglutinins. Acta Haematol 1952; 8:29–41.
7. Moeschlin S, Schmid E: Investigation of leukocyte agglutination in serum of compatible and incompatible blood groups. Acta Haematol 1954; 11:241–250.
8. Pisciotta AV: Drug induced agranulocytosis. Peripheral destruction of polymorphonuclear leukocytes and their marrow precursors. Blood Rev 1990; 4:226–237.
9. Heimpel H: Drug-induced agranulocytosis. Med Toxicol 1988; 3:449–462.
10. Vincent PC: Drug-induced aplastic anemia and agranulocytosis. Incidence and mechanisms. Drugs 1986; 31:52–63.
11. Pisciotta AV: Immune and toxic mechanisms in drug-induced agranulocytosis. Semin Hematol 1973; 10:279–310.
12. Young NS, Alter BF: Agranulocytosis. In Aplastic Anemia, Acquired and Inherited. Philadelphia, WB Saunders, 1993, pp 227–264.
13. Kaufman DW, Kelly JP, Levy M, et al: The Drug Etiology of Agranulocytosis and Aplastic Anemia. New York, Oxford University Press.
14. Strom BL, Carson JL, Schinnar R, et al: Descriptive epidemiology of agranulocytosis. Arch Intern Med 1992; 152:1475–1480.
15. Keisu M, Ekman E, Wiholm BE: Comparing risk estimates of sulphonamide-induced agranulocytosis from the Swedish Drug Monitoring System and a case-control study. Eur J Clin Pharmacol 1992; 43:211–214.
16. Shapiro S, Issaragrisil S, Kaufman DW, et al, and the Aplastic Anemia Study Group: Agranulocytosis in Bangkok, Thailand: A predominantly drug-induced disease with an unusually low incidence. Am J Trop Med Hyg 1999; 60:573–577.
17. Mink OJ, Campbell JD: Toxic effects of arsenical compounds employed in the treatment of disease in the United States Navy. US Naval Med Bull 1933; 32:383–461.
18. Jick H, Myers MW, Deam AD: The risk of sulfasalazine and mesalazine-associated blood disorders. Pharmacotherapy 1995; 15:176–181.
19. Pretty HM, Gosselin G, Colpron G, et al: Agranulocytosis: A report of 30 cases. Can Med Assoc J 1965; 93:1059–1064.
20. Bodey GP: Oral complications of the myeloproliferative diseases. Postgrad Med 1971; 49:115–121.
21. Ruvidic R, Jelíc S: Haematological aspects of drug-induced agranulocytosis. Scand J Haematol 1972; 9:18–27.
22. Heit W, Heimpel H, Fischer A, et al: Drug-induced agranulocytosis: Evidence for the commitment of bone marrow haematopoiesis. Scand J Haematol 1985; 35:459–468.
23. Ruvidic R: Haematopoiesis in drug-induced agranulocytosis. Biomed Pharmacother 1996; 50:275–278.
24. McCullough J: Granulocyte antigen systems and antibodies and their clinical significance. Hum Pathol 1983; 14:228–234.
25. Madyastha PR, Glassman AB: Neutrophil antigens and antibodies in the diagnosis of immune neutropenias. Ann Clin Lab Sci 1989; 19:146–154.
26. Shastri KA, Logue GL: Autoimmune neutropenia. Blood 1993; 81:1984–1995.
27. Cines DB, Passero F, Guerry D, IV, et al: Granulocyte-associated IgG in neutropenic disorders. Blood 1982; 59:124–132.
28. Van der Veen JPW, Hack CE, Engelfriet CP, et al: Chronic idiopathic and secondary neutropenia: Clinical and serological investigations. Br J Haematol 1986; 63:161–171.
29. Harmon DC, Weitzman SA, Stossel TP: The severity of immune neutropenia correlates with the maturational specificity of antineutrophil antibodies. Br J Haematol 1984; 58:209–215.
30. Sakaguchi M, Hattori T, Yamabe H, et al: Analysis of antibody to neutrophils associated with autoimmune neutropenia: Possible recognition of Fc-receptor–related molecules. Acta Haematol 1986; 75:236–240.
31. Victorino RMM, Maria VAJ, de Deus J: Immuno-

logic mechanism in sulphasalazine-induced agranulocytosis. Acta Haematol 1990; 84:111.
32. Schattner A, Shtalrid M, Levy R, et al: Fatal aplastic anemia due to indomethacin-lymphocyte transformation tests in vitro. Isr J Med Sci 1981; 17:433–436.
33. Ellis ME, Steed AJ, Addison GM: Neutropenia associated with dual antimalarial chemoprophylaxis—use of bone-marrow culture as an aid in further drug management. J Infect 1987; 15:147–152.
34. Ezeilo GC: Non-genetic neutropenia in Africans. Lancet 1972; 2:1003–1004.
35. Uetrecht JP: Idiosyncratic drug reactions: Possible role of reactive metabolites generated by leukocytes. Pharm Res 1989; 6:265–273.
36. Young N: Drugs and chemicals as agents of bone marrow failure. In Testa N, Gale RC (eds): Hematopoiesis. Long-term Effects of Chemotherapy and Radiation. New York, Marcel Decker, 1988, pp 131–157.
37. Kracke RR, Parker FP: The relationship of drug therapy to agranulocytosis. JAMA 1935; 105:960–966.
38. Dameshek W, Colmes A: The effect of drugs in the production of agranulocytosis with particular reference to amidopyrine hypersensitivity. J Clin Invest 1935; 15:85–97.
39. Young GAR, Croaker G, Vincent PC, et al: The CFU-C assay in patients with neutropenia and, in particular, drug associated neutropenia. Clin Lab Haematol 1987; 9:245–253.
40. Brown RD, Yuen E, Kronenberg H, et al: In vitro clonogenic assays in selective neutropenia. Scand J Haematol 1983; 30:110–116.
41. Howell A, Gumpel JM, Watts RWE: Depression of bone marrow colony formation in gold-induced neutropenia. BMJ 1975; 1:432–434.
42. Parmentier C, Tchernia G, Subtil E, et al: In vitro medullary granulocytic progenitor (CFUc) cultures from 6 cases of granulocytopenias. Scand J Haematol 1978; 21:19–23.
43. Mamus SW, Burton JD, Groat JD, et al: Ibuprofen-associated pure white-cell aplasia. N Engl J Med 1986; 314:624–625.
44. Barrett AJ, Weller E, Rozengurt N, et al: Amidopyrine agranulocytosis: Drug inhibition of granulocyte colonies in the presence of patient's serum. BMJ 1976; 2:850–851.
45. Fibbe WE, Claas FHJ, van der Star-Dijkstra W, et al: Agranulocytosis induced by propylthiouracil: Evidence of a drug dependent antibody reacting with granulocytes, monocytes and haematopoietic progenitor cells. Br J Haematol 1986; 64:363–373.
46. Levitt LJ: Chlorpropamide-induced pure white cell aplasia. Blood 1987; 69:394–400.
47. Salama A, Schütz B, Kiefel V, et al: Immune-mediated agranulocytosis related to drugs and their metabolites: Mode of sensitization and heterogeneity of antibodies. Br J Haematol 1989; 72:127–132.
48. Bilezikian SB, Laleli Y, Tsan M, et al: Immunological reactions involving leukocytes: III. Agranulocytosis induced by antithyroid drugs. Johns Hopkins Med J 1976; 138:124–129.
49. Currie MS, Weinberg JB, Rustagi PK, et al: Antibodies to granulocyte precursors in selective myeloid hypoplasia and other suspected autoimmune neutropenias: Use of HL-60 cells as targets. Blood 1987; 69:529–536.
50. Rouveix B, Coulombel L, Aymard JP, et al: Amodiaquine-induced immune agranulocytosis. Br J Haematol 1989; 71:7–11.
51. Uetrecht JP, Zahid N, Whitfield D: Metabolism of vesnarinone by activated neutrophils: Implications for vesnarinone-induced agranulocytosis. J Pharmacol Exp Ther 1994; 270:865–872.
52. Coleman MD, Simpson J, Jacobus DP: Reduction of dapsone hydroxylamine to dapsone during methaemoglobin formation in human erythrocytes in vitro IV: Implications for the development of agranulocytosis. Biochem Pharmacol 1994; 48:1349–1354.
53. Lieberman JA, Yunis J, Egea E, et al: HLA-B38, DR4, DQw3 and clozapine-induced agranulocytosis in Jewish patients with schizophrenia. Arch Gen Psychiatry 1990; 47:945–948.
54. Tamai H, Sudo T, Kimura A, et al: Association between the DRB1*08032 histocompatibilty antigen and methimazole-induced agranulocytosis in Japanese patients with Graves disease. Ann Intern Med 1996; 124:490–494.
55. Lutton JD, Hoffman R, Greenberg ML, et al: Lymphocyte mediated neutropenia in man (abstract). Blood 1976; 48:971.
56. Nagler A, Rozenbaum H, Enat R, et al: Immune basis for cimetidine-induced pancytopenia. Am J Gastroenterol 1987; 82:359–361.
57. Saal JG, Daniel PT, Berg PA: Indoprofen-induced aplastic anemia in active connective tissue disease detected by drug-specific lymphocyte transformation. Klin Wochenschr 1986; 64:481–485.
58. Turbay D, Lieberman J, Alper CA, et al: Tumor necrosis factor constellation polymorphism and clozapine-induced agranulocytosis in two different ethnic groups. Blood 1997; 89:4167–4174.
59. Pisciotta AV: Drug-induced leukopenia and aplastic anemia. Clin Pharmacol Ther 1971; 12:13–43.
60. Weetman RM, Boxer LA, Brown MP, et al: In vitro inhibition of granulopoiesis by 4-amino-4′-hydroxylaminodiphenyl sulfone. Br J Haematol 1980; 45:361–370.
61. Parent-Massin DM, Sensébé L, Léglise MC, et al: Relevance of in vitro studies of drug-induced agranulocytosis. Report of 14 cases. Drug Saf 1993; 9:463–469.
62. Palva IP, Mustala OO: Drug-induced agranulocytosis, with special reference to aminophenazone. I. Adults. Acta Med Scand 1970; 187:109–115.
63. Discombe G: Agranulocytosis caused by amidopyrine. BMJ 1952; 1:1270–1273.
64. Levy M: The epidemiology of metamizol-induced adverse reactions. Agents Actions Suppl 1986; 19:237–245.
65. Laporte J-R, Carné X: Blood dyscrasias and the

66. Moeschlin S: Immunological granulocytopenia and agranulocytosis (clinical aspects). Schweiz Med Wochenschr 1955; 84:33–50.
67. Magis CC, Barge A, Dausset J: Serological study of an allergic agranulocytosis due to noramidopyrine. Clin Exp Immunol 1968; 3:989–1003.
68. Suda T, Mizoguchi H, Miura Y, et al: Suppression of in vitro granulocyte-macrophage colony formation by the peripheral mononuclear phagocytic cells of patients with idiopathic aplastic anaemia. Br J Haematol 1981; 47:433–442.
69. Kadar D, Kalow W: Acute and latent leukopenic reaction to antipyrine. Clin Pharmacol Ther 1980; 28:820–822.
70. Uetrecht JP, Ma HM, MacKnight E, et al: Oxidation of aminopyrine by hypochlorite to a reactive dictation: Possible implications for aminopyrine-induced agranulocytosis. Chem Res Toxicol 1995; 8:226–233.
71. Inman WHW: Study of fatal bone marrow depression with special reference to phenylbutazone and oxyphenbutazone. BMJ 1977; 1:1500–1505.
72. Miescher PA, Pola W: Haematological effects of non-narcotic analgesics. Drugs 1986; 32:90–108.
73. Weissmann G, Xefteris ED: Phenylbutazone leukopenia. Arch Intern Med 1959; 103:957–961.
74. Cunningham JL, Leyland MJ, Delamore IW, et al: Acetanilide oxidation in phenylbutazone-associated hypoplastic anaemia. BMJ 1974; 3:313–317.
75. Smith CS, Chinn S, Watts RWE: The sensitivity of human bone marrow granulocyte/monocyte precursor cells to phenylbutazone, oxyphenbutazone and gamma-hydroxyphenylbutazone in vitro, with observations on the bone marrow colony formation in phenylbutazone-induced granulocytopoenia. Biochem Pharmacol 1977; 26:847–852.
76. Meyer-Gessner M, Benker G, Lederbogen S, et al: Antithyroid drug–induced agranulocytosis: Clinical experience with ten patients treated at one institution and review of the literature. J Endocrinol Invest 1994; 17:29–36.
77. Bartalena L, Bogazzi F, Martino E: Adverse effects of thyroid hormone preparations and antithyroid drugs. Drug Saf 1996; 15:53–63.
78. Tajiri J, Noguchi S, Morita M, et al: Studies on onset patterns in antithyroid drug-induced agranulocytosis. Folio Endocrinol 1993; 69:530–533.
79. Cooper DS, Goldminz D, Levin AA, et al: Agranulocytosis associated with antithyroid drugs. Ann Intern Med 1983; 98:26–29.
80. Chen B, Lang R, Jutrin Y, et al: Recurrent agranulocytosis induced by two different antithyroid agents. Med J Aust 1983; 2:38–39.
81. Wall JR, Fang SL, Kuroki T, et al: In vitro immunoreactivity to propylthiouracil, methimazole, and carbimazole in patients with Graves disease: A possible cause of antithyroid drug-induced agranulocytosis. J Clin Endocrinol Metab 1984; 58:868–872.
82. Schut NH, Wiersinga WM, Van Oers MH: Methimazole-induced agranulocytosis preceded by transient granulocytopenia. Neth J Med 1993; 43:71–73.
83. Moreb J, Shemesh O, Shilo S, et al: Transient methimazole induced bone marrow aplasia: In vitro evidence for a humoral mechanism of bone marrow suppression. Acta Haematol 1983; 69:127–131.
84. Douer D, Eisenstein Z: Methimazole-induced agranulocytosis: Growth inhibition of myeloid progenitor cells by the patient's serum. Eur J Haematol 1988; 40:91–94.
85. Toth EL, Mant MJ, Shivji S, et al: Propylthiouracil-induced agranulocytosis: An unusual presentation and a possible mechanism. Am J Med 1988; 85:725–727.
86. McCullough J, Clay ME, Priest JR, et al: A comparison of methods for detecting leukocyte antibodies in autoimmune neutropenia. Transfusion 1981; 21:483–492.
87. Lam DC, Lindsay RH: Accumulation of 2-[14C] propylthiouracil in human polymorphonuclear leukocytes. Biochem Pharmacol 1979; 28:2289–2296.
88. McCluskey WP, Esterhai JL Jr, Brighton CT, et al: Neutropenia complicating parenteral antibiotic treatment of infected nonunion of the tibia. Arch Surg 1989; 124:1309–1312.
89. Kelly JP, Kaufman DW: Anti-infective drug use in relation to the risk of agranulocytosis and aplastic anemia. Arch Intern Med 1989; 149:1036–1040.
90. Keisu M, Wiholm B-E, Palmblad J: Trimethoprim-sulphamethoxazole–associated blood dyscrasias. Ten years' experience of the Swedish spontaneous reporting system. J Intern Med 1990; 228:353–360.
91. Asmar BI, Maqbool S, Dajani AS: Hematologic abnormalities after oral trimethoprim-sulfamethoxazole therapy in children. Am J Dis Child 1981; 135:1100–1103.
92. Golde DW, Bersh N, Quan SG: Trimethoprim and sulfamethoxazole inhibition of haematopoiesis in vitro. Br J Haematol 1978; 40:363–367.
93. Schmid L, Heit W, Flury R: Agranulocytosis associated with semisynthetic penicillins and cephalosporines. Report of 7 cases. Blut 1984; 48:11–18.
94. Pisciotta AV: Agranulocytosis during antibiotic therapy: Drug sensitivity or sepsis? Am J Hematol 1993; 42:132–137.
95. Reyes MP, Palutke M, Lerner AM: Granulocytopenia associated with carbenicillin. Five episodes in two patients. Am J Med 1973; 54:413–418.
96. Allo M, Silva J, Arbor MA: Antibiotic agranulocytosis: Association with cephalothin and carbenicillin. South Med J 1977; 70:1017–1019.
97. Murphy MF, Riordan T, Minchinton RM, et al: Demonstration of an immune-mediated mechanism of penicillin-induced neutropenia and thrombocytopenia. Br J Haematol 1983; 55:155–160.
98. Neftel KA, Hauser SP, Müller MR: Inhibition of granulopoiesis in vivo and in vitro by β-lactam antibiotics. J Infect Dis 1985; 152:90–98.
99. Homayouni H, Gross PA, Setia U, et al: Leukope-

100. nia due to penicillin and cephalosporin homologues. Arch Intern Med 1979; 139:827–828.
100. Irvine AE, Morris TCM, Kelly GJ, et al: Ticarcillin-induced neutropenia corroborated by in vitro CFU-C toxicity. Acta Haematol 1983; 70:364–368.
101. Neftel KA, Müller MR, Wälti M, et al: Penicillin-G degradation products inhibit in vitro granulopoiesis. Br J Haematol 1983; 54:255–260.
102. Neftel KA, Wälti M, Schulthess HK, et al: Adverse reactions following intravenous penicillin-G relate to degradation of the drug in vitro. Klin Wochenschr 1984; 62:25–29.
103. Brodie MJ, Pellock JM: Taming the brain storms: Felbamate updated. Lancet 1995; 346:918–919.
104. Idänpään-Hekkilä J, Alhava E, Olkinuora M, et al: Agranulocytosis during treatment with clozapine. Eur J Clin Pharmacol 1977; 11:193–198.
105. Bablenis E, Weber SS, Wagner RL: Clozapine: A novel antipsychotic agent. Ann Pharmacother 1989; 23:109–115.
106. Terkelsen KG, Grosser RC: Estimating clozapine's cost to the nation. Hosp Community Psychiatry 1990; 41:863–869.
107. Alvir JMJ, Lieberman JA, Safferman AZ, et al: Clozapine-induced agranulocytosis. Incidence and risk factors in the United States. N Engl J Med 1993; 329:162–167.
108. Alvir JMJ, Lieberman JA: Agranulocytosis: Incidence and risk factors. J Clin Psychiatry 1994; 55:137–138.
109. Alvir JMJ, Lieberman JA: A reevaluation of the clinical characteristics of clozapine-induced agranulocytosis in light of the United States experience. J Clin Psychopharmacol 1994; 14:87–89.
110. Update on clozapine. Med Lett Drugs Ther 1993; 35:16–18.
111. Anger B, Reichert S, Heimpel H: Clozapine-induced agranulocytosis. Blut 1987; 55:63–64.
112. Lieberman JA, Safferman AZ: Clinical profile of clozapine: Adverse reactions and agranulocytosis. Psychiatr Q 1992; 63:51–70.
113. Krupp P, Barnes P: Clozapine-associated agranulocytosis: Risk and aetiology. Br J Psychiatry 1992; 17:38–40.
114. Pisciotta AV, Konings SA, Ciesemier LL, et al: Cytotoxic activity in serum of patients with clozapine-induced agranulocytosis. J Lab Clin Med 1992; 119:254–266.
115. Fischer V, Haar JA, Greiner L, et al: Possible role of free radical formation in clozapine (Clozaril)-induced agranulocytosis. Mol Pharmacol 1991; 40:846–853.
116. Gerson SL, Arce C, Meltzer HY: N-desmethylclozapine: A clozapine metabolite that suppresses haemopoiesis. Br J Haematol 1994; 86:555–561.
117. Pisciotta AV, Konings SA: ^{51}Cr release assay of clozapine-induced cytotoxicity: Evidence for immunogenic mechanism. J Clin Psychiatry 1994; 55:143–148.
118. de la Chapelle A, Kari C, Nurminen M, et al: Clozapine-induced agranulocytosis. A genetic and epidemiologic study. Hum Genet 1977; 37:183–194.
119. Joseph G, Nguyen V, Smith JD: HLA-B38 and clozapine-induced agranulocytosis (letter). Ann Intern Med 1992; 116:605.
120. Yunis JJ, Corzo D, Salazar M, et al: HLA associations in clozapine-induced agranulocytosis. Blood 1995; 86:1177–1183.
121. Pfister GM, Hanson DR, Roerig JL, et al. Clozapine-induced agranulocytosis in a Native American: HLA typing and further support for an immune-mediated mechanism. J Clin Psychiatry 1992; 53:242–244.
122. Lieberman JA, Johns CA, Kane JM, et al: Clozapine-induced agranulocytosis: Non-cross-reactivity with other psychotropic drugs. J Clin Psychiatry 1988; 49:271–277.
123. Frankenburg FR, Stormberg D, Gerson SL: Unsuccessful reexposure to clozapine (letter). J Clin Psychopharmacol 1994; 14:428–429.
124. Laurenson IF, Buckoke C, Davidson C, et al: Delayed fatal agranulocytosis in an epileptic taking primidone and phenytoin (letter). Lancet 1994; 344:332–333.
125. Salzman C: Mandatory monitoring for side effects. The "bundling" of clozapine. N Engl J Med 1990; 323:827–829.
126. Reid WH: Access to care: Clozapine to the public sector. Hosp Community Psychiatry 1990; 41:870–874.
127. Zhang M, Owen RR, Pope SK, et al: Cost-effectiveness of clozapine monitoring after the first 6 months. Arch Gen Psychiatry 1996; 53:954–958.
128. Cooper RA: Captopril-associated neutropenia—Who is at risk? Arch Intern Med 1983; 143:659–660.
129. Forslund T, Borgmastars H, Fyhrquist F: Captopril-associated leucopenia confirmed by rechallenge in patient with renal failure (letter). Lancet 1981; 2:166.
130. Foster AL, Coleman JW: A rat model of captopril immunogenicity. Clin Exp Immunol 1989; 75:161–165.
131. Delfraissy JF, Galanaud P, Belavoine JF, et al: Captopril and immune regulation. Int Soc Nephrol 1984; 25:925–929.
132. Meyers DG, Gonzalez ER, Peters LL, et al: Severe neutropenia associated with procainamide: Comparison of sustained-release and conventional preparations. Am Heart J 1985; 109:1393–1395.
133. Roden DM, Woosley RL: Drug therapy. Tocainide. N Engl J Med 1986; 315:41–45.
134. Ellrodt AG, Murata GH, Riedinger MS, et al: Severe neutropenia associated with sustained-release procainamide. Ann Intern Med 1984; 100:197–201.
135. Cornacchia E, Golbus J, Maybaum J, et al: Hydralazine and procainamide inhibit T cell DNA methylation and induce autoreactivity. J Immunol 1988; 140:2197–2200.
136. Symoens J, Veys E, Mielants M, et al: Adverse reactions to levamisole. Cancer Treat Rep 1978; 62:1721–1730.

137. Williams GT, Johnson SAN, Dieppe PA, et al: Neutropenia during treatment of rheumatoid arthritis with levamisole. Ann Rheum Dis 1978; 37:366–369.
138. Veys EM, Mielants H, Verbruggen G: Levamisole-induced adverse reactions in HLA B27–positive rheumatoid arthritis (letter). Lancet 1978; 1:148.
139. Hodinka L, Geher P, Meretey K, et al: Levamisole-induced neutropenia and agranulocytosis: Association with HLA B27 leukocyte agglutinating and lymphocytotoxic antibodies. Int Arch Allergy Appl Immunol 1981; 65:460–464.
140. Drew SI, Carter BM, Nathanson DS, et al: Levamisole-associated neutropenia and autoimmune granulocytotoxins. Ann Rheum Dis 1980; 39:59–63.
141. Thompson JS, Herbick JM, Klassen LW, et al: Studies on levamisole-induced agranulocytosis. Blood 1980; 56:388–396.
142. Vogel CL, Silverman MA, Mansell PW, et al: Mechanisms of levamisole-induced granulocytopenia in breast cancer patients. Am J Hematol 1980; 9:171–183.
143. Aymard J-P, Aymard B, Netter P, et al: Haematological adverse effects of histamine H2-receptor antagonists. Med Toxicol 1988; 3:430–448.
144. Carloss HW, Tavassoli M, McMillan R: Cimetidine-induced granulocytopenia. Ann Intern Med 1980; 93:57–58.
145. List AF, Beaird DH, Kummet T: Ranitidine-induced granulocytopenia: Recurrence with cimetidine administration. Ann Intern Med 1988; 108:566–567.
146. Freston JW: Cimetidine and granulocytopenia. Ann Intern Med 1979; 90:264–265.
147. Fitchen JH, Koeffler HP: Cimetidine and granulopoiesis: Bone marrow culture studies in normal man and patients with cimetidine-associated neutropenia. Br J Haematol 1980; 46:361–366.
148. Calzado MC, Garcia-Castellano JM, Manzanares RM, et al: Effects of cimetidine on haematopoiesis in vitro. Br J Pharmacol 1982; 75:301–303.
149. Amos RJ, Kirk B, Amess JAL, et al: Bone marrow hypoplasia during intensive care: Bone marrow culture studies implicating ranitidine in the suppression of haemopoiesis. Human Toxicol 1987; 6:503–506.
150. Aglietta M, Stacchini A, Sanavio F, et al: H2 receptor antagonists and human granulopoiesis. Experientia 1985; 41:375–376.
151. Neben S, Hemman S, Montgomery M, et al: Hematopoietic stem cell deficit of transplanted bone marrow previously exposed to cytotoxic agents. Exp Hematol 1993; 21:156–162.
152. Gross S, Worthington-White DA: Cimetidine suppression of CFU-C in males. Am J Hematol 1984; 17:279–286.
153. Byron JW: Mechanism for histaminine H2–receptor induced cell-cycle changes in the bone marrow stem cell. Agents Actions Suppl 1977; 7:209–213.
154. Teitelbaum AH, Bell AJ, Brown SL: Filgrastim (r-metHuG-CSF) reversal of drug-induced agranulocytosis. Am J Med 1993; 95:245–246.
155. Bradford CR, Ong EL, Hendrick DJ, et al: Use of colony stimulating factors for the treatment of drug-induced agranulocytosis. Br J Haematol 1993; 84:182–186.
156. Averns HL, Boardman, PL: Granulocyte colony stimulating factor in drug induced agranulocytosis. Br J Rheumatol 1993; 32:1029–1030.
157. Tajiri J, Noguchi S, Okamura S, et al: Granulocyte colony-stimulating factor treatment of antithyroid drug-induced granulocytopenia. Arch Intern Med 1993; 153:509–514.
158. Gullion G, Yeh H: Treatment of clozapine-induced agranulocytosis with recombinant granulocyte colony-stimulating factor. J Clin Psychiatry 1994; 55:401–405.
159. Gerson SL: G-CSF and the management of clozapine-induced agranulocytosis. J Clin Psychiatry 1994; 55:139–142.
160. Chengappa KN, Gopalani A, Haught MK, et al: The treatment of clozapine-associated agranulocytosis with granulocyte colony-stimulating factor (G-CSF). Psychopharmacol Bull 1996; 32:111–121.
161. Demuynck H, Zachée P, Verhoef GEG, et al: Risks of rhG-CSF treatment in drug-induced agranulocytosis. Ann Hematol 1995; 70:143–147.
162. Hara H, Ban Y, Sato R, et al: Change in serum G-CSF levels in patients with Graves' disease by treatment with methimazole. Nippon Naibunpi Gakkai Zasshi 1992; 68:1121–1129.
163. Fukata S, Marakami Y, Kuma K, et al: G-CSF levels during spontaneous recovery from drug-induced agranulocytosis. Lancet 1993; 342:1495.
164. Doan CA: The neutropenic state. Its significance and therapeutic rationale. JAMA 1932; 99:194–202.
165. Kastlin GJ: Agranulocytic angina. Am J Med Sci 1927; 173:799–813.
166. Jackson H, Tighe TJG: An analysis of the treatment and mortality of three hundred and ninety cases of acute agranulocytic angina. N Engl J Med 1939; 220:729–733.
167. Huguley CM Jr: Agranulocytosis induced by dipyrone, a hazardous antipyretic and analgesic. JAMA 1964; 189:938–941.
168. Böttiger LE, Westerholm B: Drug-induced blood dyscrasias in Sweden. BMJ 1973; 3:339–343.
169. Palva IP, Mustala OO: Drug-induced agranulocytosis II. The role of medication in a fatal outcome. Acta Med Scand 1972; 191:121–124.
170. Juliá A, Olona M, Revilla BE, et al: Drug-induced agranulocytosis: Prognostic factors in a series of 168 episodes. Br J Haematol 1991; 79:366–371.
171. Keisu M, Ekman E: Sulfasalazine associated agranulocytosis in Sweden 1972–1989. Clinical features, and estimation of its incidence. Eur J Clin Pharmacol 1992; 43:215–218.
172. Rosenthal N, Abel HA: The significance of the monocytes in agranulocytosis (leukopenic infectious monocytosis). Am J Clin Pathol 1936; 6:205–230.

173. Hennemann HH, Schief A: Rezidive von Agranulozytose. Dtsch Med Wochenschr 1975; 100:519–526.
174. D'Antonio D, Iacone A, Fioritoni G, et al: Patterns of infection in 41 patients with idiosyncratic drug-induced agranulocytosis. Ann Hematol 1991; 63:84–88.
175. Spaet TH, Dameshek W: Chronic hypoplastic neutropenia. Am J Med 1952; 13:35–45.
176. Butler JJ: Chronic idiopathic immunoneutropenia. Am J Med 1958; 24:145–152.
177. Cline MJ, Opelz G, Saxon A, et al: Autoimmune panleukopenia. N Engl J Med 1976; 295:1489–1493.
178. Levitt LJ, Ries CA, Greenberg PL: Pure white-cell aplasia. Antibody-mediated autoimmune inhibition of granulopoiesis. N Engl J Med 1983; 308:1141–1146.
179. Baker BL, Hendricks JB, Shahidi NT, et al: Humoral and cellular immunosuppression of granulopoiesis in a patient with neutropenia. Am J Med 1988; 85:264–267.
180. Marinone G, Roncoli B, Marinone MG Jr: Pure white cell aplasia. Semin Hematol 1991; 28:298–302.
181. Blaschke J, Goeken NE, Thompson JS, et al: Acquired agranulocytosis with granulocyte specific cytotoxic antibody. Am J Med 1979; 66:862–866.
182. Barbui T, Bassan R, Viero P, et al: Pure white cell aplasia treated by high dose intravenous immunoglobulin (letter). Br J Haematol 1984; 58:554–555.
183. Postiglione K, Ferris R, Jaffe JP, et al: Immune mediated agranulocytosis and anemia associated with thymoma. Am J Hematol 1995; 49:336–340.
184. Degos L, Faille A, Housset M, et al: Syndrome of neutrophil agranulocytosis, hypogammaglobulinemia, and thymoma. Blood 1982; 60:968–972.
185. Ackland SP, Bur ME, Adler SS, et al: White blood cell aplasia associated with thymoma. Am J Clin Pathol 1989; 89:260–263.
186. Weir AB III, Dow LW: Response of agranulocytosis to thymectomy in a patient with thymoma and chronic lymphocytic leukemia. Med Pediatr Oncol 1989; 17:58–61.
187. Mathieson PW, O'Neill JH, Durrant STS, et al: Antibody-mediated pure neutrophil aplasia, recurrent myasthenia gravis and previous thymoma: Case report and literature review. Q J Med 1990; 273:57–61.

8

Acquired Amegakaryocytic Thrombocytopenic Purpura

Stephen Rosenfeld, M.D.

Acquired amegakaryocytic thrombocytopenic purpura (AATP) is a typical bone marrow failure disorder. With minor qualifications the diagnostic criteria are well captured by the name, but time and experience have shown that the clinical findings of a low platelet count and decreased or absent megakaryocytes on bone marrow biopsy can arise from a variety of causes. Fortunately, the list of causes and also treatments is similar to that of other bone marrow failure states, and AATP is most appropriately viewed as a special case of these diseases. The disorder is very rare and incidence figures are not available. It is certainly less common than related syndromes, such as idiopathic thrombocytopenic purpura (ITP), the myelodysplastic syndromes (MDSs), and aplastic anemia. Because of its rarity, the literature on AATP consists exclusively of case reports and only an occasional small series. These provide a patchwork view of the disease, with insights into pathophysiology and treatment coming from a variety of investigators using assays that are almost never repeated from one study to the next. Although questions about the general mechanisms of disease and the best therapy remain unanswered, some general conclusions may be drawn and a rational therapeutic strategy outlined.

CLASSIFICATION

Attempts at classification of AATP divide the disorder by etiology,[1] such as idiopathic, drug-induced, or associated with other diseases. One such classification is given in Table 8–1. The small number of cases limits the utility of any nosologic scheme, and the uniqueness of some of these reports raises questions as to the relevance of observed associations. An alternative classification by disease mechanism (Table 8–2) provides insight into the relationship of AATP and other bone marrow failure states, and provides a basis for therapy.

By analogy to pure red cell aplasia (PRCA) some authors have identified "pure" AATP as a low platelet count and decreased bone marrow megakaryocytes without involvement of other hematopoietic lineages.[1] Such pure involvement of megakaryocytes seems to be an exceedingly rare and often transient phenomenon that soon broadens to involve other lineages. While it risks a loss of precision, it is useful for diagnostic purposes to

TABLE 8–1 Clinical Classification of Acquired Amegakaryocytic Thrombocytic Purpura

Drug-induced
    Acetaminophen[25]
    Oxyphenbutazone[25]
    Chemotherapeutic agents[34]
    Busulfan[3]
    Radioiodide?[16]
Associated with other disorders
    Systemic lupus erythematosus[2-5]
    Acute myeloid leukemia[34]
    Chronic myelogenous leukemia[3]
    Non-Hodgkin's lymphoma[12]
    Pregnancy[11]
    Hepatitis[11]
    Myelodysplastic syndromes[13]
    Vitamin B_{12} deficiency[24]
    Large granular lymphocyte leukemia[14]
Idiopathic

TABLE 8-2 Pathophysiologic Classification of Acquired Amegakaryocytic Thrombocytopenic Purpura

Direct bone marrow toxicity
    Drug-induced
    Radiation-induced
Immune-mediated
    Humoral
    Cellular
Clonal abnormalities of the bone marrow
Metabolic
    Vitamin B_{12} deficiency

consider AATP when involvement of the megakaryocytic lineage is clearly out of proportion to involvement of other blood elements, or when the mechanism of involvement of another lineage is clearly different.

DIFFERENTIAL DIAGNOSIS

AATP should be low on the list of differential diagnoses of a patient presenting with signs and symptoms of thrombocytopenia. The great majority of such patients will have ITP. It is not uncommon to give a therapeutic trial of steroids or intravenous (IV) immune globulin in cases of presumed ITP even before a bone marrow biopsy is performed, especially in children, and the risk of missing a case of AATP is not high enough to justify changing this practice. Patients who undergo bone marrow biopsy and are found to have decreased megakaryocyte numbers may still have ITP, but in this subset of patients AATP becomes a possible alternative diagnosis. The most practical way to distinguish the disorders in this setting is to assess platelet survival. The direct measurement of platelet survival is not generally available, but platelet survival after transfusion is a rough surrogate; in ITP transfused platelets are cleared rapidly, whereas in AATP their half-life is normal. There are other clues to the diagnosis of AATP. Unlike ITP, AATP is a failure of platelet production. It is unusual for such a process to occur without some evidence that other hematopoietic lineages are affected. Thus, macrocytosis on a peripheral smear or a high mean corpuscular volume, or mild anemia or granulocytopenia would all suggest AATP rather than ITP. AATP has been associated with systemic lupus erythematosus (SLE) in several reports,[2-5] but ITP is also associated with SLE, limiting the diagnostic utility of this association.

The designation of AATP explicitly excludes constitutional disorders. The syndrome of thrombocytopenia with absent radii (TAR) is the most common of these syndromes, is very rare, and generally presents early in life. It is unlikely that individuals with this or related constitutional thrombocytopenias would present to an internist for first diagnosis or treatment.

NATURAL HISTORY

The literature is not comprehensive enough to support the description of the "typical" natural history of primary AATP. In some cases the disorder remains stable for years.[6,7] Spontaneous remissions are rare, but have been reported.[8] A significant proportion of patients, perhaps as high as 25%, will evolve into frank aplastic anemia involving all hematopoietic lineage.[9-11] In isolated cases AATP has been the presenting sign for non-Hodgkin's lymphoma (NHL),[12] MDS,[13] large granular lymphocyte (LGL) leukemia,[14] and cyclic hematopoiesis.[15] As treatment for other bone marrow failure states has improved, so has that for AATP, and it is unusual for a patient to be reported who has not responded to one of the available modalities. The risk of relapse or evolution after therapy, a risk that may be high in other related disorders such as aplastic anemia, has not been assessed in AATP.

PATHOGENESIS

In most cases AATP appears to be immune-mediated. Involvement of the cellular immune system has been demonstrated by showing that autologous lymphocytes inhibit bone marrow colony formation.[4,8] In addition, involvement of the immune system can be inferred from the response to cyclosporine (CsA),[16-18] antithymocyte globulin (ATG),[9,19-21] or other immunosuppressive agents.[22] In other cases a serum inhibitory activity has been extracted in the IgG serum fraction,[15,23] implicating the humoral immune response. Associations with SLE, NHL, and LGL leukemia also support a pathogenic role for the immune system.

There appear to be rare cases of AATP that are not primarily immune-mediated. AATP has been associated with vitamin B_{12} deficiency,[24] although more typically megakaryocytes are increased in this disorder. One reported patient presented with AATP and normal chromosomes which evolved into MDS with a 5q- abnormality[13]; this subsequently evolved into acute myeloid leukemia (AML). AATP has been convincingly demonstrated to be drug-related in a patient taking paracetamol (acetaminophen and oxyphenbutazone),[25] as platelets returned to normal within 2 weeks of stopping the medication.

Growth factor abnormalities or deficiencies do not play a significant role in the pathogenesis of AATP. With rare exceptions, serum stimulatory activity for megakaryocyte colony formation is increased,[7,23] analogous to the increase in stimulatory factors in aplastic anemia. Where it has been measured, the serum level of thrombopoietin has been markedly elevated.[3]

THERAPY

AATP has been treated with corticosteroids,[2,5,6,9,12–14,16–22,26,27] splenectomy,[2,18,23] androgens,[9,13,19,23,28,29] vincristine,[13,14,20,23] CsA,[6,10,14,16–18] ATG,[9,10,19–21,30] cyclophosphamide,[14,17,22] lithium,[13] azathioprine,[9,14] IV immune globulin,[17,18] and plasma exchange.[16] Of these therapies, ATG and CsA were the most consistently effective. Steroids, especially in high doses, may have some efficacy; many patients will receive them before the diagnosis of AATP is made. Androgens, especially danazol, may increase platelet numbers in some cases. There is no established role for splenectomy or IV immune globulin. Given its similarity to other bone marrow failure states, it is reasonable to adopt a therapeutic strategy that builds from the experience with these related disorders. Immunosuppressive therapy with ATG or CsA should be the first line of treatment for patients definitively diagnosed with AATP. No dosing regimen has been tested systematically, but there are established regimens for both of these agents in the treatment of aplastic anemia.[31] For patients with convincing disease associations (SLE, NHL) the underlying disease process should be treated first. Platelet transfusions are effective in AATP and should be given without hesitation to any patient with hemorrhagic complications. The use of prophylactic platelet transfusions is justifiable to maintain platelet numbers over 10,000/mm^3 [32,33]; bleeding patients who have become refractory to platelet transfusions should be treated with HLA-matched platelets. Androgen therapy with danazol can be used in patients who fail or become refractory to immunosuppressive therapy, and some patients have responded to very-high-dose corticosteroid regimens. All patients should be monitored frequently for changes in their clinical condition that may herald evolution to other disorders, such as aplastic anemia or MDS.

REFERENCES

1. Boggs DR: Amegakaryocytic thrombocytopenia. Am J Hematol 20:413, 1985.
2. Griner PF, Hoyer LW: Amegakaryocytic thrombocytopenia in systemic lupus erythematosus. Arch Intern Med 125:329, 1970.
3. Mukai HY, Kojima H, Todokoro K, et al: Serum thrombopoietin (TPO) levels in patients with amegakaryocytic thrombocytopenia are much higher than those with immune thrombocytopenic purpura. Thromb Haemost 76:675, 1996.
4. Nagasawa T, Sakurai T, Kashiwagi H, et al: Cell-mediated amegakaryocytic thrombocytopenia associated with system lupus erythematosus. Blood 67:479, 1986.
5. Sakurai T, Kono I, Kabashima T, et al: Amegakaryocytic thrombocytopenia associated with systemic lupus erythematosus successfully treated by a high-dose prednisolone therapy. Jpn J Med 23:135, 1984.
6. Katai M, Aizawa T, Ohara N, et al: Acquired amegakaryocytic thrombocytopenic purpura with humoral inhibitory factor for megakaryocyte colony formation. Intern Med 33:147, 1994.
7. Podolak-Dawidziak M: Acquired amegakaryocytic thrombocytopenic purpura (AATP): A study of autologous megakaryocyte progenitors and the effect of patients' plasma on normal marrow megakaryocyte colony formation. Folia Haematol 117:347, 1990.
8. Gewirtz AM, Keefer Sacchetti M, Bien R, et al: Cell-mediated suppression of megakaryocytopoiesis in acquired amegakaryocytic thrombocytopenic purpura. Blood 68:619, 1986.
9. Chan DKY, O'Neill B: Successful trial of antithymocyte globulin therapy in amegakaryocytic thrombocytopenic purpura. Med J Aust 148:602, 1988.
10. King JAC, Elkhalifa MY, Latour LF: Rapid progression of acquired amegakaryocytic thrombocytopenia to aplastic anemia. South Med J 90:91, 1997.
11. Slater LM, Katz J, Walter B, et al: Aplastic anemia occurring as amegakaryocytic thrombocytopenia with and without an inhibitor of granulopoiesis. Am J Hematol 18:251, 1985.
12. Lugassy G: Non-Hodgkin's lymphoma presenting with amegakaryocytic thrombocytopenic purpura. Ann Hematol 73:41, 1996.
13. Geissler D, Thaler J, Konwalinka G, et al: Progressive preleukemia presenting amegakaryocytic thrombocytopenic purpura: Association of the 5q-syndrome with a decreased megakaryocyte colony formation a defective production of Meg-CSF. Leuk Res 11:731, 1987.
14. Kouides PA, Rowe JM: Large granular lymphocyte leukemia presenting with both amegakaryocytic thrombocytopenic purpura and pure red cell aplasia: Clinical course and response to immunosuppressive therapy. Am J Hematol 49:232, 1995.
15. Hoffman R, Bridell RA, van Besien K, et al: A: Acquired cyclic amegakaryocytic thrombocytopenia associated with an immunoglobulin blocking the action of granulocyte-macrophage colony-stimulating factor. N Engl J Med 321:97, 1989.
16. Hill W, Landgraf R: Successful treatment of amegakaryocytic thrombocytopenic purpura with cyclosporine. N Engl J Med 312:1060, 1985.
17. Peng CT, Kao LY, Tsai CH: Successful treatment

with cyclosporin A in a child with acquired pure amegakaryocytic thrombocytopenic purpura. Acta Paediatr 83:1222, 1994.
18. Telek B, Kiss A, Pecze K, et al: Cyclic idiopathic pure acquired amegakaryocytic thrombocytopenic purpura: A patient treated with cyclosporin A. Br J Haematol 73:128, 1989.
19. Khelif A, Ffrench M, Follea G, et al: Amegakaryocytic thrombocytopenic purpura treated with antithymocyte globulin. Ann Int Med 102:720, 1985.
20. Manoharan A, Williams NT, Sparrow R: Acquired amegakaryocytic thrombocytopenia: Report of a case and review of the literature. Q J Med 263:243, 1989.
21. Trimble MS, Glynn MFX, Brain MC: Amegakaryocytic thrombocytopenia of 4 years duration: Successful treatment with antithymocyte globulin. Am J Hematol 37:126, 1991.
22. El Saghir NS, Geltman RL: Treatment of acquired amegakaryocytic thrombocytopenic purpura with cyclophosphamide. Am J Med 81:13, 1986.
23. Hoffman R, Bruno E, Elwell J, et al: Acquired amegakaryocytic thrombocytopenic purpura: A syndrome of diverse etiologies. Blood 60:1173, 1982.
24. Ghosh K, Sarode R, Varma N, et al: Amegakaryocytic thrombocytopenia of nutritional vitamin B_{12} deficiency. Trop Geog Med 40:158, 1988.
25. Font J, Nomdedeu B, Martinez-Orozco F, et al: Amegakaryocytic thrombocytopenia and an analgesic. Ann Intern Med 95:783, 1981.
26. Rovira M, Feliu E, Florensa L, et al: Acquired amegakaryocytic thrombocytopenic purpura associated with immunoglobulin deficiency. Acta Haematol 85:34, 1991.
27. Smeets REH, Hillen HFP: Acquired amegakaryocytic thrombocytopenic purpura. Treatment with high-dose dexamethasone pulse therapy and review of the literature.Neth J Med 32:27, 1988.
28. Kayser W, Euler HH, Schmitz N, et al: Danazol in acquired amegakaryocytic thrombocytopenic purpura: A case report. Blut 51:401, 1985.
29. Koduri PR: Amegakaryocytic thrombocytopenia with a positive direct Coombs' test. Am J Hematol 44:68, 1993.
30. Faldt R: Remission of amegakaryocytic thrombocytopenia induced by antilymphocyte globulin (ALG). Br. J Haematol 63:205, 1986.
31. Rosenfeld SJ, Kimball J, Vining D, et al: Intensive immunosuppression with antithymocyte globulin and cyclosporine as treatment for severe acquired aplastic anemia. Blood 85:3058, 1995.
32. Rebulla P, Finazzi G, Marangoni F, et al: A multicenter randomized study of the threshold for prophylactic platelet transfusions in adults with acute myeloid leukemia. N Eng J Med 337:1870, 1997.
33. Wandt H, Frank M, Ehninger G, et al: Safety and cost effectiveness of a 10×10^9/L trigger for prophylactic platelet transfusions compared with the traditional 20×10^9/L trigger: A prospective comparative trial in 105 patients with acute myeloid leukemia. Blood 91:3601, 1998.
34. Worman CP, Mills HG, Linch DC, et al: Amegakaryocytic thrombocytopenia associated with an excess of Leu 2a+ suppressor cells. Scan J Haematol 28:215, 1982.

9

Human Immunodeficiency Virus–Related Bone Marrow Failure

Elaine M. Sloand and
Jaroslow P. Maciejewski

The hematologic manifestations of human immunodeficiency virus type 1 (HIV-1) infection include cytopenias; coagulopathy due to acquired factor C and factor S deficiencies, or to a lupus anticoagulant; idiopathic thrombocytopenic purpura (ITP); thrombotic thrombocytopenic purpura (TTP); and Hodgkin's (HL) and non-Hodgkin's lymphomas (NHL). HIV-associated bone marrow failure is among the commonest acquired forms of defective hematopoiesis. The pathophysiology is multifactorial, complex, and variable as the course of HIV infection evolves in the patient (Fig. 9–1). This chapter describes the epidemiology, pathophysiology, and treatment of cytopenias in HIV infection, focusing on bone marrow failure and its complications.

CLINICAL FEATURES AND CAUSES OF BONE MARROW FAILURE

Hematologic Manifestations of HIV Infection

Cytopenias are frequently observed in HIV-1–infected patients and can have important clinical sequelae. In one study, performed in the 1980s, anemia occurred in 70%, neutropenia in 50%, and thrombocytopenia in 40% of patients with a diagnosis of acquired immunodeficiency syndrome (AIDS).[1] Although immune thrombocytopenia may appear early, in general the prevalence of cytopenias increases during the course of the disease.[2] Opportunistic infections, malignancies, or HIV-1 itself all can cause suppression of hematopoiesis, and the cumulative effects of applied therapies may affect the patient's hematopoietic function (Plate 11).

Anemia

Anemia is the most frequent hematologic manifestation of AIDS. Frequently, early in the AIDS epidemic, when high doses of zidovudine (ZDV) were widely used, anemia remained common, particularly in patients with advanced disease.[3,4] Anemia was identified as an independent prognostic factor for survival by the Multi-Center AIDS Cohort Study.[5,6] Laboratory studies usually reveal normocytic, normochromic anemia with low reticulocyte counts, and iron studies are consistent with the diagnosis of anemia of chronic disease. Erythropoietin levels are usually decreased. Although ZDV-induced anemia is frequently macrocytic, it may be normocytic. A ZDV-induced decrease in erythropoietin production can be severe and may produce a clinical picture resembling pure red cell aplasia.[7]

Bone marrow failure is likely to be the most common cause of anemia in HIV infection, hemolytic anemia and anemia related to gastrointestinal bleeding accounting for a smaller proportion of cases. Hemolysis is a rare cause of anemia in AIDS patients, and antierythrocyte antibody levels are often clinically irrelevant and do not correlate with the degree of anemia; red blood cell–associated antibody can be found in a majority of

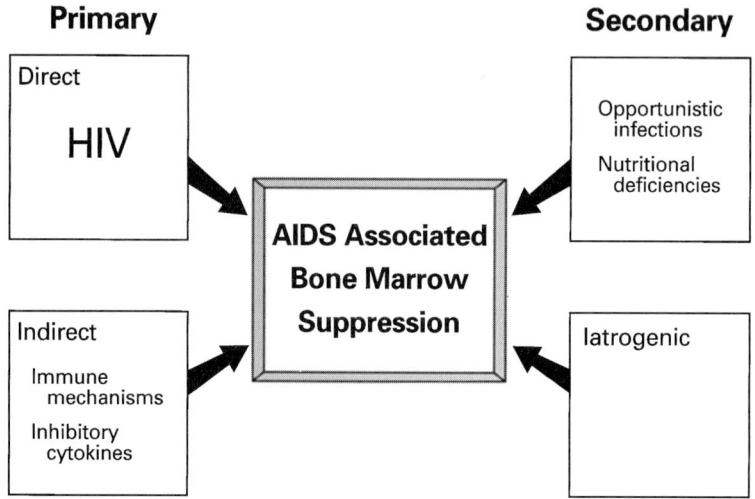

Figure 9–1 Possible mechanisms of hematopoietic inhibition in acquired immunodeficiency syndrome (AIDS). In addition to the human immunodeficiency virus type 1 (HIV-1)–triggered pathophysiologic pathways (direct or indirect), secondary mechanisms related to complications occurring in the immunosuppressed state may play a role in hematopoietic failure. In addition, iatrogenic causes contribute to hematopoietic dysfunction in AIDS.

AIDS patients but also in 44% of asymptomatic homosexual men.[8, 9] Although circulating erythropoietin is often low, the degree of anemia nevertheless is often disproportionately severe for the erythropoietin levels.[10] Suppressed erythropoiesis may be related to drug therapy or be secondary to infections with such agents as human cytomegalovirus (HCMV), parvovirus B19, and *Mycobacterium avium-intracellulare* (MAI).[11–14] Nutritional factors such as vitamin B_{12} deficiency, resulting from malabsorption or malnutrition, as well as deranged iron metabolism, have been reported as a frequent cause of anemia in patients with HIV infection.[15–17]

Thrombocytopenia

Thrombocytopenia is a common complication of HIV-1 infection, and often the presenting laboratory finding to prompt virus testing. As with the anemia, the etiology of thrombocytopenia is multifactorial. Platelet counts of less than 150,000/mL can be found in up to 11% of HIV-1–infected patients, and platelet counts of less than 50,000/mL in 1.5%.[18] Although mild thrombocytopenia is more common in patients with advanced disease, platelet counts of less than 20,000/mL occur more frequently in asymptomatic HIV-1–infected patients, implying different pathophysiologic causes.[18] Decreased platelet survival is more likely to account for thrombocytopenia in asymptomatic HIV-1–infected persons, while decreased bone marrow production of platelets is responsible in advanced disease.[17]

Factors responsible for decreased platelet survival have not been clearly defined. Platelet-associated antibodies increase during disease progression, but their role in decreasing platelet survival is unclear, as they do not correlate with thrombocytopenia.[19] TTP also occurs with increased frequency in this population, but the presence of microangiopathy facilitates differentiation from other causes of thrombocytopenia.[20] While ITP is the most frequent cause of thrombocytopenia in HIV-1–infected persons, impaired production of platelets, in combination with neutropenia and anemia, is an important part of HIV-associated marrow failure.[21] Megakaryocytes have been shown to be directly susceptible to infection with HIV-1, and megakaryocytes arising from HIV-1–infected CD34+ progenitor cells are defective in their ability to produce platelets.[22] In addition, HIV-1 strains directly cytopathic to the megakaryocytes have been isolated (see below).[23]

Neutropenia

Neutropenia also is common in HIV-1 infection. While infrequently resulting in bacterial infection alone, granulocytopenias can limit the doses of ganciclovir or cytotoxic chemotherapy. Again, antibodies associated with neutrophils are often found but do not correlate with neutropenia. As in the case of anemia and thrombocytopenia, AIDS-related bone marrow failure is thought to be the major cause of neutropenia in AIDS.

PATHOPHYSIOLOGIC MECHANISMS

Many factors have been implicated in the complex pathophysiology of the cytopenias accompanying HIV-1 infection. While bone marrow suppression may be a direct consequence of HIV-1 infection, other secondary immunologic mechanisms, including cytokine dysregulation and changes in lymphocyte subsets regulating marrow function, are also responsible (Fig. 9–1). Drug toxicity, opportunistic infection, and secondary malignancy play important roles (see Fig. 9–1; discussed above). Finally, decreased survival of peripheral blood cells contributes to the development of cytopenias, especially when the physiologic reserves of bone marrow are exhausted.

Hematologic Effects of Drug Therapy

Drug-related hematopoietic toxicity is an important clinical problem in the management of patients with AIDS (Table 9–1). ZDV is commonly associated with marrow toxicity, particularly with long-term administration. The most frequent manifestation of ZDV toxicity is anemia. In the early 1980s, when doses of ZDV in excess of 600 mg/day were used as monotherapy, anemia was common and sufficiently severe that infected patients in treatment were frequently transfusion dependent. When lower doses of ZDV were used alone or in combination with other nonmyelosuppressive antiviral drugs, anemia became less of a clinical problem. In the AIDS Clinical Trial Group, HIV-1–infected patients receiving a ZDV dose of 500 mg/day did not show any significant decrease in hemoglobin levels when compared with a similarly immunosuppressed HIV-1–infected cohort not taking the drug. However, when patients with advanced disease were studied, the incidence of ZDV-related anemia was substantial, even at the lower dose of the drug (500 mg/day). Generally, the anemia related to ZDV is reversible. Although the mechanisms of ZDV toxicity, inhibition of thymidine kinase and DNA chain termination, should apply to other hematologic lineages, neutropenia is less frequent and thrombocytopenia very uncommon. The reasons for preferential suppression of erythropoiesis are not clear. Other nucleoside analogues, didanosine (ddI) or dideoxycytidosine (zalcitabine; ddC), lamivudine (3TC), and stavudine (d4T), do not appear to have significant bone marrow toxicity.[24] Fortunately, the protease inhibitors, indinavir sulfate (Crixivan), ritonavir, and nelfinavir, alone or in combination with ZDV or other nucleoside analogues, have little or no effect on hematopoiesis.[25]

Trimethoprim-sulfamethoxazole (TMP-SMX), commonly used for the prevention of *Pneumocystis carinii* pneumonia (PCP) and has activity against toxoplasmosis. Although there is no evidence that TMP-SMX induces folate deficiency in

TABLE 9–1 Hematopoietic Effects of Drugs Frequently Used in Patients With AIDS

Drug	Activity	Hematologic toxicity
Zidovudine	Nucleoside analogues, antiviral	Anemia, neutropenia (dose-dependent)
Stavudine	Nucleoside analogues, antiviral	Anemia, neutropenia (dose-dependent)
Lamivudine	Nucleoside analogues, antiviral	Anemia, neutropenia (dose-dependent)
Saquinavir, ritonavir, indinavir	HIV protease inhibitors, antiviral	Minimal
Trimethoprim-sulfamethoxazole	Antibiotic *Pneumocystis carinii* pneumonia	Dose-related neutropenia anemia Methemoglobinemia, especially in persons with G6PD deficiency
Primaquine	Antibiotic *Pneumocystis carinii* pneumonia	Rare agranulocytoses; thrombocytopenia Methemoglobinemia, especially in G6PD deficiency
Pentamidine	*Pneumocystis carinii* pneumonia	Infrequent anemia, leukopenia, thrombocytopenia
Sulfadiazine	Toxoplasmosis	Leukopenia in 40%; thrombocytopenia in 12%
Clindamycin-pyrimethamine	Toxoplasmosis	Cytopenias in 31%
Ketoconazole, fluconazole, itraconazole	Candidiasis	Rare
Amphotericin B	Antifungal, cryptococcal meningitis	Anemia
Ganciclovir	CMV infection	Leukopenia, thrombocytopenia
Foscarnet	CMV infection	No significant toxicity
Acyclovir	Herpes simplex and herpes zoster	No significant toxicity
Rifampin, rifabutin	MAI	No significant toxicity

G6PD, glucose-6-phosphate dehydrogenase; CMV, cytomegalovirus; MAI, *Mycobacterium avium-intracellulare*.

normal persons, in patients with poor nutritional status and in combination with other hematotoxic factors, the drug may result in megaloblastic anemia, leukopenia, and thrombocytopenia on the basis of folate deficiency. In AIDS patients, a high rate of TMP-SMX–related side effects has been reported: fever, rash, malaise, and pancytopenia occurred in 8 out of 18 patients in one study, while in some series as many as 90% had ill effects.[26] Bone marrow suppression, seemingly unrelated to folate deficiency, occurs frequently with TMP-SMX. In a comparative trial with parenteral pentamidine, anemia was seen in 39% vs. 24%; mild neutropenia in 72% vs. 47%, and modest thrombocytopenia in 3% vs. 18% of patients treated with TMP-SMX and pentamidine, respectively.[27] TMP-SMX dose reduction to 20 mg/kg prevented development of neutropenia and thrombocytopenia. Dapsone (also used as prophylaxis of PCP) is associated with fewer hematologic abnormalities than TMP-SMX (but is contraindicated in the presence of glucose-6-phosphate dehydrogenase deficiency).

Ganciclovir (GCV), used for the treatment of active HCMV infection, is very myelosuppressive when administered parenterally. Leukopenia or thrombocytopenia occurs in 40% to 48% of AIDS patients receiving GCV.[28, 29] Reversible neutropenia is common after the second week of GCV administration. Concurrent administration of hematopoietic growth factors may be necessary to prevent or improve severe neutropenia. Oral ganciclovir is currently being tested in clinical trials for prophylaxis of human CMV infection. Probably because high blood levels are not achieved by this route, severe neutropenia has not been observed. However, in a recently reported trial, patients receiving oral GCV more frequently required erythropoietin and granulocyte colony-stimulating factor (G-CSF) administration than did patients who were not receiving the drug.[30] Acyclovir, frequently used for treatment of recurrent herpetic lesions, has no bone marrow toxicity.

Amphotericin B is also frequently associated with myelosuppression. Hypochromic, normocytic anemia is the most common hematopoietic toxicity. In addition to direct effects on the bone marrow, amphotericin renal toxicity may result in diminished erythropoietin production.[31]

Opportunistic Infections

Human Cytomegalovirus

Bone marrow failure is not a common complication of human CMV infection in normal persons, in whom the primary infection is usually asymptomatic. HCMV has been only infrequently associated with bone marrow failure, and the virus has been convincingly implicated as an etiologic agent for hematopoietic suppression in only a few studies.[32] Although there is substantial *in vitro* evidence that cytomegalovirus infection suppresses marrow growth, extrapolation of these results to the clinic is problematic. Certainly CMV infection is associated with graft failure in the bone marrow transplantation setting and many transplant patients with active CMV infection have cytopenias. However, these complicated patients have a myriad of other explanations for their bone marrow failure. The significance of CMV in the HIV-infected patient is even more difficult to assess. Drug therapy, other concurrent infections, and significant immunologic derangement all suppress hematopoiesis, and CMV antigen may be detected in a substantial percentage of AIDS patients without clinical signs of CMV infection.[33] However, delayed engraftment after bone marrow transplantation or graft failure suggests that HCMV may cause defective marrow function under certain circumstances.[32] There is also an association between graft-versus-host disease and evolution of HCMV disease, but the causal relationships among increased immunosuppression, graft rejection, and HCMV reactivation remain unclear.

Human CMV is a common infection in AIDS, and the virus has important clinical manifestations in this patient population. Almost all homosexual men infected with HIV-1 have antibodies to human CMV, compared to 50% seroprevalence in the general American population.[34, 35] Human CMV is shed in saliva, blood, urine, vaginal secretion, and semen. Clinically active human CMV infection occurs in 26% of all AIDS patients during their lifetime.[36] Retinitis is the most severe and frequent human CMV syndrome secondary to HIV-1–induced immunodeficiency.

Although there is agreement that human CMV infection of bone marrow progenitors suppresses hematopoiesis in vitro, the inhibitory mechanisms remain unclear.[37–42] Generally, the effects of human CMV on hematopoiesis have been attributed to direct infection of marrow progenitor cells,[37, 39–42] infection of supporting stromal cells, or interference with the ability of precursors to respond to cytokines and increased inhibitory cytokines which can suppress hematopoiesis and are produced by human CMV–infected leukocytes.[43–45] In addition, immune effector cells such as cytotoxic lymphocytes or natural killer cells activated in the course of human CMV infection can produce inhibitory cytokines, including interferons, lymphotoxin, and Fas-ligand.[46, 47]

Mycobacterium avium-intracellulare

Patients infected by MAI complex often show profound anemia. However, MAI has become infrequent as a complication of HIV infection since the institution of highly active anti-retroviral treatment (HAART). The pathophysiology of anemia in MAI infection is not clear and is unrelated to decreased survival of erythrocytes, HIV-1 load, or erythropoietin production.[48] Because of the association of MAI with low CD4+ counts, anemia in MAI infection usually coincides with late clinical stages of AIDS. Anemia, occurring in conjunction with MAI infection, is often not accompanied by other cytopenias.[49] Bone marrow examination generally demonstrates erythroid hyperplasia,[50] granulomas, and foamy histiocytes; mycobacteria can be visualized by acid-fast staining. MAI is often more readily isolated from or identified in bone marrow than in peripheral blood.

Parvovirus B19

Parvovirus B19 infection can cause pure red cell aplasia and anemia in immunosuppressed HIV-1–infected patients.[51] Although the seroprevalence of IgG antibodies against parvovirus B19 is 40% to 60% in the adult population,[52] virus can generally be detected only in patients with active early or persistent disease. Parvovirus B19 infection is associated with anemia, complete absence of reticulocytes, and pure red cell aplasia of the marrow, while leukocyte and platelet counts are unaffected. Bone marrow examination may demonstrate large vacuolated proerythrocytes or giant pronormoblasts and markedly reduced numbers of all red blood cell precursors. Typical manifestations of fifth disease are absent in AIDS patients but may be observed after treatment with immune globulin, as a result of iatrogenic immune complex formation. Persistent parvovirus B19 infection is an important, treatable cause of anemia in AIDS patients: in two studies, parvovirus B19 accounted for anemia in 17% to 31% of significantly anemic HIV-1–infected patients.[13, 53, 54] The presence of IgM to parvovirus B19 and the marrow morphology did not correlate with chronic infection.[53] A diagnosis of parvovirus B19 infection should be considered in any transfusion-dependent, HIV-1–infected patient, without other identifiable causes of anemia. Although a negative polymerase chain reaction (PCR) examination of serum excludes the diagnosis, DNA dot blot hybridization is usually adequate to establish a diagnosis of chronic infection.[53] Positive IgG serology only indicates past contact, and persistently infected AIDS patients should be negative for anti-parvovirus antibody. PCR is associated with a significant false-positive rate, and in cases of resolving infection this test also may be positive. The diagnosis of persistent parvovirus infection should be sought because treatment with commercial immune globulins is almost always associated with marked improvement in hemoglobin levels. Resolution of anemia following a course of immune globulin at 400 mg/kg/day for 5 to 10 days confirms the diagnosis.[55]

Malignancy

Involvement of the bone marrow with Kaposi's sarcoma is rare.[56] Malignant lymphoma may result in cytopenias due to the replacement of the bone marrow in advanced disease. Unlike uninfected patients with NHL, HIV-1–infected patients present with advanced stages of the lymphoproliferative disease, and 25% have bone marrow involvement at the time of diagnosis. Management of NHL in the HIV-1–infected patient is a difficult clinical problem. Compared to uninfected patients with NHL, there is a high incidence of opportunistic infection with chemotherapy, related to the neutropenia resulting from a limited bone marrow reserve.

Hematopoietic Suppression—A Component of AIDS-Related Bone Marrow Failure

HIV-1–associated inhibition of hematopoietic function may be directly mediated through the infection of bone marrow progenitor and stem cells; indirectly, by infection of marrow accessory cells; or as a result of cell- or cytokine-mediated immune effector mechanisms (Fig. 9–2).

Effects of HIV-1 on Proliferative Function of Bone Marrow Progenitors and Stem Cells

The effects of HIV-1 on colony formation have been studied, either using bone marrow cells derived from HIV-1–infected patients (Table 9–2) or after in vitro infection of hematopoietic cells from bone marrow of normal donors (Table 9–3). Results have been surprisingly divergent. Although the growth potential of committed bone marrow progenitor cells in methylcellulose cultures appears to be decreased in selected HIV-1–infected patients, normal growth frequently has also been reported (see Table 9–2). Similar disparity exists in the results of studies performed with normal bone marrow (Table 9–3). These discrepancies could be related to technical differences in assaying colony growth (total bone marrow vs. purified CD34+ cells), culture conditions (use of specific cytokines or growth factors), or patient selection. In some studies, hematopoietic progenitor cells obtained from AIDS patients or normal progenitor cells, cocultivated with infected cells, produced many fewer colonies than those from controls and dose-dependent inhibition of colony growth in the normal cultures by infected cells.[57]

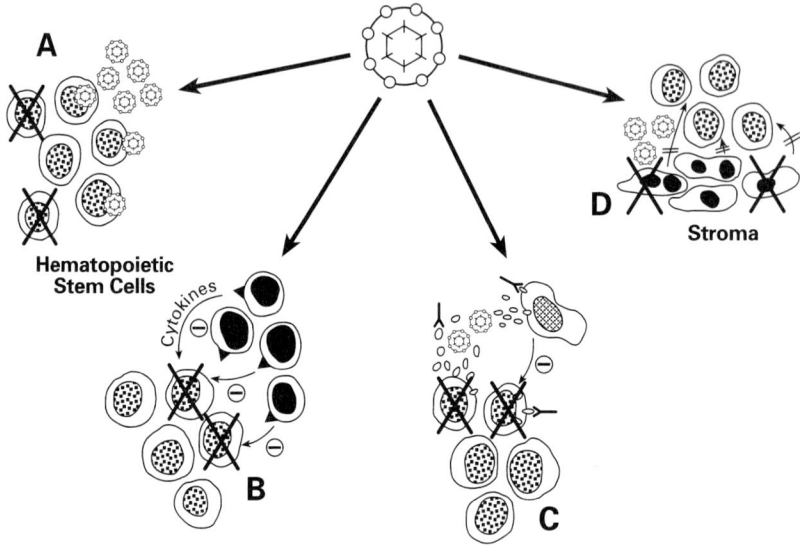

Figure 9-2 Schematic representation of possible pathophysiologic pathways leading to bone marrow failure in patients with HIV-1 infection. Portions A, B, C and D represent four hypothetical mechanisms of damage to the stem cell compartment in bone marrow of patients with HIV-1 infection. Experimental evidence supporting these mechanisms is presented in the text. **(A)** Direct virus infection leads to the destruction or inhibition of proliferation of hematopoietic progenitor and stem cells. **(B)** HIV-1-infected hematopoietic progenitor and stem cells are the target for immune cells which can kill HIV-1-infected cells, but also "innocent bystanders," that is, uninfected target cells. **(C)** HIV-1 infection leads to the destruction or defective function of stromal and accessory cells in the bone marrow, leading to defective proliferation of hematopoietic progenitors. **(D)** HIV-1 proteins released from infected cells may have a direct toxic effect on hematopoietic progenitor and stem cells or after uptake lead to an immune-mediated reaction. This reaction may include release of cytokines by accessory cells or expression of cytokine receptors on hematopoietic progenitor and stem cells.

TABLE 9-2 Hematopoiesis in Bone Marrow from HIV-Infected Patients

Study	Source of Cells	Colony Formation
Molina et al.[61]	BM	Normal
Kaczmarski et al.[62]	BM	Normal
Donahue et al.[63]	Macrophage-depleted cells	Normal
Carlo-Stella et al.[64]	BM	Decreased with depletion of T cells, increased colony formation
Leiderman et al.[65]	BM	Decreased
Lunardi-Iskandar et al.[66]	BM	Decreased
Ganser et al.[67]	BM	
Louache et al.[68]	BM	Decreased, antisense *tat* or *nof*: increased colony formation
Stanley et al.[69]	BM	Decreased
Davis et al.[70]	CD34+ cells	Normal in asymptomatic HIV-infected patients, decreased in symptomatic HIV-infected colony formation

BM, bone marrow.

TABLE 9-3 Hematopoietic Cell Proliferation After In Vitro Challenge with HIV

Study	Experimental Design	Colony Formation
Zauli et al.[80]	Effect of HIV on CD34+ cells	Decreased cell number and viability; colony formation
Donahue et al.[63]	Effect of immune globulin from HIV-infected patients on CD34+ cells	Decreased
Leiderman et al.[57]	Effect of glycoprotein inhibitor from serum of HIV-infected patients on total BM	Decreased
Balleari et al.[81]	Effect of T lymphocytes from HIV-infected patients on CD34+ cells	Decreased
Steinberg et al.[73]	Normal BM exposed to HIV-1	Decreased
Zauli et al.[82]	Normal BM exposed to HIV-1	Decreased
Cen et al.[76]	Effect of HIV on CD34+ cells	Decreased
Molina et al.[61]	Effect of HIV on BM and CD34+ cells	No effect
Maciejewski et al.[58]	Effect of HIV on BM and CD34+ cells	Reduced in BM but not with CD34+ cells
Zauli et al.[83]	Effect of 2 lympocytotropic strains on survival and proliferation of CD34+ cells (TF-1 cell line)	Increased apoptotic cell death; anti-gp120 antibody further increased apoptosis

BM, bone marrow.

In some reports, inhibition of colony formation by virus was only observed in cultures of total bone marrow cells and not with isolated CD34+ cells.[58]

While primary methylcellulose cultures can be used to study proliferation of more mature hematopoietic progenitor cells, long-term bone marrow cultures (LTBMCs) and their modifications have been applied to study more immature progenitor and stem cells. There was no effect of HIV-1 or HIV-2 on the proliferation of CD34+ cells in LTBMCs, but suppression was seen with unseparated bone marrow cells.[58, 59] However, in CD34+ cells and unseparated bone marrow cells and PB microvesicles obtained from HIV-1–infected patients with advanced disease, there was markedly decreased long-term culture initiating cell (LTC-IC) numbers, a reflection of a very primitive hematopoietic progenitor cell, when compared to asymptomatic patients and normal controls.[60] HIV-1–infected patients with neutropenia showed the greatest decreases in LTC-IC numbers.

Infection of Hematopoietic Progenitor Cells by HIV-1

Studies of the effects of HIV-1 on proliferation of hematopoietic cells do not resolve the issue of susceptibility of marrow progenitor cells. Infection of hematopoietic progenitor and stem cells with HIV-1 may immediately result in a chronic productive infection, or in latent infection. There is evidence that the CD4 receptor is weakly expressed on some CD34+ cells[77, 78] and this expression might account for the ability of immature progenitor cells to become infected under certain conditions. CD4 antigen was found only on more committed CD34+CD38+ cells, while primitive CD34+CD38− cells did not appear to express the CD4 molecule.[59] Auxiliary HIV-1 receptors have been detected on CD34+ cells. Relatively recently, two chemokine receptors, CXCR-4 (fusin) and CKR-5 (CCR-5), were identified as coreceptors required for HIV-1 infection of lymphocytes and macrophages. Both CKCR-4 and CKR-5 were present on CD4− as well as CD4+, CD34+ cells, although the number of CD34+ cells expressing CXCR-4 was relatively greater. Infection of CD34+ cells by macrophage-tropic and T cell–tropic viral stains was inhibited by the cognate ligands of CCR5 and CXCR4, respectively.[79] The identification of chemokine receptors on CD34+ cells lends further support to the possibility that CD34+ cells can be infected by HIV. Multiple studies to examine functional effects of HIV-1 on hematopoietic progenitor and stem cells have offered varying conclusions (see Tables 9–2 and 9–3). Some showed decreased growth or depletion of bone marrow progenitor cells. Infection of CD34+ cells with HIV-1 has been described.[71] Most evidence that progenitor cells are susceptible to infection with certain strains of HIV-1 comes from in vitro experiments, using purified CD34+ cells obtained from normal, uninfected donors (see Table 9–4) rather than from detection of in vivo infection in HIV-1–infected patients. Many investigators have been unable to successfully infect CD34+ cells in vitro.[61, 74, 76] In some studies, CD34+ cells could be latently infected with HIV-1, but productive infections only appeared in monocytes and macrophages.[72] The ability to infect progenitor cells may be dependent on the

TABLE 9-4 HIV Infection of Hematopoietic Progenitor Cells In Vitro

Investigator	Infection	HIV-1 isolate	Detection method
Folks et al.[71]	Yes	LAV	RT
Kitano et al.[72]	Yes	JR-FL, but not IIIB	PCR
Steinberg et al.[73]	Yes	IIIB	PCR
Zauli et al.[74]	No	IIIB	PCR
Molina et al.[75]	No	IIIB	PCR
Cen et al.[76]	No	LAV, NL-3, ICR-3	PCR

PCR, polymerase chain reaction.

strain of virus used. For example, infection of CD34+ cells generally can be induced with some monocytotropic strains of HIV-1[73]; attempts to achieve infection with lymphocytotropic HIV-1 strains, which are most commonly isolated from patients, have been less successful. A theoretical problem in the interpretation of in vitro infection experiments is the possibility that even "purified" CD34+ cells contained residual CD4+ lymphocytes.

Infection of hematopoietic stem cells could have profound pathophysiologic consequences, as integration of the HIV-1 genome might lead to the amplification of infection through stem cell proliferation and the generation of infected progeny. To test this possibility, purified CD34+ cells were infected in vitro and cultured on allogeneic stroma for extended periods of time.[59] Virus detection was possible only in the first 2 weeks of culture; a highly sensitive PCR failed to detect HIV-1 in secondary colonies generated from clonogenic cells harvested from stroma. Although some committed progenitor cells can be infected with HIV-1, the most immature stem cells appear not to be susceptible to HIV-1 infection.

Although in vitro infection of CD34+ cells with certain strains of HIV-1 has been reported, in vivo productive infection of hematopoietic progenitor cells in AIDS patients is infrequent. HIV-1 has been only occasionally isolated from CD34+ cells of patients, usually those with advanced disease (Table 9-5): HIV-1 could be detected in CD34+ cells in 14% of HIV-1–infected persons recruited in the United States and in 36% in Zaire.[69] However, in other studies, virus was not found in CD34+ bone marrow progenitor cells from any HIV-1–infected patients.[61, 84, 87]

Megakaryocytes appear to be infected with HIV-1 in vitro.[23, 88] There is circumstantial evidence that infection may be responsible, at least in part, for the thrombocytopenia seen in AIDS patients. HIV-1–infected CD34+ cells gave rise to megakaryocytes that were defective in their ability to produce platelets.[80] In an electron microscopic study of megakaryocytes obtained from an HIV-1–infected patient, budding of virus from the megakaryocyte membrane was seen.[88] A strain of HIV-1 isolated from a thrombocytopenic HIV-1–infected patient was cytopathic to normal megakaryocytes, while another virus strain obtained from a patient without thrombocytopenia did not affect megakaryocytic growth.[23]

TABLE 9-5 Detection of HIV-1 in Hematopoietic Progenitor Cells in Patients

Investigator	Patients positive	Detection method
von Laer et al[84]	1/14	PCR
Kojouharoff et al.[85]	4/6 (few positive cells)	PCR
Donahue et al.[63]	1/3	Viral isolate
Ganser et al.[86]	0/25	In situ hybridization
Stanley et al.[69]	19 of 52 Zairean	PCR
	3 of 22 American	<1 proviral copy/500 CD34+ cells
Molina et al.[61]	0/6	In situ hybridization
Davis et al.[70]	1/12	PCR
Neal et al.[87]	2/10	PCR
de Luca et al.[88a]	0/7	PCR
Kaczmarski et al.[62]	8/8	PCR
Zauli et al.[74]	2/23	PCR

PCR, polymerase chain reaction.

Loss of Progenitor Cell Numbers in HIV Infection

Although the stem cell compartment appears to be relatively well preserved early in the disease in asymptomatic patients with low CD4+ counts and few opportunistic infections, later there is a marked reduction of LTC-IC numbers.[60] Either HIV-1 spares the bone marrow early in the disease (when viral loads are lower and progenitor cell reserves are larger), or else opportunistic infections, pharmacotherapy with antiparasitic, antimicrobial, antiviral, or cytotoxic agents; vitamin deficiencies; or poorly understood virally mediated immunomodulary changes are major contributors to bone marrow failure in patients with advanced disease. Prolonged therapy with growth factors, with or without cytotoxic therapy, as in Kaposi's sarcoma, could also lead to the exhaustion of stem cell reserves.

Secondary Causes of Hematopoietic Inhibition in AIDS

Certain cells of the bone marrow microenvironment, such as bone marrow CD4+ lymphocytes and monocytes and macrophages are permissive to HIV-1 infection. When 27 patients with HIV-1 were examined, all showed decreased colony formation, but no evidence of infection.[68] However, antisense strands of DNA directed at the *tat* or *nef* genes were able to induce an increase in colony formation by total bone marrow, suggesting that infection of progenitor cells was not necessary for negative modulation of hematopoiesis and implying a role for infected accessory cells. Other studies have also suggested that infection of progenitor cells is not necessary for functional inhibition of colony formation. Exposure of CD34+ cells to HIV-1 envelope glycoprotein gp120 resulted in a dose-dependent inhibitory activity that was competitively neutralized by anti-HIV-1–neutralizing antibody.[80, 83] Similar findings have been described with gp160, as well as with inactivated virions added to cultures of total bone marrow. As no inhibition was observed when purified CD34+ cells were treated (instead of total bone marrow), it is likely that accessory cells mediated this effect.[58] Viral proteins thus may have intrinsic direct and indirect inhibitory activity in the bone marrow cell progenitors. In one study, improved colony formation was observed when the marrow was depleted of T cells, consistent with secondary immunomodulation of colony formation.[64] Finally, decreased growth potential of colony cells exposed to sera from HIV-1–infected patients has been described, and characterized as antibody by one investigator and as an 84-kD glycoprotein by another.[65]

Stromal endothelial cells obtained from HIV-1–infected patients have been shown to be susceptible to HIV-1 infection in vivo.[89] In addition, bone marrow fibroblasts were permissive to certain strains of HIV-1, suggesting that stroma can act as a reservoir for HIV-1.[90] Although stromal cells may be infected with monocytotropic strains of HIV-1, there is disagreement about the consequences of infection for hematopoiesis (Table 9–6). Decreased colony formation has been observed when HIV-1–infected stroma was used to support growth of normal uninfected bone marrow progenitor cells,[91] but in our own laboratory, when normal CD34+ cells were placed on stromal cells obtained from normal controls or HIV-1–infected persons, there was no difference in the number of secondary colonies formed (Fig. 9–3); in contrast, purified CD34+ cells from HIV-1–infected patients showed significantly decreased colony formation when cultured in LTBMCs using either normal or patient stromal cells. Unlike in previous studies, no productive infection of stroma obtained from HIV-1–infected patients was found as measured by p24 enzyme-linked immunosorbent assay (ELISA) of supernatant from stromal cultures.[91] Other data show that small infection of stromal cells appeared to be a requirement for functional inhibition of hematopoiesis related to decreased

TABLE 9–6 Infection of Stromal Elements by HIV-1

Study	Target cells	Type of infection	Effect on function
Moses et al.[89]	Stromal endothelium	In vivo	Constitutive production of hematopoietic growth factors normal, decreased IL-1α induced production of IL-6 and G-CSF
Marandin et al.[89a]	BM stroma	In vitro	Normal colony formation
Schwartz et al.[91]	BM stroma	In vitro	Decreased colony formation
Scadden et al.[90]	BM stroma	In vitro	
Sloand et al.[60]	BM stroma	In vivo	Normal colony formation

BM, bone marrow; IL, interleukin; G-CSF, granulocyte colony-stimulating factor.

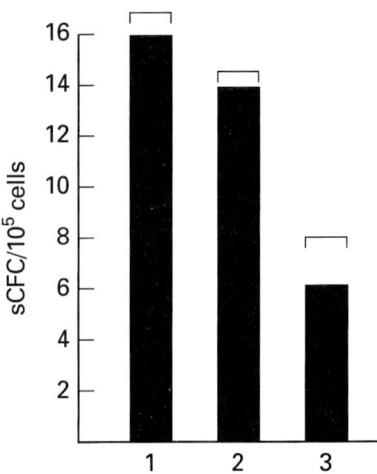

Figure 9–3 Function of stromal cells derived from patients with HIV-1 infection. Stromal cell layers were established from the bone marrow of patients with HIV-1 infection (n = 10) and normal volunteers (n = 5). CD34+ cells obtained from eight normal volunteers were plated on stromal layers prepared from normal bone marrow (1) and on stroma from five HIV-1-infected patients with advanced disease (2). CD34+ cells from these patients were also cultured on stroma from normal volunteers (3). The number of secondary colony forming cells (sCFC) per number of cells plated is shown. There was no evidence for defective function of stroma from patients infected with HIV-1, as normal CD34+ cells had comparable secondary colony formation on both controls' and patients' stroma while CD34+ cells derived from patients showed diminished colony formation on normal stromal layers.

growth factor production; normal constitutive amounts of growth factors were found after infection of stromal cells with HIV-1, but decreased levels of G-CSF and interleukin-6 (IL-6) have been observed when infected cultures were challenged with IL-1α.[89]

Cytokines and Hematopoiesis

Inconsistencies in the results of experiments attempting to demonstrate a role for direct HIV-1 infection on hematopoiesis stimulated further search for pathophysiologic mechanisms. Several cytokines that are released during the course of HIV-1 infection are potent inhibitors of hematopoiesis. Not only intact virus and productive infection of stem cells but also viral products such as gp120, gp160, and *tat* proteins induce the secretion of an array of cytokines, including tumor necrosis factor-α (TNF-α), lymphotoxin-β (TNF-β), and IL-6.[58, 61, 92–95] Although disordered cytokine production by both lymphoid tissue and bone marrow clearly occurs in HIV-1 infection, it is difficult to determine its contribution to depressed hematopoiesis. Many inhibitory cytokines are produced in greatest quantities early in the course of HIV-1 infection and their production declines as the disease progresses. In addition, increased levels of some stimulatory cytokines have been observed in HIV-1 infection. Many cytokines never reach detectable levels in the circulation, and local production of growth factors in bone marrow may be more important than systemically secreted factors.

Cytokines, released in the course of infection, may either have direct toxic effects or act indirectly by complicated metabolic cascades. Perhaps the most prominent cytokine implicated in pathophysiologic reactions in AIDS is TNF-α (or cachectin); blood levels of TNF-α are increased in AIDS.[96, 97] In addition to its effect on body metabolism and the immune system, TNF-α has intrinsic inhibitory effects on hematopoiesis.[98–101] Production of this cytokine has been demonstrated in B lymphocytes from HIV-1–infected persons after exposure to gp120,[102] in monocytic cells,[61] and by bone marrow and peripheral blood mononuclear phagocytes infected with HIV-1 or stimulated with its envelope proteins gp120 and gp160.[58]

Multiple inhibitory cytokines may act synergistically to inhibit marrow function in vitro, especially TNF-α and interferon-γ (IFN-γ).[98, 103] High levels of IFN-γ were not only associated with a poor prognosis in HIV-1 infection[104] but correlated with the degree of anemia.[105] Exposure of HIV-1–infected marrow to increasing concentrations of transforming growth factor-β (TGF-β), levels of which are also elevated in the blood of patients with HIV-1 infection, reduced the growth of all hematopoietic lineages.

Apoptosis of hematopoietic progenitor cells through the Fas-L/Fas pathway is one mechanism by which activated T cells can kill virus-infected cells (Fig. 9–4).[106] It is likely that Fas-L and other cytokine products of activated T cells contribute to the hematopoietic inhibition seen in HIV-1 infection. Increased levels of Fas-L have been reported in patients with AIDS, and triggering of Fas on lymphocytes resulted in apoptosis.[107] This effect has been clearly demonstrated for lymphocytes derived from HIV-1–infected patients but may also operate on hematopoietic progenitor and stem cells.[108–110] TNF-α and IFN-γ are both produced in increased amounts during HIV-1 infection and have been shown to upmodulate Fas on hematopoietic cells.[108] Increased expression of Fas on CD34+ cells has been found in immune-medi-

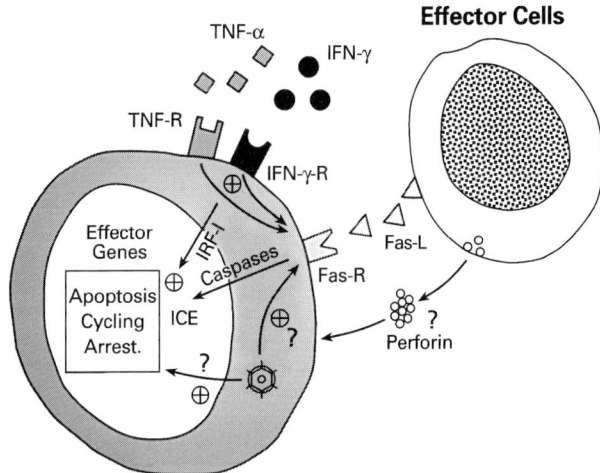

Figure 9–4 Schematic representation of possible effector mechanisms leading to hematopoietic cell inhibition in HIV-1 infection. Increased concentration of inhibitory cytokines in the bone marrow of HIV-1-infected patients or the virus itself may lead to increased expression of Fas or other cytokine receptors on hematopoietic progenitor and stem cells. Upon triggering of these receptors, diverse intracellular pathways are activated. These transduction mechanisms (such as IRF-1) may result in activation of ICE or other effector proteins leading to either cell cycling arrest or apoptosis. TNF, tumor necrosis factor; IFN-γ, interferon-γ; IRF, interferon regulatory factor; ICE, interleukin-1β converting enzyme.

ated bone marrow failure syndromes, including aplastic anemia and myelodysplastic syndromes.[108]

Intracellular Pathways in Target Cells

HIV-1 infection may directly cause toxicity to infected cells and ultimately cell death. However, other mechanisms may also negatively influence hematopoietic cell function and lead to either inhibition of cell cycling or cell destruction; these include inhibitory cytokines or direct immune cell–mediated attack (see Fig. 9–4). Activated macrophages and lymphocytes infected with HIV-1 may produce a variety of cytokines, including lymphotoxin, IFN-γ, and Fas-ligand. Effector mechanisms leading to impaired function or death of hematopoietic progenitor and stem cells have been described. After triggering of cellular receptors for IFN-γ and TNF-α, a variety of intracellular pathways can be activated. Both cytokines upregulate Fas expression on CD34+ cells.[108] Fas triggering, in turn, enhances IFN-γ-receptor expression.[111] Inhibition of IFN-γ is mediated by interferon regulatory factor-1 (IRF-1), (NF-κB) nuclear factor κB may transduce signals after tumor necrosis factor receptor triggering.[112–114] The TNF-α-mediated intracellular pathway may ultimately result in activation of CPP23 transactivating apoptotic effector genes,[115] although as yet there is no evidence that this pathway exists in hematopoietic progenitor and stem cells.

Cross-linking of the Fas by either soluble or membrane-bound Fas-ligand results in activation of a cascade of cysteine proteases (caspases). IL-1β converting enzyme (ICE, caspase-1) appears to be a key enzyme leading to activation of several effector proteins for apoptosis, and inhibition of ICE results in blockade of the apoptotic pathway.[115–117] These mechanisms operate in hematopoietic progenitor cells: ICE is activated in CD34+ cells by Fas triggering, and specific inhibitors of ICE block Fas-mediated apoptosis.[118] We and others have demonstrated that ICE messenger (mRNA) is constitutively produced by CD34+ cells of both normal and HIV-1–infected persons. Although ICE protein is not present in unstimulated CD34+ cells, Fas triggering and exposure of CD34+ cells to IFN-γ will result in generation of the active form of ICE protein in these cells. That protease inhibitors decrease CD34+ apoptosis and ICE in vitro lend support to the hypothesis that the beneficial effects of highly active anti-retroviral therapy (HAART) on the frequency of cytopenias may be related to inhibition of CD34+-programmed cell death.

Apoptosis of progenitor and stem cells can lead to depletion of these cells and inhibition of hematopoiesis. In addition to the ICE pathway, several other mechanisms can induce apoptosis. IRF-1 has been shown to activate inducible nitric oxide synthase, and inhibition of this enzyme antagonizes the inhibitory effects of IFN-γ.[107] Poly (ADP) ribose polymerase (PARP), ornithine decarboxylase, and the Jak/Stat family of proteins are modulated by both IRF-1 and ICE. All these final effector pathways may be involved in the damage to the hematopoietic progenitor and stem cells mediated by cytokines released in bone marrow in the course of HIV-1 infection.

Shortened Survival of Blood Cells

Shortened survival of mature cells of all hematopoietic lineages has been reported in conjunction with cytopenias. However, it is unclear if autoimmune factors play a role. Thrombocytopenia has most commonly been attributed to shortened platelet survival. While the frequency of autoantibodies directed against neutrophils and platelets increases with progression of HIV-1 infection, the presence of autoantibodies does not correlate with the degree of cytopenia.[18] Furthermore, if platelet samples are not handled fastidiously and autoantibodies are measured immediately after collection, even normal, unaffected platelets may factitiously demonstrate antibody binding. In addition, conditions associated with platelet injury (sepsis, infection, and TTP) promote antibody binding to the platelet membrane. In hemophiliac patients, a 7S platelet-reactive IgG capable of binding to homologous and autologous platelets was detected in serum, and an inverse relationship between the concentration of platelet-associated antibody and the platelet count demonstrated.[119] In a group of HIV-1–infected intravenous drug users presenting with ITP, immune complexes on the platelet surface also have been identified.[120] However, in an unpublished study of 10 HIV-1–infected patients with thrombocytopenia, no platelet membrane–associated antibody could be detected in any patient (Sloand, unpublished observation).

It has been postulated that while decreased survival seems to be more frequently responsible for thrombocytopenia in asymptomatic HIV-infection, decreased platelet production by the bone marrow may be more important in patients with advanced disease.[17] Decreased survival of erythrocytes and neutrophils also contributes to anemia and neutropenia in HIV-1 infection, but similar difficulties have been encountered in determining the role of red cell or neutrophil-associated antibodies.[8, 9, 18, 121]

DIAGNOSIS AND TREATMENT

The introduction of protease inhibitors, often used in combination with nucleoside analogues and viral load monitoring, has contributed significantly to the improved survival of patients with HIV-1 infection. In addition, supportive therapies, the widespread use of antibiotic prophylaxis, and better understanding and treatment of the hematologic complications of HIV-1 infection have enhanced the quality of life and outlook in AIDS.

Peripheral Blood and Bone Marrow Examination

Morphologic abnormalities can be found in the majority of bone marrow samples from HIV-1–infected patients, but most are nonspecific, except in opportunistic infection where marrow examination provides valuable diagnostic information. Substantial clinical information can be gained in the diagnosis of MAI complex, tuberculosis, or fungal infections, or as part of staging for malignancy.[122]

Histopathologic findings in the bone marrow of HIV-1–infected patients are inconsistent.[123–125] Of 216 bone marrow examinations performed in 178 HIV-1–infected patients for evaluation of cytopenia, 69% of patients exhibited hypercellular marrow, 69% showed myelodysplastic changes, and 20% had significant fibrosis[122]; only 5% of the biopsies were hypocellular; granulomas were found in 13% and lymphoid aggregates in 36% (but in other studies in up to 50%) of specimens. Higher numbers of plasma cells and elevated numbers of eosinophils can also be present, especially in conjunction with increased reticulin.[2, 50, 123–125] Hyperplasia of the granulocytic and erythrocytic lineages has been most commonly reported; the myeloid-erythroid ratio has varied from 2:1 to 5:1.[2, 125]

Morphologic changes tend to be pronounced in more immunosuppressed patients and increase in frequency as the disease progresses. All lineages can be involved.[126–130] Megaloblastic erythropoiesis and ringed sideroblasts are frequent. Using the morphologic criteria established for primary myelodysplastic syndromes, dysplasia involving at least one lineage could be diagnosed in 69% of patients.[126] Myelodysplasia increases with disease progression. However, in one study, there were significant differences in the numbers of erythroid precursors and in the morphology of megakaryocytes which clearly differentiated patients with AIDS from those with myelodysplastic syndrome.[131] The cumulative effects of drug toxicities, direct HIV-1 infection of marrow cells, and dysregulated cytokine production may be responsible for the morphologic changes that occur late in AIDS. However, there is no correlation between dysplastic changes in an individual lineage and specific peripheral blood alterations.

Marrow examination in patients with HIV-1 infection may provide valuable clinical information for the diagnosis of opportunistic infection. Foamy histiocytes and granulomas are typical of MAI infection. *Histoplasma*, cryptococcus, and mycobacteria could be identified in diagnosed patients based on the presence of granulomas, even without use of special stains.

Treatment of Anemia: Transfusion and Erythropoietin

Anemia is a common problem in AIDS patients, and a low hemoglobin is an independent factor predicting poor prognosis. Many patients with HIV-1 infection become transfusion-dependent. Blood loss, resulting from repeated phlebotomies and gastrointestinal bleeding, as well as suppression of erythropoiesis, contribute to anemia. Erythropoietin, first licensed to ameliorate the anemia associated with ZDV use, has been shown to be effective in increasing the hematocrit in HIV-1–infected patients who have low endogenous erythropoietin levels.[132] However, the hormone may still be helpful in selected individuals with high erythropoietin levels. Erythropoietin may decrease transfusion requirements or even eliminate the need for transfusions, improving the quality of life and decreasing the risk of transfusion-associated infections and viral (especially human CMV) reactivation. Transfusion requirements in HIV-infected patients appear to be decreasing due to changes in ZDV dosing or to initiation of more effective protease inhibitor regimens.

Transfusion may be associated with deleterious effects in HIV-1–infected patients.[133, 134] In one study, transfused patients with advanced disease had an increased incidence of human CMV infection and death.[133] This may be related to allogeneic lymphocytes present in the transfused product, which activate viral production by HIV-infected lymphocytes in vitro.[135] A study using quantitative PCR to measure circulating HIV-1 demonstrated increased viral loads in HIV-infected patients 5 days following transfusion.[136] A controlled clinical trial on the effects of leukodepletion of blood components in patients with HIV infection is currently in progress.

Treatment of Idiopathic Thrombocytopenic Purpura

Decreased platelet survival has been reported in conjunction with HIV-1 infection and probably is responsible for most cases of HIV-related thrombocytopenia in the early stages of disease.[17] While ITP of all causes is associated with decreased survival of platelets, most treatments appear to increase platelet production in the bone marrow.[137, 138] Antiviral therapy increases the platelet count, suggesting a direct relationship between viral load and thrombocytopenia. The effects of antiviral drugs may be at least partially related to increased production of platelets,[137] possibly related to the beneficial effects of decreased viremia. At least 50% of HIV-1–infected patients, not previously receiving antiviral agents, increase their platelet count by threefold when treated with ZDV.[139, 140] Although most published reports have examined the response of thrombocytopenia to ZDV, other antiviral agents likely have similar benefits.[139–144] The more effective antiviral activity of newer protease inhibitors, particularly when used in combination, may result in higher response rates. In addition to nucleoside analogues, IFN-α (which also has significant anti-HIV-1 activity) has demonstrated effectiveness in some cases of ITP, but the side effects of malaise, fever, and the necessity for daily injections have made patient acceptance a problem.[145]

However, since most patients currently presenting with ITP are generally receiving optimal antiviral therapy, the use of additional agents needs to be considered. Although the response of thrombocytopenic HIV-1–infected patients to corticosteroids is comparable to that of uninfected patients (60% to 80% of cases), concerns that steroids lead to further immunosuppression or may promote the growth of Kaposi's sarcoma have limited their use to brief treatment periods.[146]

As in ITP not associated with HIV, high doses of immune globulin have been effective,[147–149] but the durability of response is only 3 to 5 weeks, the therapy is quite costly, and recently the supply has been limited. Anti-Rh(D) immune globulin (Rogam) is also effective and has the advantage of greater availability and the option of subcutaneous injection. Vincristine, also a highly effective agent in HIV-related ITP, is probably underutilized.[150, 151] As with ITP of other etiologies, the use of plasmapheresis has not met with great success.[152]

Although the newly identified megakaryocyte-specific hematopoietic growth factor, thrombopoietin, has not been tested clinically in HIV-1–infected individuals with thrombocytopenia, initial studies using this drug in normal volunteers have met with unacceptable toxicity related to the development of anti-thrombopoietin antibodies.[153]

Despite concerns about its potential effect on the prognosis of HIV-1, splenectomy has been used to treat HIV-1–infected patients with refractory ITP.[154, 155] Two prospective studies showed no adverse effects on disease progression in those undergoing splenectomy for ITP.[156, 157]

Treatment of Cytopenias with Hematopoietic Growth Factors

Treatment of cytopenias has been revolutionized by the introduction of hematopoietic growth factors for clinical use.[158] Although they ameliorate leukopenia and anemia, it is not entirely clear whether growth factors significantly change the morbidity of HIV-1 infection or ultimately affect survival of patients (Table 9–7).

G-CSF is the most widely used hematopoietic growth factor in HIV-1–infected patients. When compared to granulocyte-macrophage colony-

TABLE 9–7 Hematopoietic Growth Factors and Cytokine Trials in AIDS

Drug	Dose	Therapeutic effect	Adverse effect	Effect on HIV
GM-CSF	0.25–8.0 µg/kg/day	↑ Leukocyte count, normally functioning leukocytes	Back pain, myalgia, chills, nausea, headache, fever, rash	Increases viral replication
G-CSF	150 µg/m²/day	↑ Proliferation and differentiation of committed progenitor cells	Bone pain	None
Erythropoietin	150 IU/kg 3 × weekly	↑ BFU-E colonies ↑ Hematocrit in patients with decreased erythropoietin levels	None	None
SCF[159]	In vitro studies 10 ng/mL	↑ BFU-E colonies in presence of ganciclovir or ZDV ↑ CFU_{GM} in presence of IFN-α or ganciclovir No effect with TNF-α or TNF-γ	None	None
IL-3[159]	10 ng/mL	↑ Erythroid colonies in presence of ZDV and CFU_{GM} in presence of IFN-α; no effect with TNF-α or TNF-γ	Fevers, headache, bone pain	None
IFN-α	3 × 10⁶ units SC q.o.d.	Variable response in prolonging platelet survival	Fever, myalgia, fatigue	Antiviral activity

GM-CSF, granulocyte-macrophage colony-stimulating factor; G-CSF, granulocyte colony-stimulating factor; SCF, stem cell factor; IL, interleukin; IFN, interferon; SC, subcutaneously; BFU-E, burst-forming unit—erythroid; ZDV, zidovudine; CFU_{GM}, colony-forming unit—granulocyte macrophage; TNF, tumor necrosis factor.

stimulating factor (GM-CSF), G-CSF has the advantage of fewer side effects and more rapid increases in leukocyte counts. In contrast to GM-CSF, G-CSF has not been associated with increased viral replication. In a phase I/II trial, daily G-CSF injections resulted in increased neutrophil and eosinophil counts, but did not affect hemoglobin concentrations, platelet counts, or lymphocyte subsets.[160] When used in combination with erythropoietin, G-CSF has improved both leukocyte counts and hemoglobin levels.

While GM-CSF may be associated with an increase in the replication of HIV-1,[72,161] no consistent observation of acceleration of disease progression or increase in p24 antigen levels in patients receiving GM-CSF has been demonstrated. In early clinical trials, GM-CSF increased leukocyte counts in patients receiving ZDV, without altering lymphocyte counts, hemoglobin, reticulocytes, platelets, or viral p24 levels.[162] In other preliminary studies, GM-CSF appeared to decrease the viral load and increase the CD4+ cell count. Thus, GM-CSF appears to be safe and effective when used in conjunction with antiviral therapy. In vitro, GM-CSF potentiated the antiviral effect of ZDV.[163] GM-CSF has no effect on the activities of ddI or ddC.[164] Studies using the new protease inhibitors in conjunction with GM-CSF have not been published. Long-term administration of G-CSF or GM-CSF has not been associated clinically with impairment of hematopoiesis.

IL-3 and stem cell factor (SCF) as yet have not been approved for clinical use. IL-3 stimulates myelopoiesis, erythropoiesis, and thrombopoiesis and has been used in HIV-infected patients with some success.[165] SCF alone only weakly stimulates hematopoietic colony growth in vitro but when used in combination with other growth factors exerts a potent effect on the proliferation of progenitor cells as measured in colony assays. SCF acts on the more immature multipotential progenitor cells and has the potential advantage of stimulating both erythro- and myelopoiesis.[159] Theoretically, SCF could also promote expansion of primitive progenitor and stem cells.

Growth factors may also prove useful as adjuncts in the treatment of AIDS-associated malignancies. In a prospective trial, using cyclophosphamide-doxorubicin-vincristine-prednisone combination chemotherapy, the addition of GM-CSF decreased the nadir of the absolute neutrophil count, as well as the days of hospitalization for fever and neutropenia.[166] Similarly, in treatment of Kaposi's sarcoma, growth factors allowed administration of greater and more frequent doses of chemotherapy.[167] To avoid cumulative toxicities, antiviral therapy is often discontinued during the administration of combination chemotherapy regimens. A number of modified regimens to treat NHL and HL have been developed which use smaller doses of chemotherapy (when compared to those used to treat affected patients without HIV infection); these have been successful in decreasing the extent and duration of neutropenia without seriously compromising response rates.

CONCLUSION

Although cytopenias, particularly anemia, were of import early in the AIDS epidemic, they now have a lesser impact. The recent development of much more effective antiviral agents, the protease inhibitors, has decreased viral load to a greater extent, without any significant adverse effects on hematopoiesis. With these changes, the incidence of anemia and the need for transfusion have decreased sharply (Viral Activation Trial Study, personal communication). In addition, even in the absence of formal studies most clinicians caring for HIV-1 infected patients also believe there has been a significant decrease in the frequency of ITP perhaps due to the decreased viral load resulting from more effective antiviral therapy. The development and licensing of effective hematopoietic growth factors has also had a significant impact on HIV-infected patients; of these, erythropoietin and G-CSF have been frequently and effectively used. Efforts to better control the underlying viral infection and the immunologic consequences of infection will lead to improvement in hematopoietic function of AIDS patients.

REFERENCES

1. Zon LI, Arkin C, Groopman JE: Haematologic manifestations of the human immune deficiency virus (HIV). Br J Haematol 1987; 66:251–256.
2. Zon LI, Groopman JE: Hematologic manifestations of the human immune deficiency virus (HIV). Semin Hematol 1988; 25:208–218.
3. Richman DD, Fischl MA, Grieco MH, et al: The toxicity of azidothymidine (AZT) in the treatment of patients with AIDS and AIDS-related complex: A double-blind, placebo-controlled trial. N Engl J Med 1987; 317:192–197.
4. Walker RE, Parker RI, Kovacs JA, et al: Anemia and erythropoiesis in patients with the acquired immunodeficiency syndrome (AIDS) and Kaposi sarcoma treated with zidovudine. Ann Intern Med 1988; 108:372–376.
5. Aguila HL, Weissman IL: Hematopoietic stem cells are not direct cytotoxic targets of natural killer cells. Blood 1996; 87:1225–1231.
6. Saah AJ, Munoz A, Kuo V, et al: Predictors of the risk of development of acquired immunodeficiency syndrome within 24 months among gay men seropositive for human immunodeficiency virus type 1: A report from the Multicenter AIDS Cohort Study. Am J Epidemiol 1992; 135:1147–1155.
7. Forester G: Profound cytopenia secondary to azidothymidine. N Engl J Med 1987; 317:772.
8. Toy PT, Reid ME, Burns M: Positive direct antiglobulin test associated with hyperglobulinemia in acquired immunodeficiency syndrome (AIDS). Am J Hematol 1985; 19:145–150.
9. McGinniss MH, Macher AM, Rook AH, Alter HJ: Red cell autoantibodies in patients with acquired immune deficiency syndrome. Transfusion 1986; 26:405–409.
10. Spivak JL, Barnes DC, Fuchs E, Quinn TC: Serum immunoreactive erythropoietin in HIV-infected patients. JAMA 1989; 261:3104–3107.
11. Cheong I, Flegg PJ, Brettle RP, et al: Cytomegalovirus disease in AIDS: The Edinburgh experience. Int J STD AIDS 1992; 3:324–328.
12. Snoeck R, Lagneaux L, Delforge A, et al: Inhibitory effects of potent inhibitors of human immunodeficiency virus and cytomegalovirus on the growth of human granulocyte-macrophage progenitor cells in vitro. Eur J Clin Microbiol Infect Dis 1990; 9:615–619.
13. Naides SJ, Howard EJ, Swack NS, et al: Parvovirus B19 infection in human immunodeficiency virus type 1-infected persons failing or intolerant to zidovudine therapy. J Infect Dis 1993; 168:101–105.
14. Kravcik S, Toye BW, Fyke K, et al: Impact of *Mycobacterium avium* complex prophylaxis on the incidence of mycobacterial infections and transfusion-requiring anemia in an HIV-positive population. J Acquir Immune Defic Syndr Hum Retroviral 1996; 13:27–32.
15. Markle HV: Cobalamin. Crit Rev Clin Lab Sci 1996; 33:247–356.
16. Boelaert JR, Weinberg GA, Weinberg ED: Altered iron metabolism in HIV infection: Mechanisms, possible consequences, and proposals for management. Infect Agents Dis 1996; 5:36–46.
17. Najean Y, Rain JD: The mechanism of thrombocytopenia in patients with HIV infection. J Lab Clin Med 1994; 123:415–420.
18. Sloand EM, Klein HG, Banks SM, et al: Epidemiology of thrombocytopenia in HIV infection. Eur J Haematol 1992; 48:168–172.
19. Klaassen RJL, Mulder JW, Vlekke ABJ, et al: Autoantibodies against peripheral blood cells appear early in HIV infection and their prevalence increases with disease progression. Clin Exp Immunol 1990; 81:11–17.
20. Botti AC, Hyde P, DiPillo F: Thrombotic thrombocytopenic purpura in a patient who subsequently

developed acquired immunodeficiency syndrome (AIDS). Ann Intern Med 1988; 109:242–243.
21. Blockmans D, Vermylen J: HIV-related thrombocytopenia. Acta Clin Belg 1992; 47:117–123.
22. Zauli G, Catani L, Gibellini D, et al: The CD4 receptor plays essential but distinct roles in HIV-1 infection and induction of apoptosis in primary bone marrow GPIIb/IIIa+ megakaryocytes and the HEL cell line. Br J Haematol 1995; 91:290–298.
23. Kunzi MS, Groopman JE: Identification of a novel human immunodeficiency virus strain cytopathic to megakaryocytic cells. Blood 1993; 81:3336–3342.
24. Sandstrom EG, Kaplan JC: Antiviral therapy in AIDS. Clinical pharmacological properties and therapeutic experience to date. Drugs 1987; 34:372–390.
25. Deeks SG, Smith M, Holodniy M, Kahn JO: HIV-1 protease inhibitors. A review for clinicians. JAMA 1997; 277:145–153.
26. Jaffe HS, Abrams DI, Ammann AJ, et al: Complications of co-trimoxazole in treatment of AIDS-associated *Pneumocystis carinii* pneumonia in homosexual men. Lancet 1983; 2:1109–1111.
27. Fulton B, Wagstaff AJ, McTavish D: Trimetrexate. A review of its pharmacodynamic and pharmacokinetic properties and therapeutic potential in the treatment of *Pneumocystis carinii* pneumonia. Drugs 1995; 49:563–576.
28. Kotler DP, Culpepper-Morgan JA, Tierney AR, Klein EB: Treatment of disseminated cytomegalovirus infection with 9-(1,3 dihydroxy-2-propoxymethyl) guanine: Evidence of prolonged survival in patients with the acquired immunodeficiency syndrome. AIDS Res 1986; 2:299–308.
29. Laskin OL, Cederberg DM, Mills J, et al: Ganciclovir for the treatment and suppression of serious infections caused by cytomegalovirus. Am J Med 1987; 83:201–207.
30. Spector SA, McKinley GF, Laleazri JP, et al: Oral ganciclovir for the prevention of cytomegalovirus disease in persons with AIDS. Roche Cooperative Oral Ganciclovir Study Group. N Engl J Med 1996; 334:1491–1497.
31. Wolff M, Jelkmann W: Effects of chemotherapeutic and immunosuppressive drugs on the production of erythropoietin in human hepatoma cultures. Ann Hematol 1993; 66:27–31.
32. Einsele H, Steidle M, Vallbracht A, et al: Early occurrence of human cytomegalovirus infection after bone marrow transplantation as demonstrated by the polymerase chain reaction technique. Blood 1991; 77:1104–1110.
33. Masur H, Whitcup SM, Cartwright C, et al: Advances in the management of AIDS-related cytomegalovirus retinitis. Ann Intern Med 1996; 125:126–136.
34. Spector SA, Hirata KK, Newman TR: Identification of multiple cytomegalovirus strains in homosexual men with acquired immunodeficiency syndrome. J Infect Dis 1984; 150:953–956.
35. Jackson JB, Erice A, Englund JA, et al: Prevalence of cytomegalovirus antibody in hemophiliacs and homosexuals infected with human immunodeficiency virus type 1. Transfusion 1988; 28:187–189.
36. Shepp DH, Moses JE, Kaplan MH: Seroepidemiology of cytomegalovirus in patients with advanced HIV disease: Influence on disease expression and survival. J Acquir Immune Defic Syndr Hum Retrovirol 1996; 11:460–468.
37. Maciejewski JP, Bruening EE, Donahue RE, et al: Infection of hematopoietic progenitor cells by human cytomegalovirus. Blood 1992; 80:170–178.
38. Simmons P, Kaushansky K, Torok-Storb B: Mechanisms of cytomegalovirus-mediated myelosuppression: Perturbation of stromal cell function versus direct infection of myeloid cells. Proc Natl Acad Sci USA 1990; 87:1386–1390.
39. Sing GK, Ruscetti FW: The role of human cytomegalovirus in haematological diseases. Baillieres Clin Haematol 1995; 8:149–162.
40. Rakusan TA, Juneja HS, Fleischmann WR: Inhibition of hemopoietic colony formation by human cytomegalovirus in vitro. J Infect Dis 1989; 159:127–130.
41. Sindre H, Tjoonnfjord GE, Rollag H, et al: Human cytomegalovirus suppression of and latency in early hematopoietic progenitor cells. Blood 1996; 88:4526–4533.
42. Movassagh M, Gozlan J, Senechal B, et al: Direct infection of CD34+ progenitor cells by human cytomegalovirus: Evidence for inhibition of hematopoiesis and viral replication. Blood 1996; 88:1277–1283.
43. Iwamoto GK, Monick MM, Clark BD, et al: Modulation of interleukin 1 beta gene expression by the immediate early genes of human cytomegalovirus. J Clin Invest 1990; 85:1853–1857.
44. Turtinen LW, Assimacopoulos A, Haase AT: Increased monokines in cytomegalovirus infected myelomonocytic cell cultures. Microb Pathog 1989; 7:135–145.
45. Rodgers BC, Scott DM, Mundin J, Sissons JG: Monocyte-derived inhibitor of interleukin 1 induced by human cytomegalovirus. J Virol 1985; 55:527–532.
46. Maciejewski JP, Bruening EE, Donahue RE, et al: Infection of mononucleated phagocytes with human cytomegalovirus. Virology 1993; 195:327–336.
47. Taylor-Wiedman J, Sissons JG, Borysiewicz LK, Sinclair JH: Monocytes are a major site of persistence of human cytomegalovirus in peripheral blood mononuclear cells. J Gen Virol 1991; 72:2059–2064.
48. Havlik JA, Horsburgh CR, Metchock B, et al: Disseminated *Mycobacterium avium* complex infection: Clinical identification and epidemiologic trends. J Infect Dis 1992; 165:577–580.
49. Sathe SS, Gascone P, Lo W, et al: Severe anemia is an important negative predictor for survival with disseminated *Mycobacterium avium-intracellulare* in acquired immunodeficiency syndrome. Am Rev Respir Dis 1990; 142(6 Pt 1):1306–1312.

50. Castella A, Croxson TS, Mildvan D, et al: The bone marrow in AIDS. A histologic, hematologic, and microbiologic study. Am J Clin Pathol 1985; 84:425–432.
51. Brown KE, Young NS: Parvovirus B19 infection and hematopoiesis. Blood Rev 1995; 9:176–182.
52. Kerr JR: Parvovirus B19 infection. Eur J Clin Microbiol Infect Dis 1996; 15:10–29.
53. Abkowitz JL, Brown KE, Wood RW, et al: Clinical relevance of parvovirus B19 as a cause of anemia in patients with human immunodeficiency virus infection. J Infect Dis 1997; 176:269–273.
54. Frickhofen N, Abkowitz JL, Safford M, et al: Persistent B19 parvovirus infection in patients infected with human immunodeficiency virus type 1 (HIV-1): Treatable cause of anemia in AIDS. Ann Intern Med 1990; 113:926–933.
55. Fuller A, Moaven L, Spelman D, et al: Parvovirus B19 in HIV infection: A treatable cause of anemia. Pathology 1996; 28:277–280.
56. Little BJ, Spivak JL, Quinn TC, Mann RB: Kaposi's sarcoma with bone marrow involvement: Occurrence in a patient with the acquired immunodeficiency syndrome. Am J Med Sci 1986; 292:44–46.
57. Leiderman IZ, Greenberg ML, Adelsburg BR, Siegal FP: Defective myelopoiesis in acquired immune deficiency syndrome (AIDS). In Gottlieb MS, Groopman JE (eds): AIDS. New York, Alan Liss, 1984, pp 281–289.
58. Maciejewski JP, Weichold FF, Young NS: HIV-1 suppression of hematopoiesis in vitro mediated by envelope glycoprotein and TNF-alpha. J Immunol 1994; 153:4303–4310.
59. Weichold FF, Zella D, Dunn D, et al: Neither HIV-1 nor HIV-2 infect most primitive human hematopoietic stem cells as assessed in long-term bone marrow cultures. Blood 1997, in press.
60. Sloand EM, Young NS, Sato T, et al: Secondary colony formation after long-term bone marrow culture using peripheral blood and bone marrow of HIV-infected patients. AIDS 1997; 11:1547–1553.
61. Molina JM, Schindler R, Ferriani R, et al: Production of cytokines by peripheral blood monocytes/macrophages infected with human immunodeficiency virus type 1 (HIV-1). J Infect Dis 1990; 161:888–893.
62. Kaczmarski RS, Davison F, Blair E, et al: Detection of HIV in haemopoietic progenitors. Br J Haemat 1992; 82:764–769.
63. Donahue RE, Johnson MM, Zon LI, et al: Suppression of in vitro haematopoiesis following human immunodeficiency virus infection. Nature 1987; 326:200–203.
64. Stella CC, Ganser A, Hoelzer D: Defective in vitro growth of the hemopoietic progenitor cells in the acquired immunodeficiency syndrome. J Clin Invest 1987; 80:286–293.
65. Leiderman IZ, Greenberg ML, Adelsburg BR, Siegal FP: A glycoprotein inhibitor of in vitro granulopoiesis associated with AIDS. Blood 1987; 70:1267–1272.
66. Koka PS, Jamieson BD, Brooks DG, Zack JA: Human immunodeficiency virus type 1-induced hematopoietic inhibition is independent of productive infection of progenitor cells in vivo. J Virol 1999; 73:9089–9097.
67. Ganser A, Greher J, Voklers B, et al: Inhibitory effect of azidothymidine, 2′-3′-dideoxyadenosine and 2′-3′-dideoxycytidine on in vitro growth of hematopoietic progenitor cells from normal persons and from patients with AIDS. Exp Hematol 1989; 17:321–325.
68. Louache F, Henri A, Bettajeb A, et al: Role of human immunodeficiency virus replication in defective in vitro growth of hematopoietic progenitors. Blood 1992; 80:2991–2999.
69. Stanley SK, Kessler SW, Justement JS, et al: $CD34^+$ bone marrow cells are infected with HIV in a subset of seropositive individuals. J Immunol 1992; 149:689–697.
70. Davis BR, Zauli G: Effect of human immunodeficiency virus infection on haematopoiesis. Baillieres Clin Haematol 1995; 8:113–130.
71. Folks TM, Kessler SW, Orenstein JM, et al: Infection and replication of HIV-1 in purified progenitor cells of normal human bone marrow. Science 1988; 242:919–922.
72. Kitano K, Abboud CN, Ryan DH, et al: Macrophage-active colony-stimulating factors enhance human immunodeficiency virus type I infection in bone marrow stem cells. Blood 1991; 77:1699–1705.
73. Steinberg HN, Crumpacker CS, Chatis PA: In vitro suppression of normal human bone marrow progenitor cells by human immunodeficiency virus. J Virol 1991; 65:1765–1769.
74. Zauli G, Re MC, Giovannini M, et al: Effect of human immunodeficiency virus Type 1 on $CD34^+$ cells. Ann NY Acad Sci 1991; 628:273–278.
75. Molina JM, Scadden DT, Sakaguchi M, et al: Lack of evidence for infection of or effect on growth of hematopoietic progenitor cells after in vivo or in vitro exposure to human immunodeficiency virus. Blood 1990; 76:2476–2482.
76. Cen D, Zauli G, Szarnicki R, Davis BR: Effect of different human immunodeficiency virus type-1 (HIV-1) isolates on long-term bone marrow hemopoiesis. Br J Haematol 1993; 85:596–602.
77. Louache F, Debili N, Marandin A, et al: Expression of CD4 by human hematopoietic progenitors. Blood 1994; 84:3344–3355.
78. Zauli G, Furlini G, Vitale M, et al: A subset of human CD34 + hematopoietic progenitors express low levels of CD4, the high-affinity receptor for human immunodeficiency virus-type 1. Blood 1994; 84:1896–1905.
79. Ruiz ME, Cicala C, Arthos J, et al: Peripheral blood-derived $CD34^+$ progenitor cells: CXC chemokine receptor 4 and CC chemokine receptor 5 expression and infection by HIV. J Immunol 1998; 16:4169–4176.
80. Zauli G, Re MC, Davis B, et al: Impaired in vitro growth of purified ($CD34^+$) hematopoietic progenitors in human immunodeficiency virus-1

seropositive thrombocytopenic individuals. Blood 1992; 79:2680–2687.
81. Balleari E, Timitilli S, Puppo F, et al: Impaired in vitro growth of peripheral blood hematopoietic progenitor cells in HIV-infected patients: Evidence of an inhibitory effect of autologous T lymphocytes. Ann Hematol 1991; 63:320–325.
82. Zauli G, Re MC, Furlini G, et al: Human immunodeficiency virus type 1 envelope glycoprotein gp120-mediated killing of human haematopoietic progenitors (CD34+ cells). J Gen Virol 1992; 73:417–421.
83. Zauli G, Vitale M, Re MC, et al: In vitro exposure to human immunodeficiency virus type 1 induces apoptotic cell death of the factor-dependent TF-1 hematopoietic cell line. Blood 1994; 83:167–175.
84. von Laer D, Hufert FT, Fenner TE, et al: CD34+ hematopoietic progenitor cells are not a major reservoir of the human immunodeficiency virus. Blood 1990; 76:1281–1286.
85. Kojouharoff G, Ottmann OG, von Briesen H, et al: Infection of granulocyte/monocyte progenitor cells with HIV 1. Res Virol 1991; 142:151–157.
86. Ganser A, Ottmann OG, von Briesen H, et al: Changes in the haematopoietic progenitor cell compartment in the acquired immunodeficiency syndrome. Res Virol 1990; 141:185–193.
87. Neal TF, Holland HK, Baum CM, et al: CD34+ progenitor cells from asymptomatic patients are not a major reservoir for human immunodeficiency virus-1. Blood 1995; 86:1749–1756.
88. Zucker-Franklyn D, Seremetis S, Zheng ZY: Internalization of human immunodeficiency virus type 1 and other retroviruses by megakaryocytes and platelets. Blood 1990; 75:1920–1923.
88.a DeLuca A, Teofili L, Antinori A, et al: Haemopoietic CD34+ progenitor cells are not infected by HIV-1 in vivo but show clonogenesis. Br J Haematol 1993; 85:20–24.
89. Moses AV, Williams S, Heneveld ML, et al: Human immunodeficiency virus infection of bone marrow endothelium reduces induction of stromal hematopoietic growth factors. Blood 1996; 87:919–925.
89a. Marandin A, Canque B, Coulombee L, et al: In vitro infection of bone marrow–adherent cells by human immunodeficiency virus type 1 (HIV-1) does not alter their ability to support hematopoiesis. Virology 1995; 213:245–248.
90. Scadden DT, Zeira M, Woon A, et al: Human immunodeficiency virus infection of human bone marrow stromal fibroblasts. Blood 1990; 76:317–322.
91. Schwartz GN, Kessler SW, Rothwell SW, et al: Inhibitory effects of HIV-1-infected stromal cell layers on the production of myeloid progenitor cells in human long-term bone marrow cultures. Exp Hematol 1994; 22:1288–1296.
92. Roux-Lombard P, Modoux C, Chruchaud A, Dayer JM: Purified blood monocytes from HIV-1 infected patients produce high levels of TNF-alpha and IL-1. Clin Immunol Immunopathol 1989; 50:374–384.
93. Clouse KA, Cosentino LM, Weih KA, et al: The HIV-1 gp120 envelope protein has the intrinsic capacity to stimulate monokine secretion. J Immunol 1991; 147:2892–2901.
94. Oyaizu N, Chirmule N, Ohnishi Y, et al: Human immunodeficiency virus type 1 envelope glycoproteins gp120 and gp160 induce IL-6 production in CD4+ T-cell clones. J Virol 1991; 65:6277–6282.
95. Sugiura K, Oyaizu N, Pahwa R, et al: Effect of human immunodeficiency virus-1 envelope glycoprotein on in vitro hematopoiesis of umbilical cord blood. Blood 1992; 80:1463–1469.
96. Lau AS, Williams BR: The role of interferon and tumor necrosis factor in the pathogenesis of AIDS. J Exp Pathol 1990; 5:111–122.
97. Odeh M: The role of tumor necrosis factor-alpha in acquired immunodeficiency syndrome. J Intern Med 1990; 228:549–556.
98. Selleri C, Sato T, Anderson S, et al: Interferon-gamma and tumor necrosis factor-alpha suppress both early and late stages of hematopoiesis and induce programmed cell death. J Cell Physiol 1995; 165:538–546.
99. Rusten LS, Jacobsen FW, Lesslauer W, et al: Bifunctional effects of TNF-α on the growth of mature and primitive human hematopoietic progenitor cells. Blood 1994; 83:3152–3159.
100. Rusten LS, Smeland EB, Jacobsen FW, et al: Tumor necrosis factor-α inhibits stem cell factor-induced proliferation of human bone marrow progenitor cells in vitro. J Clin Invest 1994; 94:165–172.
101. Roodman GD, Bird A, Hutzler D, Montgomery W: Tumor necrosis factor-alpha and hematopoietic progenitors: Effects of tumor necrosis factor on the growth of erythroid progenitors CFU-E and BFU-E and the hematopoietic cell lines K562, HL60 and HEL cells. Exp Hematol 1987; 15:928–935.
102. Rieckmann P, Poli G, Fox CH, et al: Recombinant gp120 specifically enhances tumor necrosis factor-alpha production and Ig secretion in B lymphocytes from HIV-infected individuals but not from seronegative donors. J Immunol 1991; 147:2922–2927.
103. Broxmeyer HE, Williams DE, Lu L, et al: The suppressive influences of human tumor necrosis factors on bone marrow progenitor cells from normal donors and patients with leukemia: Synergism of tumor necrosis factor and interferon-gamma. J Immunol 1986; 136:4487–4495.
104. Kramer A, Biggar RJ, Hampl H, et al: Immunologic markers of progression to acquired immunodeficiency syndrome are time-dependent and illness-specific. Am J Epidemiol 1992; 136:71–80.
105. Fuchs D, Reibnegger G, Werner ER, et al: Low haemoglobin in haemophilia children is associated with chronic immune activation. Acta Haematol 1991; 85:62–65.
106. Kagi D, Vignaux F, Ledermenn B, et al: Fas and perforin pathways as major mechanisms of T-cell mediated cytotoxicity. Science 1994; 265:528.

107. Maciejewski JP, Selleri C, Sato T, et al: Nitric oxide suppression of human hematopoiesis in vitro. Contribution to inhibitory action of interferon-gamma and tumor necrosis factor-alpha. J Clin Invest 1995; 96:1085–1092.
108. Maciejewski J, Selleri C, Anderson S, Young NS: Fas antigen expression on CD34+ human marrow cells is induced by interferon γ and tumor necrosis factor α and potentiates cytokine-mediated hematopoietic suppression in vitro. Blood 1995; 85:3183–3190.
109. Maciejewski JP, Selleri C, Sato T, et al: Increased expression of Fas antigen on bone marrow CD34+ cells of patients with aplastic anemia. Br J Hematol 1995; 91:245–252.
110. Nagafuji K, Shibuya T, Harada M, et al: Functional expression of Fas antigen (CD95) on hematopoietic progenitor cells. Blood 1995; 86:883–889.
111. Sato T, Selleri C, Anderson S, et al: Expression and modulation of cellular receptors for interferon-gamma, tumour necrosis factor, and Fas on human bone marrow CD34+ cells. Br J Haematol 1997; 97:356–365.
112. Taniguchi T, Harada H, Lamphier M: Regulation of the interferon system and cell growth by the IRF transcription factors. J Cancer Res Clin Oncol 1995; 121:516–520.
113. Sen GC, Lengyel P: The interferon system. J Biol Chem 1992; 267:5017–5020.
114. Lenardo MJ, Baltimore D: NF-kappa B: A pleiotropic mediator of inducible and tissue-specific gene control. Cell 1989; 58:227–229.
115. Nagata S: Apoptosis by death factor. Cell 1997; 88:355–365.
116. Los M, Van de Craen M, Penning LC, et al: Requirement of an ICE/CED-3 protease for Fas/APO-1 mediated apoptosis. Nature 1995; 375:81–83.
117. Enari M, Hase A, Nagata S: Apoptosis by a cytosolic extract from Fas-activated cells. EMBO J 1995; 14:5201–5208.
118. Sloand EM, Young NS, Sato T, et al: Inhibition of interleukin-β converting enzyme in human hematopoietic progenitor cells results in blockade of cytokine-mediated apoptosis and expansion of their proliferative potential. Exp Hematol 1998; 26:1093–1099.
119. Karpatkin S, Nardi MA, Hymes KB: Immunologic thrombocytopenic purpura after heterosexual transmission of human immunodeficiency virus (HIV). Ann Intern Med 1988; 109:190–193.
120. Savona S, Nardi MA, Lennette ET, Karpatkin S: Thrombocytopenic purpura in narcotics addicts. Ann Intern Med 1985; 102:737–741.
121. Murphy MF, Metcalfe P, Waters AH, et al: Incidence and mechanism of neutropenia and thrombocytopenia in patients with human immunodeficiency virus infection. Br J Haematol 1987; 66:337–340.
122. Karcher DS, Frost A: The bone marrow in human immunodeficiency virus (HIV)-related disease. Am J Clin Pathol 1991; 95:63–71.
123. Mir N, Costello C, Luckit J, Lindley R: HIV-disease and bone marrow changes: A study of 60 cases. Eur J Haematol 1989; 42:339–343.
124. Osborne BM, Guarda LA, Butler JJ: Bone marrow biopsies in patients with the acquired immunodeficiency syndrome. Hum Pathol 1984; 15:1048–1053.
125. Perkocha LA, Rodgers GM: Hematologic aspects of human immunodeficiency virus infection: Laboratory and clinical considerations. Am J Hematol 1988; 29:94–105.
126. Harris CE, Biggs JC, Concannon AJ, Dodds AJ: Peripheral blood and bone marrow findings in patients with acquired immune deficiency syndrome. Pathology 1990; 22:206–211.
127. Franco CM, Hendrix LE, Lokey JL: Bone marrow abnormalities in the acquired immunodeficiency syndrome. Ann Intern Med 1984; 101:275–276.
128. Geller SA, Muller R, Greenberg ML, Siegal FP: Acquired immunodeficiency syndrome. Distinctive features of bone marrow biopsies. Arch Pathol Lab Med 1985; 109:138–141.
129. Hromas RA, Murray JL: Bone marrow in the acquired immunodeficiency syndrome. Ann Intern Med 1984; 101:877.
130. Schneider DR, Picker LJ: Myelodysplasia in the acquired immune deficiency syndrome. Am J Clin Pathol 1985; 84:144–152.
131. Thiele J, Zirbes TK, Wiemers P, et al: Incidence of apoptosis in HIV-myelopathy, myelodysplastic syndromes and non-specific inflammatory lesions of the bone marrow. Histopathology 1997; 30:307–311.
132. Henry DH, Beall GN, Benson CA: Recombinant human erythropoietin in the treatment of anemia associated with human immunodeficiency virus (HIV) infection and zidovudine therapy. Ann Intern Med 1992; 117:739–748.
133. Sloand E, Kumar P, Klein HG, et al: Transfusion of blood components to persons infected with human immunodeficiency virus type 1: Relationship to opportunistic infection. Transfusion 1994; 34:48–53.
134. Vamvakas E, Kaplan HS: Early transfusion and length of survival in acquired immune deficiency syndrome: Experience with a population receiving medical care at a public hospital. Transfusion 1993; 33:111–118.
135. Busch MP, Lee TH, Heitman J: Allogeneic leukocytes but not therapeutic blood elements induce reactivation and dissemination of latent human immunodeficiency virus type 1 infection: Implications for transfusion support of infected patients. Blood 1992; 80:2128–2135.
136. Mudido PM, Georges D, Dorazio D, et al: Human immunodeficiency virus type 1 activation after blood transfusion. Transfusion 1996; 36:860–865.
137. Ballem PJ, Belzberg A, Devine DV, et al: Kinetic studies of the mechanism of thrombocytopenia in patients with human immunodeficiency virus infection. N Engl J Med 1992; 327:1779–1784.
138. Gernsheimer T, Stratton J, Ballem PJ, Slichter SJ: Mechanisms of response to treatment in autoim-

mune thrombocytopenic purpura. N Engl J Med 1989; 320:974–980.
139. Hymes KB, Greene JB, Karpatkin S: The effect of azidothymidine on HIV-related thrombocytopenia. N Engl J Med 1988; 318:516–517.
140. Oksenhendler E, Bierling P, Ferchal F, et al: Zidovudine for thrombocytopenic purpura related to human immunodeficiency virus (HIV) infection. Ann Intern Med 1989; 1110:365–368.
141. Ratner L: Human immunodeficiency virus-associated autoimmune thrombocytopenic purpura: A review. Am J Med 1989; 86:194–198.
142. Pottage JC, Benson CA, Spear JB, et al: Treatment of human immunodeficiency virus-related thrombocytopenia with zidovudine. JAMA 1988; 260:3045–3048.
143. Gottlieb MS, Wolfe PR, Chafey S: Response of AIDS-related thrombocytopenia to intravenous and oral azidothymidine (3′-azido-3′-deoxythymidine). AIDS Res Hum Retroviruses 1987; 3:109–114.
144. Fischl MA, Parker CB, Pettinelli C, et al: A randomized controlled trial of a reduced daily dose of zidovudine in patients with the acquired immunodeficiency syndrome. The AIDS Clinical Trials Group. N Engl J Med 1990; 323:1009–1014.
145. Ellis ME, Neal KR, Leen CL, Newland AC: Alfa-2a recombinant interferon in HIV associated thrombocytopenia. Br Med J 1987; 295:1519.
146. Guo WX, Antakly T: Aids-related Kaposi's sarcoma: Evidence for direct stimulatory effect of glucocorticoid on cell proliferation. Am J Pathol 1995; 146:727–734.
147. Beard J, Savidge GF: High-dose intravenous immunoglobulin and splenectomy for the treatment of HIV-related immune thrombocytopenia in patients with severe haemophilia. Br J Haematol 1988; 68:303–306.
148. Pollak AN, Janinis J, Green D: Successful intravenous immune globulin therapy for human immunodeficiency virus-associated thrombocytopenia. Arch Intern Med 1988; 148:695–697.
149. Bussel JB, Haimi JS: Isolated thrombocytopenia in patients infected with HIV: Treatment with intravenous gammaglobulin. Am J Hematol 1988; 28:79–84.
150. Oksenhendler E, Bierling P, Brossard Y, et al: Anti-RH immunoglobulin therapy for human immunodeficiency virus-related immune thrombocytopenic purpura. Blood 1988; 71:1499–1502.
151. Biniek R, Malessa R, Brockmeyer NH, Luboldt W: Anti-Rh(D) immunoglobulin for AIDS-related thrombocytopenia. Lancet 1986; 2:627.
152. Mintzer DM, Real FX, Jovino L, Krown SE: Treatment of Kaposi's sarcoma and thrombocytopenia with vincristine in patients with the acquired immunodeficiency syndrome. Ann Intern Med 1985; 102:200–202.
153. Yang C, Xia Y, Li J, Kutner DJ: The appearance of anti-thrombopoietin antibody and circulating thrombopoietin-IgG complexes in a patient developing thrombocytopenia after the injection of PEG-rHuMGDF. Blood 1999; 94:681a.
154. Barbui T, Cortelazzo S, Minetti B, et al: Does splenectomy enhance risk of AIDS in HIV-positive patients with chronic thrombocytopenia. Lancet 1987; 2:342–343.
155. Schneider PA, Abrams DI, Rayner AA, Hohn DC: Immunodeficiency-associated thrombocytopenic purpura (IDTP). Response to splenectomy. Arch Surg 1987; 122:1175–1178.
156. Morlat P, Dequae-Merchadou L, Dabis F, et al: Splenectomy and prognosis of HIV infection. AIDS 1996; 10:1170–1172.
157. Brown SA, Majumdar G, Harrington C, et al: Effect of splenectomy on HIV-related thrombocytopenia and progression of HIV infection in patients with severe haemophilia. Blood Coagul Fibrinolysis 1994; 5:393–397.
158. Groopman JE: Granulocyte-macrophage colony-stimulating factor in human immunodeficiency virus disease. Semin Hematol 1990; 27(3 Suppl 3):8–14.
159. Scadden DT, Zon LI, Groopman JE: Pathophysiology and management of HIV-associated hematologic disorders. Blood 1989; 74:1455–1463.
160. Groopman JE, Feder D: Hematopoietic growth factors in AIDS. Semin Oncol 1992; 19:408–414.
161. Pluda JM, Mitsuya H, Yarchoan R: Hematologic effects of AIDS therapies. Hematol Oncol Clin North Am 1991; 5:229–248.
162. Levine JD, Allan JD, Tessitore JH, et al: Recombinant human granulocyte-macrophage colony-stimulating factor ameliorates zidovudine-induced neutropenia in patients with acquired immunodeficiency syndrome (AIDS)-AIDS-related complex. Blood 1992; 78:3148–3154.
163. Hammer SM, Gillis JM, Pinkston P, Rose RM: Effect of zidovudine and granulocyte-macrophage colony-stimulating factor on human immunodeficiency virus replication in alveolar macrophages. Blood 1990; 75:1215–1219.
164. Perno CF, Cooney DA, Gao WY, et al: Effects of bone marrow stimulatory cytokines on human immunodeficiency virus replication and the antiviral activity of dideoxynucleosides in cultures of monocyte/macrophages. Blood 1992; 80:995–1003.
165. Scadden DT, Wang A, Zsebo KM, Groopman JE: *In vitro* effects of stem-cell factor or interleukin-3 on myelosuppression associated with AIDS. AIDS 1994; 8:193–196.
166. Kaplan LD, Kahn JO, Crowe S, et al: Clinical and virologic effects of recombinant human granulocyte-macrophage colony-stimulating factor in patients receiving chemotherapy for human immunodeficiency virus-associated non-Hodgkin's lymphoma: Results of a randomized trial. J Clin Oncol 1991; 9:929–940.
167. Sloand E, Kumar PN, Pierce PF: Chemotherapy for patients with pulmonary Kaposi's sarcoma: Benefit of filgrastim (G-CSF) in supporting dose administration. South Med J 1993; 86:1219–1224.

10

T Cell Large Granular Lymphocyte Lymphoproliferative Disorder

Jeffrey Molldrem, M.D.

HISTORY

For many years it has been recognized that increased numbers of circulating large granular lymphocytes (LGLs) in the peripheral blood are associated with neutropenia with or without anemia or thrombocytopenia.[1] We have only recently recognized this relationship as a separate clinical and pathophysiologic entity, as laboratory tools necessary for diagnosis have become more readily available. However, because of uncertainty over the etiology, the classification of this syndrome as leukemia is controversial. Normal LGLs are the morphologic equivalents of reactive lymphocytes, although controversy still exists as to the malignant nature of this disease. In fact, as we discuss later, the proximal cause of the abnormal proliferation of LGLs will likely dictate whether we ultimately should consider this disorder a leukemia.

Many terms have been used to describe the disease, such as T cell chronic lymphocytic leukemia (CLL), T suppressor cell CLL, neutropenia with T lymphocytosis, and Tγ-lymphocytosis.[2] The French-American-British (FAB) classification proposed in 1989 separated out T cell CLL or LGL leukemia.[3] It was agreed upon by the Morphologic, Immunologic, Cytogenetic (MIC) Cooperative Study Group 1 year later that the term LGL leukemia should replace T cell CLL, in order to consolidate the number of names given to this constellation of clinical and pathologic findings into a single disease category. Based on the phenotype of the LGL, we can separate LGL lymphoproliferative (LPD) disorder into T cell (CD3+) and natural killer (NK) cell-(CD3−) types, as first proposed by Chan et al. in 1986[4] and reviewed by Loughran in 1993.[2] Furthermore, because of the clonal nature of the LGLs and the potentially aggressive clinical course, we have come to classify this disease as leukemia. Both T-LGL leukemia and NK-LGL leukemia are now recognized as distinct diseases, based on clonality, phenotype, and common clinical features. T-LGL leukemia is much more common in Europe and the United States, while NK-LGL leukemia is prevalent in Asia. In this chapter, we limit our discussion to T-LGL leukemia.

DIAGNOSIS

There is no broad consensus on the exact criteria to establish the diagnosis of T-LGL leukemia. However, this new entity is recognized as a distinct disease and there is now general agreement that three requirements must be met to establish the diagnosis: (1) evidence of a clonal population of T cells based on T cell receptor (TCR) gene rearrangement studies, (2) an abnormal number of phenotypic T-LGLs based on flow cytometry, and (3) the proper clinical scenario of prolonged cytopenia.[2,5] Determination of clonality is central to the diagnosis, since polyclonal proliferations of T-LGLs can occur, often transiently and associated with infections.[6–12]

The diagnosis is often suspected when isolated neutropenia is found with circulating large granular lymphocytes in the patient's peripheral blood, as shown in Plate 12. These lymphocytes are morphologically heterogeneous, varying in appearance from the usual large and granular, to small and granular, to quite large and agranular.[13] Importantly, however, all share the same phenotype as measured by flow cytometry.

CLINICAL AND HEMATOLOGIC FEATURES

T-LGL leukemia is an indolent disease characterized by prolonged periods of neutropenia. Treatment has generally been unsatisfactory. Patients may be of any age when diagnosed, although they are often over the age of 50 years. Since the molecular tools used to diagnose T-LGL leukemia were not in widespread use until recently, this historically led to underdiagnosis, so the median age may in fact be much younger. The male-to-female distribution is approximately equal.[2]

Patients are typically not diagnosed until after several months to years of neutropenia and recurrent fevers. The neutropenia may not be sustained but can instead be periodic. Recurrent bacterial infections are quite common, although fungal and viral infections are rare. In addition to neutropenia, the blood smear shows both an increased number and percentage of LGLs. LGLs are larger than normal lymphocytes, typically 10 to 20 μm in diameter. They contain abundant pale cytoplasm, with prominent azurophil granules (Plate 13). Although the total number of lymphocytes may not be elevated, the number of circulating LGLs is increased, usually between 500/μL and 50,000/μL, with an average number near 5000/μL. While original descriptions of the disease included a granular lymphocytosis of greater than 2000/μL lasting for more than 6 months, more recent reports have recognized the heterogeneity of the granular lymphocytosis, and an absolute number is no longer used to define the disease.[5] Although modest overall lymphocytosis is not universal, it is observed in over 70% of patients and is rarely in excess of 50,000/μL. A very careful survey of the blood smear is therefore necessary in order to suggest the diagnosis.

The clinical and blood count findings suggest the diagnosis, which must then be confirmed by lymphocyte phenotyping and TCR gene rearrangement studies for T cell clonality. In rare circumstances, when there are very few granular lymphocytes on peripheral blood smear, phenotyping for screening purposes establishes diagnosis. Although most patients do not have a constant number of granular lymphocytes in the peripheral blood over time, and the amount of cytoplasmic granulation may vary over time as well, the phenotypic and clonal abnormalities persist.[13]

Splenomegaly is found in half of all patients, although the spleen is rarely greatly enlarged, and hepatomegaly occurs in 25% of cases.[14, 15] Lymphadenopathy is very rare in T-LGL leukemia, and more common in NK-LGL leukemia. The LGLs usually infiltrate the sinusoids of the liver as well as the splenic red pulp, resulting in the organomegaly. Skin rashes are quite rare, and their presence should suggest an alternative diagnosis.[16-18]

Bone marrow involvement is nearly universal, and the pattern is usually small focal areas of infiltration. More diffuse involvement is seen much less often. The degree of lymphocyte infiltration in the marrow is never enough to account for the degree of cytopenia, however. Maturation arrest is observed in the myeloid series, usually at or before the promyelocyte stage of development. Erythroid hyperplasia may be present in patients with a normal hemoglobin, and megakaryocytes decreased in number, although morphologically normal. Quite often clusters of granular lymphocytes surrounding myeloid precursors can be seen on marrow aspirates (see Plate 15). These lymphocytes may appear polarized, with their cytoplasm, tightly folded around the larger myeloid cells, giving the impression of a darker appearance near the point of contact with the myeloid cells. The morphology may reflect a process of antigen recognition of hematopoietic precursors by the abnormal lymphocytes and gives the suggestion of ongoing inhibition of these progenitor cells, which would contribute to cytopenia.

The neutropenia that is observed in 90% to 100% of patients with T-LGL leukemia is generally moderate with an absolute neutrophil count (ANC) between 500 and 1000/μL. Neutropenia may be present for months before an infection occurs, finally bringing the patient to medical attention. Severe neutropenia, with an ANC below 500/μL, is present in about half of patients at diagnosis. Tests for neutrophil survival may reveal a decreased survival, but this is not a consistent finding. Antineutrophil antibodies are present in 30% to 40% of patients; the antibody titer does not correlate with the degree of neutropenia or the T-LGL burden.[19] Immune complexes of all types are found in greater than half of patients, and polyclonal hypergammaglobulinemia occurs in nearly half. Serologic abnormalities are frequent, including autoantibodies such as rheumatoid factor and antinuclear antibody; frank rheumatoid arthritis is present in 25% to 30% of patients.[20, 21]

Patients with T-LGL leukemia and rheumatoid arthritis resemble cases of Felty's syndrome, blurring the distinction between these disorders.[21, 22] The clinical triad of rheumatoid arthritis, splenomegaly, and neutropenia defines Felty's syndrome.

Most of these patients also have clonal CD3+ LGL populations present in peripheral blood, although the true prevalence is not known. T-LGL leukemia usually develops prior to the onset of rheumatoid arthritis or Felty's syndrome.

Patients with adult-onset cyclic neutropenia often have clonal CD3+ LGLs present at diagnosis or at some time during their illness.[23, 24] Especially as the disease tends to "burn out," cycling becomes less evident, and the patients develop sustained neutropenia.

Other hematologic abnormalities in T-LGL leukemia include normocytic, normochromic anemia (less than 10 g/dL), which is observed in half of all patients and sometimes may be the only cytopenia. The anemia is usually chronic and present for months or years before transfusions are required. Direct or indirect Coomb's test may be positive. The anemia usually resembles pure red cell aplasia with pronounced bone marrow erythroid hypoplasia, except that granular lymphocytes are prominent in the marrow and peripheral blood.

Mild to moderate thrombocytopenia (less than 100,000/μL) is observed in 25% of patients, usually in conjunction with neutropenia. Platelet counts rarely fall below 20,000/μL, except after many years of the disease, and pancytopenia is frequent when platelet counts are significantly low. Megakaryocytes are usually reduced in number but are morphologically normal.

IMMUNOLOGIC AND MOLECULAR FEATURES

After prominent granular lymphocytes are identified in the blood and marrow, the lymphocyte immunophenotype must be assessed by flow cytometry. The essential feature of T-LGL leukemia is the presence of a discrete clonal population of cells, often suspected and sometimes confirmed after phenotypic analysis. Table 10–1 summarizes the phenotypic pattern of patients with T-LGL and NK leukemia. A homogeneous population of CD3+ CD16+ lymphocytes is present in virtually all cases of T-LGL leukemia.[25] This subset accounts for fewer than 5% of normal cells in healthy subjects, and any increase in this population is highly suggestive of T-LGL leukemia.[25] It is important to emphasize the requirement of using recently produced monoclonal antibodies against CD16 (KD1 or VD4), which are able to identify the totality of CD16 cells.[2, 25]

Although early descriptions of T-LGL leukemia classified these lymphocytes as Tγ-lymphoproliferations, the lymphocytes are actually TCR-αβ+ in greater than 95% of cases. T-LGL leukemia may involve rearranged expressed TCR-γδ, but these rare cases are clinically indistinguishable from the most common TCR-αβ+ lymphocytes. The lymphocytes are CD8+ in almost all cases, although a few cases of CD4+ cells have been described as well. Three-parameter flow cytometry usually reveals a homogeneous population of CD3+CD16+CD57+cells.

Finally, to establish the diagnosis of T-LGL leukemia, clonality needs to be demonstrated molecularly. Analysis is based on Southern blot hybridization using complementary DNA (cDNA) probes to the TCR genes. Most laboratories make use of primers and probes directed against the TCR-γ gene, since the number of probes needed is smaller and this locus undergoes rearrangement prior to reassortment of either the α or β genes, and would therefore also be rearranged in T-LGL leukemia. The use of the polymerase chain reaction (PCR) to uncover small populations of T cell clones has not been adequately evaluated, but this technique is probably too sensitive for clinical use.

PATHOGENESIS

Neither the clonal expansion of CD3+ granular lymphocytes in T-LGL leukemia nor the mechanism of cytopenia, the clinical hallmark of this disease, is fully understood. CD3+ LGLs have many characteristics of antigen-activated cytotoxic T lymphocytes. They may use a restricted Vβ and Vα TCR repertoire, but some show a diverse Jα usage.[26] These findings suggest an immune-mediated selection process affecting the TCR-α chain occurring after the event that established the clone. In addition, the LGL phenotype is similar to normally activated cells, as shown in Figure 10–1, and they constitutively express perforin, CD95, and CD95L.[27] T-LGLs likely proliferate to

TABLE 10–1 Phenotype of Clonal Large Granular Lymphocyte (LGL) Leukemia Populations

Surface Antigen	T-LGL Leukemia	NK-LGL Leukemia
TCR-αβ	+	−
CD3	+	−
CD8	+	−
CD16	+	+
CD56	−	+
CD57	+	±
IL-2R p75	+	+

NK, natural killer cell, TCR-αβ, T cell receptor αβ; IL-2R p75, interleukin-2 receptor p75 subunit.

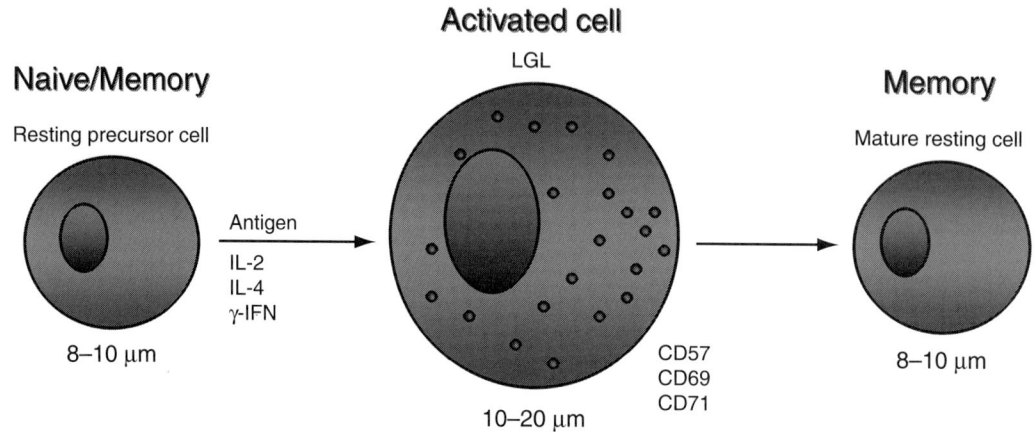

Figure 10–1 Immunophenotype in normal T cell development. The activated state is usually transient in normal lymphocytes and occurs after antigen recognition. T-LGL leukemia cells are morphologically and phenotypically similar to these normal cells. LGL, large granular lymphocyte; IL, interleukin; IFN, interferon.

abnormal levels after antigen stimulation. However, their persistence might be the result of either chronic antigen stimulation or inhibition of normal apoptosis mechanisms. Recent evidence suggests that a defect in post-CD95 signaling exists in T-LGL cells.[28]

The mechanism by which neutropenia develops is not clear. However, based on the similarity of T-LGL leukemia cells to activated cytotoxic T lymphocytes (CTLs) and the response to immunosuppressive therapy, it is tempting to speculate that T-LGLs contribute to cytopenia by suppressing normal hematopoiesis. Normal granular lymphocytes have been shown to inhibit colony-forming units—granulocyte macrophage (CFU_{GM}), but this effect was not observed when granular lymphocytes from patients with T-LGL leukemia were cocultured with marrow from normal donors or with autologous marrow.[29] However, in early studies incomplete HLA matching and the absence of proper coincubation of the LGLs with marrow cells prior to plating in methylcellulose (necessary for appropriate antigen recognition by T cells) might explain the observed lack of inhibition of myeloid progenitor cells.

Since shortened neutrophil survival, the presence of antigranulocyte antibodies, and antibody-dependent cell-mediated cytotoxicity have all been demonstrated in patients with T-LGL leukemia, immune destruction by granulocyte antibodies has been postulated as a mechanism of neutropenia.[30, 31] This pathophysiology would not explain the anemia and thrombocytopenia that are often observed, however, and antigranulocyte antibodies persist even after neutrophil counts normalize in response to therapy.

Granular lymphocytes from T-LGL leukemia patients produce a variety of cytokines that might play a role in producing cytopenia. Both interferon-γ (IFN-γ) and tumor necrosis factor-α (TNF-α) are made by LGLs, and inhibition of myeloid colony growth by IFN-γ has been demonstrated.[32] Increased levels of IFN-γ in the marrow microenvironment might also contribute to the cytopenia of aplastic anemia (AA),[32] and clonal T cells capable of secreting IFN-γ and that suppress myeloid precursors have been isolated from AA patients.

Interestingly, elevations of clonal T cells with granular lymphocyte morphology and immunophenotype are a common occurrence in many marrow failure syndromes. Some patients with myelodysplastic syndrome (MDS) have activated clonal CTLs that suppress CFU_{GM} and that are eliminated following treatment with antithymocyte globulin (ATG),[33, 34] a drug also active in patients with AA. In addition, increased numbers of clonal CD3+ LGLs have been found in a majority of patients with pure red cell aplasia, who responded more often to immunosuppressive therapy.[35–37] A separate report also details the case of a patient with pure red cell aplasia, parvovirus B19 infection, and the presence of clonal CD3+ LGLs.[38] Thus, there may be a final common pathway of marrow failure and cytopenia in these diseases, characterized by an antigen-driven autoimmune process directed toward marrow progenitors.

Although not proven, the connection between oligoclonal expansions of CD3+ LGLs in patients after allogeneic bone marrow transplant[39, 40] and the possible antileukemic effect of these cells is intriguing in light of the connection of T-LGL

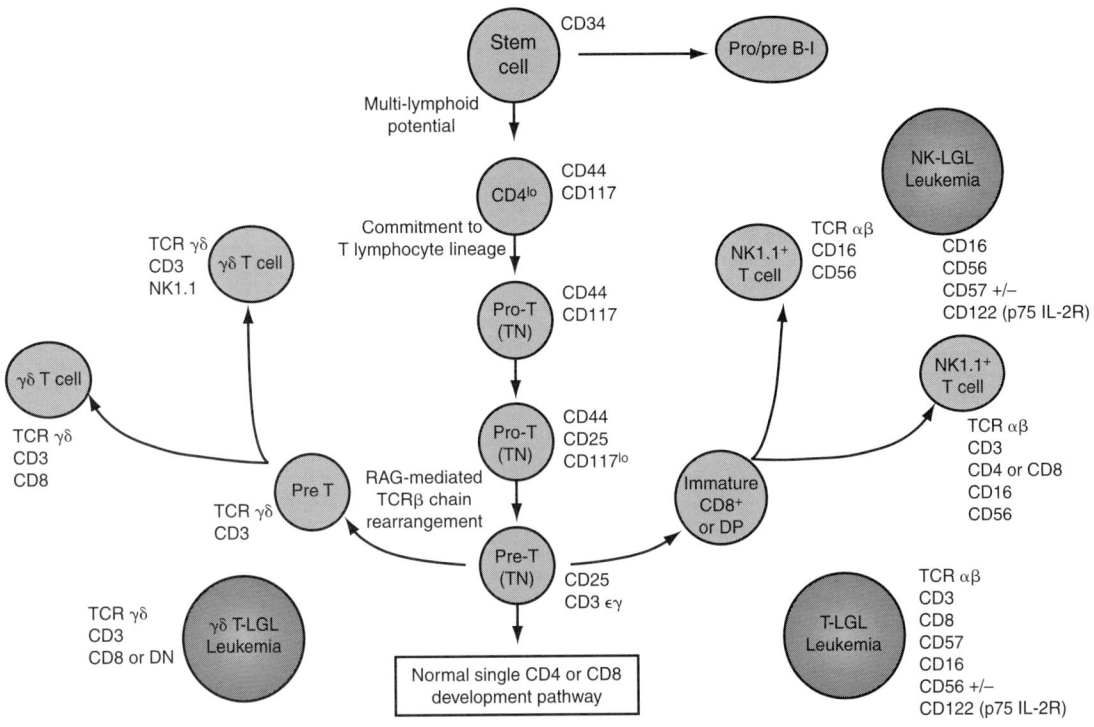

Figure 10–2 Normal lymphocyte development and corresponding large granular lymphocyte (LGL) development. Hematopoietic stem cells give rise to triple-negative (TN) precursors and branch off to give rise to lymphocytes with phenotype similar to the three dominant forms of LGL leukemia (also shown). TCR, T cell receptor; NK, natural killer cell.

leukemia to other acquired marrow failure syndromes. Hematopoietic and leukemic progenitors may share common antigens recognized by CD3+ LGL cells. One interesting case report documents the expansion of a clonal CD3+ LGL population that proliferated in response to the patient's own acute myeloid leukemia (AML) cells. CD3+ LGL cells decreased at the time of relapse of her AML but increased during disease remission, suggesting the CD3+ LGLs responded to a leukemia-associated antigen.[41]

The inciting event that triggers the proliferation of CD3+ LGLs might be an intrinsic abnormality of hematopoietic precursors, an extrinsic event such as a viral infection, or perhaps an abnormality inherent in the LGLs themselves. However, the normal phenotype of the leukemic LGL as shown in Figure 10–2, suggests a sustained reactive process of essentially normal lymphocyte proliferation.

While clonality is central to T-LGL leukemia, clonality alone does not establish the diagnosis. Clonal populations of lymphocytes have been detected during autoimmune processes, in bone marrow transplant recipients, after viral infections, and in otherwise healthy persons (Table 10–2). These observations underscore that lymphocyte expansions frequently arise in response to environmental exposures, and that the border between normal and pathologic clonal lymphocyte expansions is narrow and often blurred. In order to make the diagnosis of T-LGL leukemia, the proper clinical setting of sustained cytopenia must be present.

Recent advances in immunology have allowed the easy enumeration of antigen-specific lymphocytes by using specific "tetramer" reagents, where peptide antigen is combined with major histocompatibility complex (MHC) class I heavy chains that are linked to a fluorochrome via steptavidin.[42] Using this technology, as many as 50% of all peripheral blood lymphocytes in patients acutely infected with the Epstein-Barr virus (EBV) are specific for a single viral epitope.[43] These cells are usually derived from a single lymphocyte clone or a small number of distinct clones, which gradually diminish with time.[44] When clonal CD3+ LGLs emerge in T-LGL leukemia, tetramer technology

TABLE 10–2 Clinical Syndromes Associated With Clonal Cytotoxic T Lymphocytes (CTLs)

Clinical Syndrome	Clinical Findings	In Vitro Characteristics of Clonal CTL Population
Normal healthy persons	Clonal populations increase with age Present in up to 40% of population Constitute up to 15% of total PBL population	Inhibit CTL proliferation Inhibit B cell and antibody production
HIV disease	Increase in late-stage disease	Some secrete an inhibitor of CTL proliferation Some are specific for HIV-derived peptides
Other viral infections	CMV, EBV, HSV acute infection Represents the dominant peripheral blood T cell clone for 6 mo to 3 yr following acute infection	Display CTL activity toward virally infected targets
Postallogeneic bone marrow transplant	CTL clones correlate with CMV status, immune status, and chronic GvHD Presence of clonal CTL inversely correlates with relapse risk of leukemia Clone may decrease after 6 yr	Secrete soluble inhibitor of CTL proliferation Homology of TCR Vβ_{16} family noted in some patients
Rheumatoid arthritis	Usually restricted to joints and areas of acute inflammation	50% of clones may show TCR Vβ_3 family restriction
Solid tumors	Clones increased at sites of tumor (present in peripheral blood, but only slightly increased)	Represent up to 15% of tumor-infiltrating lymphocyte population

PBL, peripheral blood lymphocyte; HIV, human immunodeficiency virus; CMV, cytomegalovirus; EBV, Epstein-Barr virus; HSV, herpes simplex virus; GvHD, graft-versus-host disease; TCR, T cell receptor.

might also be useful to demonstrate antigen-specificity and allow determination of the nature of such antigens.

PROGNOSIS AND TREATMENT

Because the defining features of T-LGL leukemia have only recently been elucidated, the natural history of the disease has not been adequately studied. In perhaps the largest single-institution cohort of patients, 61 (90%) of 68 patients were alive at 3½ years, with the majority of patients (70%) requiring therapy during the period of study.[45] At diagnosis, most patients were symptomatic with fatigue, B symptoms and recurrent infections occurred in 15%, and only 28% were asymptomatic. A separate multicenter study reported 20% mortality at 4 years. Spontaneous remissions are rare, if they occur at all.

Although the disease is commonly thought of as indolent, most patients eventually require therapy.[2] The primary indication for treatment is recurrent infections secondary to neutropenia, although other severe cytopenias may lower the threshold for therapeutic intervention. Immunosuppression remains the mainstay of therapy. Traditional induction chemotherapy regimens used to treat AML do not eradicate the CD3+ clone, and cytopenia persists after this kind of treatment. Splenectomy is usually of limited benefit and may lead to partial recovery of anemia more often than improvement in neutropenia. In addition, the number of CD3+ LGLs increases post-splenectomy, which may have the unwanted effect of eventually worsening cytopenia.

The major objective of therapy is to increase the number of neutrophils in order to decrease the incidence of life-threatening infections. Because most immunosuppressive treatments do not result in the total disappearance of the CD3+ LGL clone, therapy may be required lifelong in most patients. However, generally only low doses of immunosuppressive drugs are required to maintain neutrophil counts above 500/µL, and periods of "drug holiday" are often possible. Exceptions to this rule include patients with adult-onset cyclic neutropenia or patients with "transformed" T-LGL leukemia, who develop additional cytogenetic abnormalities that require an aggressive treatment approach.[2]

A majority of patients, as many as 60% to 70%, respond to intermittent cyclophosphamide at 25 to 100 mg/day with or without prednisone at 40 to 60 mg/day initiated for 6 to 12 months, and intermittent therapy is often effective for maintenance. Lower toxicity and longer duration of response are associated with the combination, although the treatment-related toxicity is predominantly related to long-term corticosteroid use. Long-term use of alkylators is associated with secondary leukemia and myelodysplasia.

Low-dose oral methotrexate has also been useful. In a study of 10 patients treated with 5 mg weekly up to 10 mg/m^2, five had a complete clinical remission and one a partial remission.[46] Many of the patients also received prednisone, although it was tapered while methotrexate was administered. The abnormal CD3+ clone was no longer detectable in three of the patients, as assessed by TCR gene rearrangement and Southern blot analyses. Responses were seen after 2 weeks to 4 months of treatment, the patients could be maintained on therapy, and toxicity was minimal.

Growth factors such as granulocyte-macrophage colony-stimulating factor (GM-CSF) and granulocyte colony-stimulating factor (G-CSF) have been successful in reversing neutropenia in a small number of patients, but continuous therapy is required.[47–49] Although G-CSF appears to be more effective than GM-CSF, the combined use of either of these agents with a form of immunosuppressive treatment may be additive.[50, 51]

Purine nucleosides appear to be very effective at eliminating the CD3+ LGL clone, but toxicity from these drugs is often greater than that seen with other low-dose immunosuppressive regimens.[52, 53] Only three to four cycles of therapy with fludarabine or 2-chloro-2′-deoxyadenosine may be required to achieve complete molecular remission. Since very few patients in separate small series have been treated with purine analogues, larger studies are needed to assess their impact on the disease. However, because these drugs act primarily on T cells, it is hoped that such selectivity will translate into improved long-term responses.

Recently, cyclosporine (CsA) has been used to treat T-LGL leukemia, and in a small study involving five subjects, four attained normal neutrophil counts on CsA alone, the longest responder has been maintained for 8½ years.[54] We also used CsA to treat 10 patients with clonal T-LGL leukemia, and eight patients have responded with normal neutrophil counts. An advantage of this type of therapy is that the dose of CsA necessary to maintain normal neutrophil counts is as little as 1 to 2 mg/kg/day orally. However, despite resolution of neutropenia, increased populations of the CD3+ LGLs have persisted in all patients during CsA therapy in both studies.

For patients with aggressive or transformed variants of the disease, allogeneic bone marrow transplant can be curative.[55] However, the risks of this therapy need to be carefully balanced with the severity of the T-LGL leukemia, the age of the patient, and the degree of HLA matching. Experimental approaches such as the use of monoclonal antibodies directed against the interleukin-2 (IL-2) receptor or the CD7 surface marker are also in clinical trial, but the results of these studies have not yet been published.

With an improved understanding of the initiating events of T-LGL leukemia, we will be able to design more specific and effective therapy. If, for instance, a target antigen of the CD3+ LGL were uncovered, vaccine strategies aimed at induction of tolerance might be useful. Likewise, if a mechanism of resistance to apoptosis could be clarified, treatment with various cytokines or targeted biologic agents could be designed. In the meantime, future comparative treatment studies performed at multiple centers would be helpful in determining the best choice of therapy among the many forms of immunosuppressive treatments.

REFERENCES

1. McKenna RW, Parkin J, Kersey JH, et al: Chronic lymphoproliferative disorder with unusual clinical, morphologic, ultrastructural and membrane surface marker characteristics. Am J Med 1977; 62:588–596.
2. Loughran TP Jr: Clonal diseases of large granular lymphocytes. Blood 1993; 82:1–14.
3. Bennett JM, Catovsky D, Daniel MT, et al: Proposals for the classification of chronic (mature) B and T lymphoid leukaemias. French-American-British (FAB) Cooperative Group. J Clin Pathol 1989; 42:567–584.
4. Chan WC, Link S, Mawle A, et al: Heterogeneity of large granular lymphocyte proliferations: Delineation of two major subtypes. Blood 1986; 68:1142–1153.
5. Semenzato G, Zambello R, Starkebaum G, et al: The lymphoproliferative disease of granular lymphocytes: updated criteria for diagnosis. Blood 1997; 89:256–260.
6. Arras M, Contu L: Heterogeneity of the CD8 lymphocytes in healthy and HIV 1 infected subjects. Allergol Immunopathol (Madr) 1991; 19:79–84.
7. Borthwick NJ, Bofill M, Gombert WM, et al: Lymphocyte activation in HIV-1 infection. II. Functional defects of CD28-T cells. AIDS 1994; 8:431–441.
8. Kern F, Ode-Hakim S, Vogt K, et al: The enigma of CD57+CD28- T cell expansion—anergy or activation? Clin Exp Immunol 1996; 104:180–184.
9. Asada H, Okada N, Tei H, et al: Epstein-Barr virus–associated large granular lymphocyte leukemia with cutaneous infiltration. J Am Acad Dermatol 1994; 31:251–255.

10. Lynne JE, Schmid I, Matud JL, et al: Major expansions of select CD8+ subsets in acute Epstein-Barr virus infection: Comparison with chronic human immunodeficiency virus disease. J Infect Dis 1998; 177:1083–1087.
11. Gratama JW, Langelaar RA, Oosterveer MA, et al: Phenotypic study of CD4+ and CD8+ lymphocyte subsets in relation to cytomegalovirus carrier status and its correlate with pokeweed mitogen–induced B lymphocyte differentiation. Clin Exp Immunol 1989; 77:245–251.
12. Wang EC, Moss PA, Frodsham P, et al: CD8^{high}CD57+ T lymphocytes in normal, healthy individuals are oligoclonal and respond to human cytomegalovirus. J Immunol 1995; 155:5046–5056.
13. Gonzales-Chambers R, Przepiorka D, Winkelstein A, et al: Lymphocyte subsets associated with T cell receptor beta-chain gene rearrangement in patients with rheumatoid arthritis and neutropenia. Arthritis Rheum 1992; 35:516–520.
14. Ahern MJ, Roberts-Thomson PJ, Bradley J, et al: Phenotypic and genotypic analysis of mononuclear cells from patients with Felty's syndrome. Ann Rheum Dis 1990; 40:103–106.
15. Bowman SJ, Bhavnani M, Geddes GC, et al: Large granular lymphocyte expansions in patients with Felty's syndrome: Analysis using anti-T cell receptor V beta–specific monoclonal antibodies. Clin Exp Immunol 1995; 101:18–24.
16. Adachi M, Maeda K, Takekawa M, et al: High expression of CD56 (N-CAM) in a patient with cutaneous CD4- positive lymphoma. Am J Hematol 1994; 47:278–282.
17. Daskalova M, Taskov H, Dimitrova E, et al: Humoral and cellular immune response to elastin in patients with systemic sclerosis. Autoimmunity 1997; 25:233–241.
18. Haeffner AC, Zepter K, Elmets CA, et al: Analysis of tumor-infiltrating lymphocytes in cutaneous squamous cell carcinoma. Arch Dermatol 1997; 133:585–590.
19. Loughran TP Jr., Starkebaum G: Large granular lymphocyte leukemia. Report of 38 cases and review of the literature. Medicine (Baltimore) 1987; 66:397–405.
20. Loughran TP Jr, Starkebaum G, Kidd P, et al: Clonal proliferation of large granular lymphocytes in rheumatoid arthritis. Arthritis Rheum 1988; 31:31–36.
21. Starkebaum G, Loughran TP Jr, Gaur LK, et al: Immunogenetic similarities between patients with Felty's syndrome and those with clonal expansions of large granular lymphocytes in rheumatoid arthritis. Arthritis Rheum 1997; 40:624–626.
22. Bowman SJ, Corrigall V, Panayi GS, et al: Hematologic and cytofluorographic analysis of patients with Felty's syndrome. A hypothesis that a discrete event leads to large granular lymphocyte expansions in this condition. Arthritis Rheum 1995; 38:1252–1259.
23. Loughran TP Jr, Hammond WP 4th: Adult-onset cyclic neutropenia is a benign neoplasm associated with clonal proliferation of large granular lymphocytes. J Exp Med 1986; 164:2089–2094.
24. Loughran TP Jr, Clark EA, Price TH, et al: Adult-onset cyclic neutropenia is associated with increased large granular lymphocytes. Blood 1986; 68:1082–1087.
25. Lanier LL, Le AM, Civin CI, et al: The relationship of CD16 (Leu-11) and Leu-19 (NKH-1) antigen expression on human peripheral blood NK cells and cytotoxic T lymphocytes. J Immunol 1986; 136:4480–4486.
26. Kasten-Sportes C, Zaknoen S, Steis RG, et al: T-cell receptor gene rearrangement in T-cell large granular leukocyte leukemia: Preferential V alpha but diverse J alpha usage in one of five patients. Blood 1994; 83:767–775.
27. Perzova R, Loughran TP Jr: Constitutive expression of Fas ligand in large granular lymphocyte leukaemia. Br J Haematol 1997; 97:123–126.
28. Lamy T, Liu JH, Landowski TH, et al: Dysregulation of CD95/CD95 ligand-apoptotic pathway in CD3(+) large granular lymphocyte leukemia. Blood 1998; 92:4771–4777.
29. Loughran TP Jr, Kadin ME, Starkebaum G, et al: Leukemia of large granular lymphocytes: association with clonal chromosomal abnormalities and autoimmune neutropenia, thrombocytopenia, and hemolytic anemia. Ann Intern Med 1985; 102:169–175.
30. Currie MS, Weinberg JB, Rustagi PK, et al: Antibodies to granulocyte precursors in selective myeloid hypoplasia and other suspected autoimmune neutropenias: Use of HL-60 cells as targets. Blood 1987; 69:529–536.
31. Gentile TC, Wener MH, Starkebaum G, et al: Humoral immune abnormalities in T-cell large granular lymphocyte leukemia. Leuk Lymphoma 1996; 23:365–370.
32. Gascon P, Zoumbos N, Young N: Analysis of natural killer cells in patients with aplastic anemia. Blood 1986; 67:1349–1355.
33. Molldrem JJ, Jiang YZ, Stetler-Stevenson M, et al: Haematological response of patients with myelodysplastic syndrome to antithymocyte globulin is associated with a loss of lymphocyte-mediated inhibition of CFU-GM and alterations in T-cell receptor Vbeta profiles. Br J Haematol 1998; 102:1314–1322.
34. Molldrem JJ, Caples M, Mavroudis D, et al: Antithymocyte globulin for patients with myelodysplastic syndrome. Br J Haematol 1997; 99:699–705.
35. Dhodapkar MV, Lust JA, Phyliky RL: T-cell large granular lymphocytic leukemia and pure red cell aplasia in a patient with type I autoimmune polyendocrinopathy: Response to immunosuppressive therapy. Mayo Clin Proc 1994; 69:1085–1088.
36. Motoji T, Yamada O, Takahashi M, et al: Granular lymphocyte leukemia with pure red cell aplasia: Usefulness of gene analysis in assessing therapeutic effect. Am J Hematol 1992; 39:212–219.
37. Lacy MQ, Kurtin PJ, Tefferi A: Pure red cell aplasia: Association with large granular lymphocyte

leukemia and the prognostic value of cytogenetic abnormalities. Blood 1996; 87:3000–3006.
38. Ergas D, Resnitzky P, Berrebi A: Pure red blood cell aplasia associated with parvovirus B19 infection in large granular lymphocyte leukemia (letter). Blood 1996; 87:3523–3524.
39. Autran B, Leblond V, Sadat-Sowti B, et al: A soluble factor released by CD8+CD57+ lymphocytes from bone marrow transplanted patients inhibits cell-mediated cytolysis. Blood 1991; 77:2237–2241.
40. Fukuda H, Nakamura H, Tominaga N, et al: Marked increase of CD8+S6F1+ and CD8+CD57+ cells in patients with graft-versus-host disease after allogeneic bone marrow transplantation. Bone Marrow Transplant 1994; 13:181–185.
41. Suzushima H, Asou N, Eto K, et al: CD4+ CD8+ granular lymphocytic leukemia arising in a patient with acute myeloblastic leukemia. Leukemia 1994; 8:1884–1889.
42. Altman JD, Moss PAH, Goulder PJR, et al: Phenotypic analysis of antigen-specific T lymphocytes. Science 1996; 274:94–96.
43. Callan MF, Tan L, Annels N, et al: Direct visualization of antigen-specific CD8+ T cells during the primary immune response to Epstein-Barr virus in vivo. J Exp Med 1998; 187:1395–1402.
44. Ufret-Vincenty RL, Quigley L, Tresser N, et al: In vivo survival of viral antigen-specific T cells that induce experimental autoimmune encephalomyelitis. J Exp Med 1998; 188:1725–1738.
45. Dhodapkar MV, Li CY, Lust JA, et al: Clinical spectrum of clonal proliferations of T-large granular lymphocytes: A T-cell clonopathy of undetermined significance? Blood 1994; 84:1620–1627.
46. Loughran TP Jr, Kidd PG, Starkebaum G: Treatment of large granular lymphocyte leukemia with oral low-dose methotrexate. Blood 1994; 84:2164–2170.
47. Genvresse I, Spath-Schwalbe E, Lukowsky A, et al: Delayed response to granulocyte colony-stimulating factor (G-CSF) in a case of severe neutropenia associated with large granular lymphocyte (LGL) leukemia. Eur J Haematol 1998; 60:133–134.
48. Weide R, Heymanns J, Koppler H, et al: Successful treatment of neutropenia in T-LGL leukemia (T gamma-lymphocytosis) with granulocyte colony-stimulating factor. Ann Hematol 1994; 69:117–119.
49. Lang DF, Rosenfeld CS, Diamond HS, et al: Successful treatment of T-gamma lymphoproliferative disease with human-recombinant granulocyte colony stimulating factor. Am J Hematol 1992; 40:66–68.
50. Jakubowski A, Winton EF, Gencarelli A, et al: Treatment of chronic neutropenia associated with large granular lymphocytosis with cyclosporine A and filgrastim. Am J Hematol 1995; 50:288–291.
51. Bargetzi MJ, Wortelboer M, Pabst T, et al: Severe neutropenia in T-large granular lymphocyte leukemia corrected by intensive immunosuppression. Ann Hematol 1996; 73:149–151.
52. Edelman MJ, O'Donnell RT, Meadows I: Treatment of refractory large granular lymphocytic leukemia with 2-chlorodeoxyadenosine. Am J Hematol 1997; 54:329–331.
53. Witzig TE, Weitz JJ, Lundberg JH, et al: Treatment of refractory T-cell chronic lymphocytic leukemia with purine nucleoside analogues. Leuk Lymphoma 1994; 14:137–139.
54. Sood R, Stewart CC, Aplan PD, et al: Neutropenia associated with T-cell large granular lymphocyte leukemia: Long-term response to cyclosporine therapy despite persistence of abnormal cells. Blood 1998; 91:3372–3378.
55. Seebach J, Speich R, Gmur J: Allogeneic bone marrow transplantation for CD3+/TCR gamma delta+ large granular lymphocyte proliferation. Blood 1995; 85:853.

Index

Note: Page numbers in *italics* refer to illustrations; page numbers followed by t refer to tables.

A

Abscesses, agranulocytosis with, 160
Acetaminophen, thrombocytopenic purpura induced by, 184
Aciclovir (acyclovir), 189t
Acquired immunodeficiency syndrome. See *HIV infection*.
Age, agranulocytosis incidence related to, 158
  aplastic anemia incidence and, 5, 5–6
  myelodysplastic syndrome correlation with, 71
Agglutinins, leukocyte, agranulocytosis role of, 157, 161
Agnogenic myeloid metaplasia (AMM). See *Myelofibrosis*.
Agranulocytosis, 156–177
  age association of, 158
  antibodies in, 161–162, 165–166, 166t
  clinical features of, 156, *158*, 160t, 160–162
  course and prognosis of, 175–176
  differential diagnosis of, 162t, 162–163
  drug-induced, 156, *158*, 160t, 164t, 167–175, 168t, 169t, *170*
  epidemiology of, 158–160
  etiology of, 156, *158*, 160t, 160–161
  experimental induction of, 164, *165*
  growth factor therapy in, 175
  historical aspects of, 156–158, *157–159*
  immune-mediated, 160, 164t, 164–167, 166t
  laboratory studies of, 161–162, 164
  mechanisms of, 163–167, 164t, *165*

Agranulocytosis *(Continued)*
  pure white cell aplasia and, 176–177
  treatment of, 175
AIDS. See *HIV infection*.
Alcohol, neutropenia induction by, 163
ALG (antilymphocyte globulin), aplastic anemia treated with, 1, *3*, 23–24, 26t
Alkylating agents, myelodysplastic syndrome caused by, 72–73
Amegakaryocytosis, acquired, 183t, 183–185, 184t
  thrombocytopenic purpura of, 183t, 183–185, 184t
Aminopyrine, agranulocytosis role of, 156, *158*, 164, *165*, 169, *170*
  chemical structure of, *170*
AMM (agnogenic myeloid metaplasia). See *Myelofibrosis*.
Amphotericin, 189t, 190
Analgesics, agranulocytosis role of, 156, *158*, 164, *165*, 167–169
Androgens, aplastic anemia treated with, 27
  Fanconi's anemia therapy using, 59
  thrombocytopenic purpura therapy using, 185
Anemia, 1–4
  aplastic, 1–32
    acquired, 4t, 6t, 6–7
    age distribution of, 5, 5–6
    androgen therapy for, 27
    bleeding associated with, 4, 7–8, 28–30
    blood count in, 8, *21*, 30–31
    bone marrow transplant for, *3*, 19t, 19–23, 26t, 26–27
    classification of, 4t, 9t, 15t

Anemia *(Continued)*
    clonality in, *12*
    late, 32
    definition of, 1, 3–4
    differential diagnosis of, 8–9, 9t
    drug-induced, 1, 6t, 14–19, 15t
    environmental risk factors in, 6t, 6–7
    epidemiology of, 4–7, *5*, 5t, 6t
    etiology of, 1, 6t, 6–7, 14–19, 15t
    genetic factors in, 7, *12*
    geographic distribution of, 6
    growth factors in, 9–10, 27–28
    hematopoiesis in, 9–13, *11*, *12*
    historical aspects of, 1–3, *2*
    immune-mediated, 2–3, 10–13, *11*, *12*
    immunosuppression therapy for, *3*, 21, 23–27, 26t
    incidence of, 4–5, *5*, 5t
    infection and, 8, 18, 30–31
    inherited, 4t, 46–62
    laboratory findings in, 8, 10–13, *21*, 30–31
    myelodysplastic syndrome vs., *70*, 70–71, 76t
    pathophysiology of, 9–19, *11*, *12*, 15t
    platelet transfusion therapy for, 28–29
    prognosis in, 31–32
    radiation-induced, 13–14
    supersevere, 31
    survival in, *3*, 19t, *20*, 26t
    symptoms and signs in, 1, 7–8
    transfusion therapy for, *3*, *20*, 29–30

217

Anemia *(Continued)*
    treatment of, 3, 19t, 19–31, 20, 21, 26t
    viruses and, 4t, 12, 18–19
  Diamond-Blackfan (congenital), 141–147, 142t, 144t, 145, 146t, 147
  Fanconi's, 46–62
    androgen therapy for, 59
    apoptosis in, 57–58
    bone marrow transplant therapy for, 58t, 58–59
    cancer association with, 48, 49
    cell cycle disturbances in, 52–53, 53, 57–58
    chromosome analysis in, 47, 48–52, 50
    clinical features of, 47, 48–49
    complementation studies in, 50, 50–51
    diagnosis of, 47, 48–52, 50
    DNA repair mechanisms of, 53–56, 54, 56
    genetic factors in, 49–58, 50
      therapy using, 60–62, 61
    growth factors in, 58, 59–60
    hematopoiesis in, 49, 52–58, 53, 54, 56
    historical aspects of, 47–48
    mutations related to, 50, 51
    oxygen reactivity role for, 52–53, 53
    pathophysiology of, 52–58, 53, 54, 56
    severity index for, 49
    symptoms and signs of, 47, 48–49
    treatment of, 58t, 58–62, 61
    umbilical cord blood therapy for, 59
  hemoglobinuria with, 100–101. See also *Hemoglobinuria, paroxysmal nocturnal.*
  HIV infection with, 187–188, 189t, 198–201, 200t
  leukemia of large granular lymphocytes with, 209
  myelofibrosis with, 124–126, 125. See also *Myelofibrosis.*
  parvovirus B19 associated with, 139–141, 141
  pure red cell aplasia with, 135–138, 141, 141–143
  refractory, 69–71, 70, 71t. See also *Myelodysplastic syndrome.*
  sideroblastic, 69–71, 70, 71t
Antibiotics, agranulocytosis role of, 167, 168t, 171–172
Antibodies, in agranulocytosis, 161–162, 165–166, 166t
  in aplastic anemia, 2–3, 10–13, 11, 12
  in myelodysplastic syndrome, 80, 80–81
  in pure red cell aplasia, 136–137, 144, 148
Anticoagulation therapy, paroxysmal nocturnal hemoglobinuria treated with, 114
Antigens, aplastic anemia and, 7
  HLA, agranulocytosis association with, 160, 166t, 166–167

Antihistamines, agranulocytosis and, 168t, 174–175
Antilymphocyte globulin (ALG), aplastic anemia treated with, 1, 3, 23–24, 26t
Antipsychotropic drugs, agranulocytosis and, 167, 168t, 172–173
Antithymocytic globulin (ATG), aplastic anemia treated with, 1, 20–21, 21, 23–24, 26t
Antithyroid drugs, agranulocytosis and, 164, 168t, 171
Antiviral drugs, 189, 189t
Aplasia. See *Anemia, aplastic; Pure red cell aplasia; Pure white cell aplasia.*
Apoptosis, aplastic anemia and, 2–3, 12
  Fanconi's anemia modulation of, 57–58
  HIV infection mechanisms for, 196–198, 197
  myelodysplastic syndrome mechanisms of, 80, 80, 89–90
  treatment aimed at, 89–90
Arsenic, aplastic anemia associated with, 18
Arthritis, sulfa therapy for, hematologic effects of, 160, 160t
Aspirin, "Mexican," 169
ATG (antithymocytic globulin), aplastic anemia treated with, 1, 20–21, 21, 23–24, 26t
Autoimmunity, aplastic anemia mediated by, 2–3, 10–13, 11, 12
  myelodysplastic syndrome and, 80, 80–81
  neutropenia and, 161, 162t, 164–166, 166t
  pure red cell aplasia and, 136–137, 144, 148

B

Benzene, aplastic anemia linked to, 1, 14, 15t, 16–17
  industrial sources of, 16–17
  myelodysplastic syndrome caused by, 71
Blast-forming units (BFUs). See *Hematopoietic progenitor cells.*
Bleeding, aplastic anemia with, 4, 7–8, 28–30
  myelodysplastic syndrome with, 73, 81, 85
  myelofibrosis with, 126
  thrombocytopenic purpura with, 183–185
Blood, peripheral. See also *Transfusion.*
  stem cell transplant from, 86–87, 88–89
Blood count, agranulocytosis and, 156, 158, 160, 164, 165
  aplastic anemia effect on, 8, 21, 30–31
  Fanconi's anemia and, 49
  myelodysplastic syndrome effect on, 71t, 74, 75t, 81, 85
  thrombocytopenia and, 29
Blood smear, agranulocytosis in, 161

Blood smear *(Continued)*
  aplastic anemia effect on, 8
  Fanconi's anemia and, 49
  leukemia of large granular lymphocytes in, 208–209
  myelodysplastic syndrome and, 74, 75t, 81
  paroxysmal nocturnal hemoglobinuria and, 99–100
Bone marrow, agranulocytic morphology in, 161
  aplastic anemia affecting, 3–4, 8–9
  CMV infection of, 190
  Fanconi's anemia and, 47, 49, 58
  HIV suppression of, 187–201, 188, 192, 192t–195t, 196, 197, 200t
  hypocellular, 9t
  malignant diseases affecting, 124t, 137t
  myelodysplastic syndrome affecting, 71t, 74–75, 75t, 86–89
  myelofibrosis affecting, 123t, 123–124, 124t
  pancytopenia and, 9t
  paroxysmal nocturnal hemoglobinuria role of, 99–101
  pure red cell aplasia affecting, 135–139, 143–144, 148
  thrombocytopenic purpura diagnosis and, 184
Bone marrow transplant therapy, aplastic anemia treatment with, 3, 19t, 19–23, 26t, 26–27
  Fanconi's anemia treatment with, 58t, 58–59
  hemoglobinuria treated with, 104–105, 105t, 114–115
  myelodysplastic syndrome treated with, 86–87, 88
  myelofibrosis treated with, 130–131
  pure red cell aplasia treated with, 145–147, 146t

C

Cancer. See *Leukemia; Neoplasia.*
Captopril, agranulocytosis and, 173–174
  chemical structure of, 170
Cardiac drugs, agranulocytosis and, 168t, 173–174
CD34 cells, HIV infection role of, 191, 192t, 193–195
Cell cycle, Fanconi's anemia effect on, 52–53, 53, 57–58
  oxygen sensitivity of, 52–53, 53
Cell death. See *Apoptosis.*
CFUs (colony-forming units). See *Hematopoietic progenitor cells.*
Chelation therapy, iron excess treated with, 85
Chemicals, 6t, 15t, 137t, 168t, 169t, 183t. See also *Drugs.*
  aplastic anemia associated with, 1, 6t, 6–7, 14–19, 15t
  myelodysplastic syndrome associated with, 71–73
Chemotherapy, agents used in, 88t
  aplastic anemia due to, 10, 14–16, 15t

Chemotherapy *(Continued)*
  Diamond-Blackfan anemia treated with, 138, 144–145, 146t
  leukemia of large granular lymphocytes treated with, 212–213
  myelodysplastic syndrome relation to, 71–72, 87
    etiology of, 72–73, 77
    treatment modes for, 87–88, 88t, 89
  myelofibrosis treated with, *129*, 129–130
  pure red cell aplasia treated with, 138, 144–145, 146t
Chloramphenicol, aplastic anemia linked to, 1, 15t, 17–18
Chlorpromazine, agranulocytosis and, 167, 168t
  chemical structure of, *170*
Chromosome(s), Fanconi's anemia and, 47, 48–52, *50*
  myelodysplastic syndrome and, 75, 77–80
  myelofibrosis and, 122, 123t
  Philadelphia, 128
  pure red cell aplasia and, 135, 143
  X, paroxysmal nocturnal hemoglobinuria gene on, 99
    lyonization inactivation of, 78
Ciliated neurotrophic factor (CNTF), 109
Cimetidine, agranulocytosis and, 168t, 174–175
Clindamycin-pyrimethamine, 189t
Clonality, aplastic anemia role of, *12*, 32
  leukemia of large granular lymphocytes role of, 209–212, 212t
  myelodysplastic syndrome role of, 78
Clozapine, *170*
  agranulocytosis and, 166, 166t, 168t, 172–173
CMV (cytomegalovirus), HIV infection and, 190
CNTF (ciliated neurotrophic factor), 109
Coal tar derivatives, agranulocytosis associated with, 156, *159*
Collagen, bone marrow fibrosis role of, 123–124, *125*
  pure red cell aplasia association with, 137t
Colony-forming units (CFUs). See *Hematopoietic progenitor cells.*
Complement, Fanconi's anemia and, *50*, 50–51
  paroxysmal nocturnal hemoglobinuria and, 103–104
Corticosteroid therapy, aplastic anemia treated with, 25, 27
  Diamond-Blackfan anemia treated with, 144t, 144–145, *145*, 146t
  Fanconi's anemia treated with, 59
  myelodysplastic syndrome treated with, 89–90
  myelofibrosis treated with, 130
  paroxysmal nocturnal hemoglobinuria treated with, 113–114
  pure red cell aplasia treated with, 138, 144–145, *145*, 146t

Corticosteroid therapy *(Continued)*
  thrombocytopenic purpura treated with, 185
Cyclosporine, aplastic anemia treatment using, *21*, 24–25
  leukemia of large granular lymphocytes therapy with, 213
  myelodysplastic syndrome treated with, 90
Cytokines, aplastic anemia and, 10–13, *11*, *12*, 27–29
  HIV infection and, *192*, 196–197, *197*
Cytomegalovirus (CMV), HIV infection and, 190
Cytopenia. See also *Blood count*; specific cell type deficiencies.
  conditions associated with, 9t
  HIV infection with, 187–188, 198–201, 200t

D

Dapsone, agranulocytosis and, 167, 168t
Deoxyribonucleic acid. See *DNA (deoxyribonucleic acid).*
Di Guglielmo syndrome, 70
Diamond-Blackfan anemia, 141–147
  bone marrow in, 143–147, 146t
  chemotherapy for, 146t
  clinical features of, 142t, 142–143
  corticosteroid therapy for, 144t, 144–147, *145*, 146t
  immunosuppression therapy for, 144t, 144–145, *145*, 146t
  malformations associated with, 142t, 142–143
  pathogenesis of, 143–144
  pure red cell aplasia of, 141–147, 142t, 144t, *145*, 146t, *147*
  survival in, 146t, 147, *147*
  transfusion therapy for, 144t, 144–145, 146t
  transplant therapy for, 145–147, 146t
  treatment of, 144t, 144–147, *145*, 146t
Differentiation therapy, 90
Dipyrone, *170*
  agranulocytosis and, 159, 167, 168t, 169, 169t
DNA (deoxyribonucleic acid), *54*, *56*
  Fanconi's anemia role of, 53–56, *54*, *56*
  repair of, 53–56, *54*, *56*
Drugs, 6t, 15t, 137t, 168t, 169t, 183t. See also *Chemicals.*
  agranulocytosis induced by, 156, *158*, 160t, 167–175, 168t, 169t, *170*
  aplastic anemia caused by, 1, 6t, 14–19, 15t
  HIV infection treated with, 189t, 189–190, 200t
  pure red cell aplasia association with, 136, 137t
  thrombocytopenic purpura induced by, 183, 183t

E

EGF (epidermal growth factor), 124, *125*
Ehrlichiosis, neutropenia with, 163
Environment. See also *Chemicals*; *Drugs.*
  aplastic anemia due to, 6t, 6–7
  myelodysplastic syndrome due to, 71–73
  risk factors in, 6t, 6–7, 71–73
Epidermal growth factor (EGF), 124, *125*
Erythroblastopenia (of childhood), 147–149
  transient, 147–149
    clinical features of, 147–148
    epidemiology of, 147–148
    familial, 148–149
    laboratory studies in, 148
    pathophysiology of, 148–149
    treatment of, 149
Erythrocytes, aplastic anemia and, 3–4, 8, 29–30
  Fanconi's anemia affecting, 49
  GPI-deficient, 99–103
  hemoglobinuria and, 100–101
  myelodysplastic syndrome effect on, 71t, 74, 75t, 81, 86
  myelofibrosis affecting, 123t, 124–126
  pure red cell aplasia affecting, 135–149
  transfusion therapy using, 29–30
Erythropoiesis, HIV infection role of, 187–189
  pure red cell aplasia affecting, 135–139, *139*, *141*, 143–144, 148
Erythropoietin, HIV infection treated with, 198–199
  myelodysplastic syndrome treated with, 86
  myelofibrosis treated with, 130

F

FAB (French-American-British) classification, myelodysplastic syndromes of, 70–71, 71t, *82*, 82–83, 83t
  refractory anemia in, 70–71, 71t
Facies, Cathie's, 142, 142t
  Diamond-Blackfan anemia affecting, 142, 142t
  Fanconi's anemia affecting, 47, 48
FANC genes, *50*, 50–52, 55–58, *56*
Fanconi's anemia. See *Anemia, Fanconi's.*
Fibroblasts, myelofibrosis role of, 124, *125*
Flow cytometry, aplastic anemia lymphocytes in, *11*
  myelodysplastic syndrome in, 75–76
  PNH lymphocytes in, 111, *112*
Foscarnet, 189t
French-American-British (FAB) classification, myelodysplastic syndrome in, 70–71, 71t, *82*, 83, 83t

French-American-British (FAB) classification *(Continued)*
  refractory anemia in, 70–71, 71t

G

Ganciclovir, HIV infection treated with, 189t, 190
Gangrene, agranulocytosis associated with, 156, 160
  throat affected by, 156, 160
Gene(s), cancer, myelodysplastic syndrome and, 79–80
  FANC, *50,* 50–52, 55–58, *56*
  PIG-A, *102,* 103–112, *109–113*
Genetic factors, in aplastic anemia, 7, 12
  in Fanconi's anemia, 49–58, *50*
  gene therapy and, 60–62, *61*
  in myelodysplastic syndrome, 75, 77–80
  in myelofibrosis, 122, 123t
  in paroxysmal nocturnal hemoglobinuria, 99–113, *109–111*
Geography, aplastic anemia relation to, 6
Glycosylphosphatidylinositol (GPI), 99
  anchored protein (GPI-AP) associated with, 99
  paroxysmal nocturnal hemoglobinuria and, 101–112, *102, 109–113*
GM-CSF (granulocyte-macrophage colony-stimulating factor). See *Growth factors.*
Gold, agranulocytosis and, 167, *170*
  aplastic anemia induced by, 4t, 6, 6t, 15t, 18
GPI (glycosylphosphatidylinositol), 99
  anchored protein (GPI-AP) associated with, 99–103
  deficiency of, 99–103
  hemoglobinuria role of, 101–112, *102, 109–113*
Graft-vs.-host disease (GVHD), 19–21
  aplastic anemia and, 1, 19t, 19–21
  Fanconi's anemia and, 58t, 58–59
  hemoglobinuria treatment and, 114–115
  pure red cell aplasia treatment and, 145–147, 146t
Granules, alpha, myelofibrosis role of, 124, *125*
  platelet origin of, 124, *125*
Granulocytes, aplastic anemia and, 10–13
  colony-stimulating factors for. See *Growth factors.*
  decreased or absent. See *Agranulocytosis; Neutropenia.*
  Fanconi's anemia affecting, 49, 58
  myelodysplastic syndrome affecting, 74, 75t, 81
Gray platelet syndrome, 124t, 129
Growth factors, agranulocytosis role of, 164, 175
  AIDS treated with, 199–201, 200t
  aplastic anemia role of, 9–10, 27–28
  Fanconi's anemia role of, 58, 59–60
  HIV infection treated with, 199–201, 200t

Growth factors *(Continued)*
  leukemia of large granular lymphocytes therapy with, 213
  myelodysplastic syndrome treated with, 85–86
  myelofibrosis role of, 123–124, *125*
GVHD (graft-vs.-host disease), 19–21
  aplastic anemia and, 1, 19t, 19–21
  Fanconi's anemia and, 58t, 58–59
  hemoglobinuria treatment and, 114–115
  pure red cell aplasia treatment and, 145–147, 146t

H

Hematopoiesis. See also *Bone marrow; Growth factors; Progenitor cells; Stem cells.*
  agranulocytosis role of, 164, 175
  aplastic anemia affecting, 9–13, *11,* 12
  extramedullary, myelofibrosis with, 122, 124
  Fanconi's anemia affecting, 49, 52–58, *53, 54, 56*
  HIV infection and, 187–201, *188, 192,* 192t–195t, *196,* 197, 200t
  myelodysplastic syndrome and, 74, 81
  paroxysmal nocturnal hemoglobinuria relation to, 109–110, *110, 111,* 114
  pure red cell aplasia role of, 135–138, *141,* 144, 148
Hematopoietic progenitor cells, aplastic anemia and, 9
  pure red cell aplasia and, 136–139, *139,* 143–144, 148
Hemoglobin, parviroral anemia effect on, *141*
Hemoglobinuria, 99
  paroxysmal nocturnal, 99–115
    anticoagulation therapy for, 114
    bone marrow transplant therapy for, 104–105, 105t, 114–115
    case definition of, 99–100
    clinical manifestations of, 100–101
    corticosteroid therapy for, 113–114
    epidemiology of, 100
    genetic factors in, 99–113, *109–111*
    glycosylphosphatidylinositol (GPI) role in, 101–112, *102, 109–113*
    hematopoiesis in, 109–110, *110, 111,* 114
    historical aspects of, 99
    immune factors in, 108–112, *109–113*
    immunosuppression therapy for, 114
    laboratory studies in, 105–107
    modelling of, 107–112, *109–113*
    murine, 107
    pathophysiology of, 101–112, *102, 109–113*
    PIG-A gene role in, *102,* 103–112, *109–113*

Hemoglobinuria *(Continued)*
  T cell role in, 110–112, *111–113*
  thrombosis in, 114
  treatment of, 112–115
  virus in, 109, *110*
Hemorrhage. See *Bleeding.*
HIV infection, 187–201
  anemia in, 187–188, 189t, 198–201, 200t
  bone marrow failure in, 187–201
  clinical features of, 187–188
  pathophysiologic mechanisms of, *188,* 188–198
  treatment of, 189t, 189–190, 198–201, 200t
  CMV infection accompanying, 190
  drug therapy in, 189t, 189–190, 200t
  growth factor therapy in, 199–201, 200t
  hematopoiesis affected by, 187–191, *188,* 189t, *192,* 193–201, 192t–195t, *196, 197,* 200t
  mycobacterium avium–intracellulare infection with, 190–191
  myelodysplastic syndrome due to, 77
  neoplasia with, 191
  neutropenia in, 187, 188
  parvovirus infection with, 191
  progenitor cells role in, 191, *192,* 192t–194t, 193–194
  prognosis in, 198
  stem cells in, 191, *192,* 192t–194t, 193–194, *197*
  stromal cells role in, *192,* 195t, *196,* 195–196
  thrombocytopenia in, 187, 188, 189t, 199, 200t
  treatment of, 189t, 189–190, 198–201, 200t
HSC (hematopoietic stem cells). See *Stem cells.*
Human immunodeficiency virus infection. See *HIV infection.*
Hydrocarbons, aromatic, aplastic anemia caused by, 17
Hydrogen peroxide, Fanconi's anemia and, 52, *53*

I

IFN (interferon), aplastic anemia and, 10–13, *11,* 12
Immunity, agranulocytosis and, 160, 164t, 164–167, 166t
  aplastic anemia mediated by, 2–3, 10–13, *11,* 12
  myelodysplastic syndrome and, 80, 80
  paroxysmal nocturnal hemoglobinuria and, 108–112, *109–113*
  pure red cell aplasia and, 136–137, 144, 148
  thrombocytopenic purpura mediated by, 184, 184t
Immunodeficiency. See specific type, e.g., *HIV infection.*
Immunoglobulin, pure red cell aplasia therapy with, 140–141, *141*
Immunosuppression therapy, for aplastic anemia, *3,* 21, 23–27, 26t

Immunosuppression therapy
    (Continued)
  for Diamond-Blackfan anemia, 144t, 144–145, *145*, 146t
  for hemoglobinuria, 114
  for leukemia of large granular lymphocytes, 212–213
  for myelodysplastic syndrome, 89–90
  for myelofibrosis, 130
  for pure red cell aplasia, 138, 144–145, *145*, 146t
  for thrombocytopenic purpura, 185
Impotence, paroxysmal nocturnal hemoglobinuria related to, 100
Infection. See also specific infection or organism.
  aplastic anemia relation to, 8, 18–19, 30–31
  neutropenia associated with, 162t, 163
Inflammatory bowel disease, sulfa therapy for, hematologic effects of, 160, 160t
Insecticides, aplastic anemia caused by, 17
Interferon (IFN), aplastic anemia and, 10–13, *11*, *12*
Interleukin. See *Growth factors*.
IPPS (International Prognostic Scoring System), 69
  in myelodysplastic syndrome, *82*, 83, 83t
Iron, chelation therapy and, 85
  in myelodysplastic syndrome, 71t, 74, 81, 85

J

Jaundice, paroxysmal nocturnal hemoglobinuria with, 100

K

Ketoconazole, 189t

L

Lamivudine, 189t
Leukemia. See also *Neoplasia*.
  large granular lymphocytic, 207–213
    clinical features of, 208–209
    diagnosis of, 207–208
    disorders associated with, 211–212, 212t
    historical aspects of, 207
    immunologic and molecular features of, 209, 209t
    NK cell, 207, 209t, *211*
    pathogenesis of, 209–212, *210*, *211*, 212t
    prognosis in, 212
    T cell, 207–213, 209t, *211*, 212t
    treatment of, 212–213
  myelodysplastic syndrome and, 69–70, *70*, 71t, 77, 79, 82, *82*
Leukocytes. See also *Granulocytes*; *Lymphocytes*.

Leukocytes *(Continued)*
  absent or decreased. See *Agranulocytosis*; *Neutropenia*.
  agglutinins affecting, 157, 161
  aplastic anemia and, 9–13
  Fanconi's anemia affecting, 49, 58
  GPI-deficient, 99–103
  hemoglobinuria and, 100
  myelodysplastic syndrome affecting, 74, 75t, 81
  pure white cell aplasia affecting, 176–177
  sulfa drug effect on, 160t
Levamisole, agranulocytosis role of, 166, 166t, 168t, 174
  chemical structure of, *170*
LGL (large granular lymphocyte). See *Leukemia, large granular lymphocytic*.
Lipid bilayer, GPI anchored protein on, 101–103, *102*
Lymphocytes, aplastic anemia and, 10–13, *11*, *12*
  Fanconi's anemia affecting, 49, 58
  hemoglobinuria role of, 103–111, *110*, *111*
  large granular, 207–213. See also *Leukemia, large granular lymphocytic*.
  lymphoblastoid cell line of, 103–111
  pure red cell aplasia and, 137–138, 148
  T. See *T cells*.
Lyonization, X chromosome inactivation by, 78

M

Macrophages, colony-stimulating factors for. See *Growth factors*.
MAI (mycobacterium avium-intracellulare) infection, HIV infection with, 190–191
Malformations, Fanconi's anemia with, 47, 48
  pure red cell aplasia associated with, 142t, 142–143
Megakaryocytes. See also *Platelets*.
  HIV infection of, 188, 194
  myelodysplastic syndrome with, 75, 76t
  myelofibrosis affecting, 123t, 123–124, *125*
  thrombocytopenic purpura role of, 183t, 183–185, 184t
Metals, agranulocytosis and, 168t
  aplastic anemia caused by, 14, 15t, 18
Methimazole, agranulocytosis and, 166, 166t, 168t, 171
Modelling, hemoglobinuria etiology shown in, 107–112, *109*–*113*
Monocytes, myelodysplastic syndrome affecting, 74, 75t
Mosaicism, Fanconi's anemia and, 48
Mutations, Fanconi's anemia role of, 50, 51
  myelodysplastic syndrome role of, 79–80

Mutations *(Continued)*
  of PIG-A gene, 104–105, 109, *109*
Mycobacterium avium-intracellulare (MAI) infection, HIV infection with, 190–191
Myelodysplastic syndrome, 69–90
  age correlation of, 71
  aplastic anemia vs., *70*, 70–71, 76t
  apoptosis in, 80, *80*
  blood count in, 71t, 74–75, 75t, 76t, 81
  bone marrow in, effects seen in, 75t
    transplant therapy using, 86–89
  case overlap related to, *70*, 70–71, 76t
  chemicals causing, 71–73
  chemotherapy relationship to, 71–72, 87
  causative factors found in, 72–73
    high-dose, 87–88, 88t
    low-dose, 89
    treatment and, 87–88, 88t, 89
  chromosomes in, 75, 77–80
  classification of, 70–71, 71t
  clinical course of, 81–84, *82*
  clonality in, 78
  diagnostic approach in, *72*, 73t, 73–77, 75t, 76t
  differential diagnosis of, *72*, 73t, 73–74
  epidemiology of, 70–73
  etiology of, 71–73, 77–81, *80*
  genetic factors in, 75, 77–80
  hematopoiesis in, 74, 81
  historical aspects of, 69–70
  HIV disease with, 77
  immune mechanisms in, *80*, 80
  incidence of, 71
  laboratory testing for, *72*, 73–77, 76t
  leukemia and, 69–70, *70*, 71t, 77, 79, 82, *82*
  myeloproliferative disorders vs., 69–71, *70*, 71t
  pathophysiology of, 77–81, *80*
  prognosis in, 81–84, *82*, 83t
  radiation causing, 71
  refractory anemia vs., 69–71, *70*, 71t
  stem cell transplant therapy for, 86–87, 88–89
  survival in, *82*, 82–85, 83t
  symptoms and signs in, 73
  transfusion therapy for, 85–86
  treatment of, 84–90, *84*
Myelofibrosis, 122–131
  acute, 128
  anemia of, 124–126, *125*
  clinical features of, 123t, 126–127, *128*
  cytopenias of, 123t, *125*, 126
  diagnosis of, 123t, 126–127
  differential diagnosis of, 123t, 127–129
  epidemiology of, 122–123
  etiology of, 122–127, *125*, 129
  genetic factors in, 122, 123t
  growth factors role in, 123–124, *125*
  hematopoiesis in, 122–124
    extramedullary, 122, 124
  historical aspects of, 122
  natural history of, 123t, 127, *128*

Myelofibrosis *(Continued)*
 pathophysiology of, 123–126, *125*
 prognosis and survival in, 131
 thorium exposure role in, 122
Myeloid metaplasia. See *Myelofibrosis.*
Myeloproliferative disorder(s), 123t
 feature comparison of, 122, 123t
 myelodysplastic syndrome vs., 69–71, *70*, 71t
 myelofibrosis as, 122
Myelosclerosis. See *Myelofibrosis.*

N

Natural killer (NK) cells, leukemia of large granular lymphocytes and, 207, 209t, *211*
Neoplasia. See also *Leukemia.*
 aplastic anemia and, 21–22
 bone marrow fibrosis association with, 124t
 Fanconi's anemia and, 48, 49
 HIV infection and, 191
 myelodysplastic syndrome and, 71t, 77, 79, 82, *82*
 pure red cell aplasia with, 136, 136t, 137t
 pure white cell aplasia with, 177
Neuroleptic drugs, aplastic anemia caused by, 18
Neutropenia. See also *Agranulocytosis.*
 aplastic anemia with, 3–4, 8–9
 causes and forms of, 162, 162t
 differential diagnosis of, 162t, 162–163
 drug-mediated, 156, *158*, 160t, 164t, 167–175, 168t, 169t, *170*
 Fanconi's anemia with, 49, 58
 hemoglobinuria with, 100
 HIV infection with, 187, 188
 immune-mediated, 160–162, 162t, 164t, 164–167, 166t
 infections accompanied by, 162t, 163
 leukemia of large granular lymphocytes with, 208
 myelodysplastic syndrome and, 74, 81
Nezeloff's syndrome, 140
NK (natural killer) cells, leukemia of large granular lymphocytes and, 207, 209t, *211*
Nocturnal hemoglobinuria. See *Hemoglobinuria.*
NSAIDs (nonsteroidal anti-inflammatory drugs), 18, 167
 agranulocytosis and, 167, 168t, 169–171
 aplastic anemia associated with, 4t, 6, 6t, 14, 15t, 18

O

Oncogenes, myelodysplastic syndrome and, 79–80
OPC-8212 (drug), chemical structure of, *170*
Oxygen reactivity, cell cycle sensitivity to, 52–53, *53*

Oxyphenbutazone, thrombocytopenic purpura induced by, 184

P

Pancytopenia, aplastic anemia with, 3–4, 8–9
 conditions associated with, 9t
 differential diagnosis of, 9t
 Fanconi's anemia with, 49
 myelodysplastic syndrome with, 74, 81
 myelofibrosis with, *125*, 126
 paroxysmal nocturnal hemoglobinuria with, 100
Paroxysmal nocturnal hemoglobinuria (PNH). See *Hemoglobinuria, paroxysmal nocturnal.*
Parvovirus B19 infection, 139–141
 clinical manifestations of, 139–140
 epidemiology of, 139–140
 HIV infection and, 191
 pathophysiology in, 140
 pure red cell aplasia related to, 135, 136t, 139–141, *141*
 "slapped cheek disease" due to, 139
 treatment of, 140–141, *141*
PDGF (platelet-derived growth factor). See also *Platelets.*
 myelofibrosis and, 123–124, *125*, 129
Pelger-Huët anomalies, myelodysplastic syndrome with, 74
Penicillin, agranulocytosis and, 168t, 172
Pentamidine, 189t
Peripheral blood. See also *Transfusion.*
 stem cell transplant from, 86–87, 88–89
Peroxide, Fanconi's anemia and, 52, *53*
Pharyngitis, agranulocytosis associated with, 156, 160
Phenothiazine, agranulocytosis and, 164t, 167, 168t, 172
Phenylbutazone, agranulocytosis and, 169t, 169–171
Philadelphia chromosome, 128
PIG-A gene, hemoglobinuria and, *102*, 103–112, *109–113*
 mutations of, 104–105, *109*, *109*
Pigmentation, Fanconi's anemia affecting, 47, 48
Platelet transfusion, aplastic anemia treated with, 28–29
 thrombocytopenic purpura treated with, 185
Platelets, alpha granules of, 124, *125*
 aplastic anemia and, 28–29
 decreased. See *Thrombocytopenia.*
 Fanconi's anemia affecting, 49
 giant, 74
 gray platelet syndrome affecting, 124t, 129
 hemoglobinuria and, 100–101
 HIV infection affecting, 187, 188, 189t, 198, 199
 myelodysplastic syndrome and, 74, 81, 85
 myelofibrosis affecting, 123t, 123–124, *125*

Platelets *(Continued)*
 thrombocytopenic purpura and, 183t, 183–185, 184t
Pluripotent cells. See also *Progenitor cells.*
 myelodysplastic syndrome and, 69, 75t
PNH. See *Hemoglobinuria, paroxysmal nocturnal.*
Polycythemia vera, clinical features of, 122, 123t, 129
 myelofibrosis vs., 120, 123t, 129
Precursor cells. See *Progenitor cells*; *Stem cells.*
Primaquine, 189t
Procainamide, agranulocytosis and, 168t, 174
Progenitor cells. See also *Stem cells.*
 aplastic anemia and, 9–10
 Fanconi's anemia and, 60–62, *61*
 hemoglobinuria related to, 106
 HIV infection of, 191, *192*, 192t–194t, 193–194
 leukemia of large granular lymphocytes and, 210, *211*
 myelodysplastic syndrome and, 69, 75t
 myelofibrosis and, 123–124, *125*
 pure red cell aplasia affecting, 135–139, *139*, 143–144, 148
Propylthiouracil, agranulocytosis and, 164, 168t, 171
 chemical structure of, *170*
Protease inhibitors, 189, 199
Protein(s), encoding of, by FANC gene, 50, 50–52, 55–58, *56*
Psychotropic drugs, 168t
 agranulocytosis and, 167, 168t, 172–173
 aplastic anemia and, 18
Pure red cell aplasia, 135–149
 antibodies in, 136–137, 144, 148
 bone marrow in, 135–139, 143–147, 146t, 148
 chemotherapy in, 138, 144–145, 146t
 clinical features of, 135, 139–140, 142t, 142–143, 147–148
 congenital, 141–147, 142t, 144t, *145*, 146t, *147*
 corticosteroid therapy in, 144t, 144–147, *145*, 146t
 Diamond-Blackfan anemia as, 141–147, 142t, 144t, *145*, 146t, *147*
 differential diagnosis of, 136t, 148t
 disorders associated with, 135–136, 137t
 epidemiology of, 135, 139, 142, 147–148
 etiologic agent classification for, 137t
 fetal, 136t
 immunoglobulin therapy for, 140–141, *141*
 immunosuppression therapy for, 144t, 144–145, *145*, 146t
 parvovirus B19 and, 139–141, *141*
 pathophysiology of, 136–138, 137t, 140, 143–144, 148
 survival in, 146t, 147, *147*
 T cells role in, 137–138, 148
 thymoma association with, 136, 137t

Pure red cell aplasia *(Continued)*
  transfusion therapy for, 138, 140, 144t, 144–145, 146t
  transient, of childhood, 147–148, 148t
  treatment of, 138–141, *139*, *141*, 144t, 144–147, *145*, 146t, 149
Pure white cell aplasia, 176–177
  thymoma with, 177
Purpura. See also *Bleeding*; *Thrombocytopenia*.
  acquired amegakaryocytic thrombocytopenic, 183t, 183–185, 184t
  idiopathic thrombocytopenic, 183t, 183–184
Pyrazolone, agranulocytosis and, 169

R

Radiation, aplastic anemia due to, 10, 13–14
  lethal dose calculation for, 13–14
  myelodysplastic syndrome caused by, 71, 77
  myelofibrosis and, 122
Ranitidine, agranulocytosis role of, 168t, 174–175
Red blood cells. See *Erythrocytes*.
Refractory anemia, 69–71, *70*, 71t. See also *Myelodysplastic syndrome*.
Reticulocytes, aplastic anemia decrease in, 98
  parvoviral infection and, 140, *141*
Rickettsial diseases, neutropenia with, 163
Rifampin, 189t

S

Saquinavir, 189t
Sideroblasts. See also *Myelodysplastic syndrome*.
  anemia with, 69–71, *70*, 71t, 81
  ringed, *70*, 70–71, 71t, 81
"Slapped cheek disease," parvovirus infection causing, 139
Solvents, aplastic anemia linked to, 1, 14, 15t, 16–17
  myelodysplastic syndrome caused by, 71
Sore throat, agranulocytosis associated with, 156, 160
Splenectomy, myelofibrosis treated with, *129*, 130
Stavudine, 189t
Stem cells. See also *Progenitor cells*.
  aplastic anemia effect on, 10
  extramedullary seeding by, 124, *125*
  Fanconi's anemia and, 60–62, *61*
  hemoglobinuria etiology in, 103–104, 109–110, *110*, *111*
  HIV infection of, 191, *192*, 192t–194t, 193–194, *197*
  leukemia of large granular lymphocytes and, 210–211, *211*
  myelodysplastic syndrome and, 69, 86–87, 88–89
  myelofibrosis and, 123–124, *125*
  transplant of, 86–87, 88–89

Steroids. See *Corticosteroid therapy*.
Stromal cells, aplastic anemia and, 10
  HIV infection of, *192*, 195t, 195–196, *196*
Sulfa drugs, *170*
  agranulocytosis associated with, 160, 160t, 168t, *170*
  aplastic anemia associated with, 4t, 6, 6t
Sulfadiazine, 189t
Sulfasalazine, chemical structure of, *170*
Superoxide, Fanconi's anemia and, 52
Syphilis, drug therapies for, agranulocytosis due to, 159–160

T

T cells, activated, 209–210, *210*
  cytotoxic, 212t
  in aplastic anemia, 10–13, *11*, *12*
  in hemoglobinuria, 110–112, *111*–*113*
  in leukemia of large granular lymphocytes, 207–213, 209t, *211*
  in pure red cell aplasia, 137–138, 148
  resting, 210, *210*
TGF (transforming growth factor), in myelofibrosis, 124, *125*
Thorium, myelofibrosis role of, 122
Thrombocytes. See *Platelets*.
Thrombocytopenia, 122, 123t, 183–185
  aplastic anemia with, 28–29
  blood count in, 29
  essential, clinical features of, 122, 123t
  myelofibrosis vs., 123t, 129
  sulfa drug induction of, 160t
  HIV infection with, 187, 188, 189t, 199, 200t
  leukemia of large granular lymphocytes with, 209
  purpuric, 183–185
    acquired amegakaryocytic, 183–185
    androgen therapy for, 185
    classification of, 183t, 183–184, 184t
    differential diagnosis of, 183t, 183–184, 184t
    disorders associated with, 183, 183t
    drug-induced, 183, 183t
    immune-mediated, 184, 184t
    immunosuppression therapy for, 185
    natural history of, 184
    pathogenesis of, 184t, 184–185
    platelet transfusion for, 185
    treatment of, 185
    idiopathic, 183t, 183–185
Thrombosis, hemoglobinuria accompanied by, 114
Thymocytes, antiserum against, 1, 20–21, *21*, 23–24, 26t
Thymoma, pure red cell aplasia association with, 136, 137t
  pure white cell aplasia with, 177
Thyrostatic drugs, aplastic anemia caused by, 14, 15t

TMP-SMX (trimethoprim-sulfamethoxazole), HIV infection treated with, 189t, 189–190
TNF (tumor necrosis factor), Fanconi's anemia and, 52–53
Transforming growth factor (TGF), in myelofibrosis, 124, *125*
Transfusion, aplastic anemia treated with, *3*, *20*, 28–30
  Diamond-Blackfan anemia treated with, 144t, 144–145, 146t
  myelodysplastic syndrome treated with, 85–86
  pure red cell aplasia treated with, 138, 140, 144t, 144–145, 146t
  thrombocytopenic purpura treated with, 185
Transplantation, bone marrow used for. See *Bone marrow transplant therapy*.
  umbilical cord blood used for, 59
Trimethoprim-sulfamethoxazole (TMP-SMX), HIV infection treated with, 189–190, 189t
Trisomy, myelofibrosis and, 122, 123t
Tuberculosis, bone marrow failure in, 9t
Tumor necrosis factor (TNF), Fanconi's anemia and, 52–53

U

Ulcers, throat, agranulocytosis with, 160
Umbilical cord blood, Fanconi's anemia treatment using, 59
  transplantation of, 59
Urine, dark-colored, 100
  hemoglobin in, 99. See also *Hemoglobinuria, paroxysmal nocturnal*.

V

Virus(es), AIDS caused by, 187–201
  cytomegalovirus, 190
  in aplastic anemia, 4t, *12*, 18–19
  in pure red cell aplasia, 136, 137t, 139–141, *141*, 149
  parvovirus B19, 139–141, 191
Vitamin B_{12}, thrombocytopenic purpura and, 184, 184t

W

White cells. See *Leukocytes*.

X

X chromosome, hemoglobinuria gene on, 99
  inactivation of, 78
  lyonization of, 78

Z

Zidovudine (ZDV), anemia caused by, 187–188, 189t
  HIV infection treated with, 187–189, 189t

ISBN 0-7216-7174-8

90038